Improving Mental Well-Being at the Intersection of Mindfulness, Meditation, and Yoga

Shubhangni Jain
https://orcid.org/0009-0006-0160-9960
Amity University, India

Shweta Sharma
Amity University, Gurugram, India

Akanksha Singh
https://orcid.org/0000-0001-7784-1826
Chitkara School of Psychology and Counselling, Chitkara University, Punjab, India

IGI Global
Scientific Publishing
Publishing Tomorrow's Research Today

Vice President of Editorial	Melissa Wagner
Director of Acquisitions	Mikaela Felty
Director of Book Development	Jocelynn Hessler
Production Manager	Mike Brehm
Cover Design	Jose Rosado

Published in the United States of America by
IGI Global Scientific Publishing
701 East Chocolate Avenue
Hershey, PA, 17033, USA
Tel: 717-533-8845 | Fax: 717-533-7115
Website: https://www.igi-global.com E-mail: cust@igi-global.com

Library of Congress Cataloging-in-Publication Data

LCCN: 2025028973 (CIP Data Pending)
ISBN13: 9798337341873
Isbn13Softcover: 9798337341880
EISBN13: 9798337341897
British Cataloguing in Publication Data
A Cataloguing in Publication record for this book is available from the British Library.

Table of Contents

Detailed Table of Contents

scientifically backed way through which a person can actively carve out his or her own neural structure.

This chapter explores the relevance of Swami Vivekananda's Practical Vedanta in addressing contemporary mental health challenges. Drawing from core Vedantic principles, such as Atman (the Self), Brahman (ultimate reality), and Advaita (non-dualism), the chapter examines how self-awareness, detachment (Vairagya), and Karma Yoga can transform emotional distress into inner strength. It integrates philosophical insights with psychological concepts like emotional regulation, mindfulness, and resilience, offering a spiritually grounded framework for mental well-being. Through Vivekananda's reinterpretation of Vedanta as a lived philosophy, the chapter argues for inward-directed approaches that transcend symptom management and foster deeper self-realization. This synthesis provides an inclusive, non-sectarian path to emotional clarity and inner freedom in an age of psychological fragmentation.

This chapter explores the profound integration of body and mind achieved through yoga, emphasizing its role in harmonizing physiological, psychological, and cognitive functions. It highlights how practices such as breath regulation, postures, meditation, and mindfulness foster neural synchronization, enhance autonomic balance, and promote emotional stability and stress resilience. Drawing upon both ancient philosophy and contemporary scientific evidence, the discussion demonstrates yoga's capacity to optimize attention regulation, cognitive flexibility, and overall well-being. By bridging traditional wisdom with modern research, the chapter underscores yoga's potential as a holistic approach to health, performance enhancement, and comprehensive mind-body synchronization across diverse populations.

The global mental health crisis, characterized by escalating rates of anxiety, depression, and existential distress, has exposed the limitations of conventional biomedical approaches. This chapter explores the integrative potential of mindfulness, meditation, and yoga as a synergistic triad for promoting comprehensive mental well-being. Grounded in both ancient contemplative traditions and contemporary empirical research, the triad fosters emotional regulation, neuroplastic adaptability, embodied awareness, and a deeper sense of meaning. Rather than focusing solely on symptom reduction, these practices support psychological resilience and spiritual growth. The chapter further investigates their increasing application across therapeutic, educational, and occupational domains, highlighting their adaptability, scientific credibility, and cross-cultural relevance. It calls for a paradigm shift toward person-centered, developmental models of care that recognize contemplative practices as foundational tools for long-term healing and flourishing.

Breath and emotion are intricately connected, forming continuous waves that shape our inner experiences and outward expressions. This chapter explores the physiological, psychological, and cultural ties between breathing patterns and emotional states, demonstrating how breath acts as both a mirror and a regulator of emotion. Insights from neuroscience, somatic psychology, and cultural traditions reveal that conscious breath practices—such as mindfulness, breathwork, and pranayama—enhance emotional resilience, interoceptive awareness, and self-regulation. Breath also holds symbolic significance in art, literature, and spiritual traditions, where it serves as a non-verbal language of expression and transformation. By developing breath literacy—the awareness and intentional modulation of breathing—we gain tools not only for personal well-being but also for fostering presence, connection, and

Foreword

The contemporary world is witnessing an unprecedented paradox: despite remarkable advancements in science, technology, and connectivity, individuals and societies are grappling with rising levels of stress, anxiety, emotional imbalance, and a pervasive sense of inner disquiet. Mental well-being, once considered a peripheral concern, has now become central to discussions on health, education, productivity, and sustainable human development. It is within this broader context that the present volume, Improving Mental Well-Being at the Intersection of Mindfulness, Meditation, and Yoga, finds its deepest relevance and purpose.

Mindfulness, meditation, and yoga are time-tested disciplines rooted in ancient contemplative traditions, particularly those of the East, yet their resonance today is unmistakably global. Far from being mere techniques for relaxation, these practices represent comprehensive systems of self-regulation, self-awareness, and self-transformation. They address the human being as an integrated whole—where mental health is inseparable from physical vitality, emotional balance, ethical living, and inner meaning. This book thoughtfully acknowledges that integration and offers a multidimensional exploration of mental well-being that transcends reductionist approaches.

The themes presented in this volume collectively reflect a progressive journey. Beginning with a holistic understanding of mental well-being, the chapters lay a conceptual foundation that recognizes mental health as a dynamic interplay of cognitive, emotional, behavioral, and social dimensions. The exploration of mindfulness and meditation introduces readers to practices of present-moment awareness, attentional stability, and reflective clarity—capacities that are increasingly essential in an era of distraction and information overload. The inclusion of yoga and the mind–body connection further enriches this discourse by highlighting the role of embodied awareness, breath regulation, and disciplined movement in fostering psychological resilience and inner harmony.

Equally noteworthy is the book's strong emphasis on application and lived experience. By addressing practical tools for everyday practice, emotional regulation, trauma-informed mindfulness and yoga, and therapeutic interventions for mental health challenges, this volume bridges the often-observed gap between theory and practice. These chapters underscore that inner transformation is not confined to retreats or clinical settings but unfolds gradually through conscious choices, daily discipline, and compassionate engagement with oneself and others.

The later themes—focusing on spiritual psychology, inner transformation, compassion, self-care, and self-evaluation—invite readers to reflect more deeply on the purpose and direction of personal growth. They remind us that mental well-being is not merely the absence of distress but the presence of meaning, connection, and ethical sensitivity. The emphasis on community, lifestyle, and the lifelong journey of learning reinforces the idea that well-being is both an individual and collective responsibility.

What makes this volume particularly valuable is its integrative spirit. By bringing together perspectives from psychology, neuroscience, health sciences, education, and contemplative traditions, it contributes to an emerging interdisciplinary paradigm that honors both empirical rigor and experiential wisdom.

It is hoped that this book will serve not only as an academic contribution indexed in global scholarly platforms but also as a guiding light for reflective practice and compassionate living. Ultimately, this volume stands as an invitation—to pause, to reflect, and to rediscover the profound potential of inner awareness in shaping a healthier, more humane world.

Shivam Bhardwaj
Sharda University, Greater Noida, India

Preface

INTRODUCTION

The contemporary world is characterized by unprecedented speed, complexity, and transformation. Rapid social change, technological acceleration, urbanization, shifting family structures, and evolving work cultures have fundamentally altered the ways individuals live, relate, and make meaning of their experiences. While these changes have brought remarkable advancements and opportunities, they have also intensified psychological demands on individuals across age groups, socioeconomic strata, and cultural contexts. Mental well-being, once considered a peripheral concern, has now emerged as a central issue for individuals, families, communities, organizations, and societies at large.

Across the globe, there is a visible rise in stress-related disorders, anxiety, depression, emotional burnout, sleep disturbances, attentional difficulties, and lifestyle-related psychological challenges. Children and adolescents grapple with academic pressure, digital overexposure, identity confusion, and social comparison; adults struggle with work–life imbalance, relational stress, economic uncertainty, and role overload; and older adults often face loneliness, declining health, and existential concerns. The COVID-19 pandemic further exposed the fragility of psychological health systems worldwide, underscoring the urgent need for preventive, promotive, and sustainable approaches to mental well-being rather than crisis-driven or symptom-focused interventions alone.

Within this broader context, mental health is increasingly being understood not merely as the absence of illness, but as a dynamic state of emotional balance, cognitive clarity, psychological resilience, and meaningful engagement with life. Contemporary psychological discourse now emphasizes well-being, flourishing, self-regulation, and resilience alongside traditional diagnostic frameworks. However, despite advances in psychotherapy, pharmacology, and clinical interventions, many individuals continue to experience a sense of inner fragmentation, chronic stress, and disconnection from self and others. This gap has led scholars and practitioners alike to look beyond conventional models and explore integrative approaches that address the whole person i.e. *mind, body, and consciousness.*

It is within this evolving landscape that mindfulness, meditation, and yoga have gained renewed attention as powerful, complementary pathways to mental well-being. Although these practices originated in ancient contemplative and philosophical traditions, particularly within Eastern cultures, their relevance has expanded far beyond their historical and cultural origins. Over the past few decades, mindfulness-based interventions, meditative practices, and yogic techniques have been systematically examined through the lens of modern psychology, neuroscience, and behavioral science. This growing body of evidence highlights their effectiveness in reducing stress, enhancing emotional regulation, improving attention and cognitive flexibility, fostering self-awareness, and promoting overall psychological well-being.

Improving Mental Well-Being at the Intersection of Mindfulness, Meditation, and Yoga brings together these interconnected domains to offer a comprehensive, interdisciplinary exploration of how contemplative and embodied practices can enrich mental health in contemporary contexts. Rather than treating mindfulness, meditation, and yoga as isolated techniques, this volume views them as mutually reinforcing practices that collectively cultivate present-moment awareness, mind–body integration, and inner stability. At their core, all three emphasize conscious awareness, intentionality, and the cultivation of a balanced relationship with one's internal experiences.

Mindfulness, as conceptualized in both classical and contemporary frameworks, involves paying attention to present-moment experiences with openness, curiosity, and non-judgment. Within psychology, mindfulness has been operationalized as a trainable mental skill that enhances awareness of thoughts, emotions, bodily sensations, and environmental stimuli. Extensive research has demonstrated its utility in reducing rumination, emotional reactivity, and stress, while promoting psychological flexibility, self-compassion, and emotional resilience. Mindfulness-based approaches such as Mindfulness-Based Stress Reduction (MBSR) and Mindfulness-Based Cognitive Therapy (MBCT) have been successfully applied across clinical, educational, and organizational settings.

Meditation, while closely related to mindfulness, encompasses a broader range of practices aimed at cultivating concentration, insight, emotional balance, and self-transcendence. From focused attention and loving-kindness meditation to insight-oriented and contemplative practices, meditation offers structured methods for training the mind and deepening self-awareness. Contemporary research suggests that regular meditative practice can lead to measurable changes in brain functioning, emotional regulation, stress physiology, and subjective well-being. Beyond symptom reduction, meditation invites individuals to develop a more reflective, compassionate, and integrated sense of self.

Yoga, often misunderstood as merely a physical exercise, represents a holistic system of self-development that integrates posture (āsana), breath regulation (prā āyāma), ethical principles, concentration, and meditative awareness. Rooted in ancient yogic philosophy, yoga emphasizes harmony between body, mind, and consciousness. Modern adaptations of yoga have shown significant benefits for mental health, including reductions in anxiety and depression, improved emotional regulation, enhanced body awareness, and greater stress resilience. Importantly, yoga offers an embodied pathway to mental well-being, recognizing that psychological states are deeply catalysed by the bodily experience, breath, and movement.

By positioning mindfulness, meditation, and yoga within a shared conceptual framework, this volume emphasizes a holistic model of mental well-being that acknowledges the inseparable and reciprocal relationship between psychological processes, physiological states, and conscious awareness. Rather than privileging cognition alone, this integrative approach recognizes the role of embodiment, breath, emotion, and lived experience in shaping mental health. Such a perspective aligns with emerging trends in psychology that emphasize embodied cognition, affective neuroscience, and person-centered care.

The primary aim of this edited volume is to provide an interdisciplinary platform for researchers, mental health professionals, educators, counselors, yoga practitioners, and scholars to engage with both the theoretical foundations and applied dimensions of mindfulness-based practices, meditative techniques, and yogic philosophies. The chapters bring together diverse disciplinary perspectives, including psychology, counseling, education, health sciences, neuroscience, philosophy, and cultural studies. This interdisciplinary approach allows for a richer, more nuanced understanding of mental well-being that transcends disciplinary silos.

The contributions in this book address a wide range of themes relevant to contemporary mental health discourse. These include stress reduction and coping, emotional resilience, self-regulation, mental health promotion, and prevention of psychological distress. Several chapters explore clinical and counseling applications of mindfulness, meditation, and yoga in addressing anxiety, depression, trauma, and psychosomatic concerns. Others examine their relevance in educational settings, highlighting how contemplative practices can support students' emotional development, attention, and academic engagement. The volume also engages with workplace well-being, exploring how mindfulness and yoga-based interventions can mitigate burnout, enhance emotional intelligence, and foster healthier organizational cultures.

CHAPTER OVERVIEWS

Chapter 1: Inward Journeys: Philosophical Maps for Mindfulness, Meditation, and Yogic Practice

The essay explores the philosophical foundations of Indian contemplative traditions, offering a comprehensive understanding of yoga, meditation, and mindfulness in both traditional and modern settings. It reestablishes the connection between these disciplines and their original philosophical, ethical, and existential purposes, using ancient sources like Patañjali's Yoga Sutras, Advaita Vedanta, and Buddhist teachings. The essay emphasizes the importance of lived experiences in achieving freedom from pain and illusion, rather than just academic concepts. The essay criticizes the commercialization of yoga and mindfulness in contemporary contexts, advocating for more morally sound and culturally sensitive methods. The research offers valuable insights for educators, practitioners, therapists, and academics seeking a deeper connection to contemplative life. Inner Journeys presents mindfulness as a transformative path towards ethical simplicity, existential insight, and holistic well-being, rather than a self-optimization method.

Chapter 2: Mindfulness Meditation Yoga Mantra and Spiritual Practices for Mental Well-Being

Mindfulness, meditation, yoga, mantra recitation, and spiritually oriented reading are increasingly combined to support mental well-being. This chapter reports an integrative review with systematic searches (2010–2025) across major databases, following PRISMA 2020 guidance and using established appraisal tools. Evidence from randomized and non-randomized studies indicates consistent small-to-moderate improvements in stress, anxiety, depressive symptoms, sleep, quality of life, and spiritual well-being. Converging mechanisms include attention and emotion regulation, interoception and autonomic balance, compassion, and meaning-making. Distil pragmatic guidance for brief, blended programs with opt-in spiritual elements and validated measurement. Key gaps concern comparative effectiveness of integrated protocols, dose reporting, mediator testing, long-term maintenance, active controls, and equity. We conclude with priorities for rigorous, culturally sensitive trials and implementation studies in community, clinical, educational, and workplace contexts. Guidance for design & practice.

Chapter 3: Neuroplasticity and the Breath: Unpacking the Brain Mechanisms Behind Yogic Pranayama

Pranayama, the Yogic discipline of regulated breathing, has evolved from a spiritual practice into a scientifically recognized method for supporting mental and neurological health. This chapter examines its neuroplastic potential by outlining effects on major brain regions and networks, while summarizing key Pranayama techniques and their physiological signatures. Evidence indicates improvements in parasympathetic activation, heart rate variability, cortisol modulation, and emotional–cognitive regulation. Integrating recent advances in contemplative and clinical neuroscience, the chapter highlights technology-supported breathwork, trauma-responsive approaches informed by polyvagal theory, and individualized applications based on autonomic profiling. It also clarifies distinctions between established neural biomarkers and emerging theoretical claims of structural change. Overall, the chapter positions Pranayama as an accessible, non-invasive, and increasingly personalized neuromodulatory tool within the broader "Neuro-Yogic Paradigm."

Chapter 4: Rewiring the Anxious Brain A Psychospiritual Exploration of Mindfulness and Yogic Practices in Emotion Regulation

In today's world of rising psychological stress and emotional imbalance, mindfulness and yoga have become highly relevant for mental health care. This chapter explores their impact on emotional regulation from both spiritual and neuropsychological perspectives, highlighting therapeutic mechanisms and practical applications. Based on cognitive-affective theory and supported by recent neurobiology, it explains how breath and awareness practices influence brain regions linked with anxiety and mood disorders, with consistent use leading to neuroplastic changes. By combining psychology, evidence-based research, and traditional wisdom, it shows that mindfulness and yoga enhance resilience, self-awareness, and healthy brain function. The chapter reviews theoretical models, neuroimaging, clinical trials, and longitudinal studies, and discusses integration with standard treatments like CBT and medication. It concludes with structured, evidence-based protocols for professionals, addressing practical use, cultural factors, and contraindications in diverse clinical settings.

Chapter 5: Rewiring the Brain - The Science of Neuroplasticity and the Power of Mindfulness

This chapter explores the intersection of neuroplasticity and mindfulness, highlighting how contemplative practices can induce structural and functional changes in the brain. It outlines the science of neuroplasticity, describing mechanisms like synaptogenesis, dendritic branching, and functional reorganization. The chapter traces mindfulness from its roots in Hindu and Buddhist traditions to its integration into modern therapeutic models such as MBSR, ACT, and DBT. It categorizes formal, informal, and clinical mindfulness practices and examines evidence from neuroscience that demonstrates their role in enhancing emotional regulation, attention, and cognitive flexibility through neuroplastic adaptation

Chapter 6: Rewiring the Brain for Resilience: The Role of Neuroplasticity in Mindfulness, Meditation, and Yoga

One of the most intriguing findings of neuroscience is the ability of contemplative practice to transform the human brain. This chapter explores how neuroplasticity can use mindfulness, meditation, and yoga to strengthen psychological resilience to help us understand how ancient wisdom can be used in combination with new brain science. The chapter introduces clinical studies that demonstrate practical applications across trauma recovery, educational settings, and workplace wellness programs. A holistic implementation model is used to transfer knowledge gathered during the research to practical programs by looking into the training needs, cultural appropriateness, and sustainability questions. The chapter concludes by examining future research priorities, including methodological innovations, cultural inclusivity, precision medicine approaches, and clinical translation challenges. By integrating contemplative neuroscience with practical application, this synthesis offers a scientifically backed way through which a person can actively carve out his or her own neural structure.

Chapter 7: Swami Vivekananda and Practical Vedanta: Transforming Mental Health Through Ancient Wisdom

This chapter explores the relevance of Swami Vivekananda's Practical Vedanta in addressing contemporary mental health challenges. Drawing from core Vedantic principles, such as Atman (the Self), Brahman (ultimate reality), and Advaita (non-dualism), the chapter examines how self-awareness, detachment (Vairagya), and Karma Yoga can transform emotional distress into inner strength. It integrates philosophical insights with psychological concepts like emotional regulation, mindfulness, and resilience, offering a spiritually grounded framework for mental well-being. Through Vivekananda's reinterpretation of Vedanta as a lived philosophy, the chapter argues for inward-directed approaches that transcend symptom management and foster deeper self-realization. This synthesis provides an inclusive, non-sectarian path to emotional clarity and inner freedom in an age of psychological fragmentation.

Chapter 8: Synchronization through Yoga: Connecting the Physical and Mental Realms

This chapter explores the profound integration of body and mind achieved through yoga, emphasizing its role in harmonizing physiological, psychological, and cognitive functions. It highlights how practices such as breath regulation, postures, meditation, and mindfulness foster neural synchronization, enhance autonomic balance, and promote emotional stability and stress resilience. Drawing upon both ancient philosophy and contemporary scientific evidence, the discussion demonstrates yoga's capacity to optimize attention regulation, cognitive flexibility, and overall well-being. By bridging traditional wisdom with modern research, the chapter underscores yoga's potential as a holistic approach to health, performance enhancement, and comprehensive mind-body synchronization across diverse populations.

Chapter 9: The Triad of Transformation Exploring the Synergistic Landscape of Mindfulness, Meditation, and Yoga in Contemporary Mental Health Enhancement

The global mental health crisis, characterized by escalating rates of anxiety, depression, and existential distress, has exposed the limitations of conventional biomedical approaches. This chapter explores the integrative potential of mindfulness, meditation, and yoga as a synergistic triad for promoting comprehensive mental well-being. Grounded in both ancient contemplative traditions and contemporary empirical research, the triad fosters emotional regulation, neuroplastic adaptability, embodied awareness, and a deeper sense of meaning. Rather than focusing solely on symptom reduction, these practices support psychological resilience and spiritual growth. The chapter further investigates their increasing application across therapeutic, educational, and occupational domains, highlighting their adaptability, scientific credibility, and cross-cultural relevance. It calls for a paradigm shift toward person-centered, developmental models of care that recognize contemplative practices as foundational tools for long-term healing and flourishing.

Chapter 10: Undulations: The Flow of Breath and Emotions

Breath and emotion are intricately connected, forming continuous waves that shape our inner experiences and outward expressions. This chapter explores the physiological, psychological, and cultural ties between breathing patterns and emotional states, demonstrating how breath acts as both a mirror and a regulator of emotion. Insights from neuroscience, somatic psychology, and cultural traditions reveal that conscious breath practices—such as mindfulness, breathwork, and pranayama—enhance emotional resilience, interoceptive awareness, and self-regulation. Breath also holds symbolic significance in art, literature, and spiritual traditions, where it serves as a non-verbal language of expression and transformation. By developing breath literacy—the awareness and intentional modulation of breathing—we gain tools not only for personal well-being but also for fostering presence, connection, and adaptability in a fast-paced world. Ultimately, breath emerges as a tide, guiding us back to equilibrium amidst life's emotional undulations.

Chapter 11: Yoga and the Mind-Body Connection – Integrative Perspectives on Neurophysiology, Mental Health, and Embodied Awareness

The chapter presents a unified examination of yoga and its body-mind approach by exploring neural mechanisms, psychological and philosophical aspects. It examines how yoga facilitates the body-mind connection through yogic texts and scientific study, such as breath regulation (pranayama), postural awareness (asana) and meditative focus (dhyana). This study applies polyvagal theory, interoceptive awareness, neuroplasticity and the biopsychosocial framework. Research in neuroscience and mental health shows yoga's efficacy in addressing anxiety, depression, trauma and stress. The chapter highlights yoga as an evidence-based non-drug intervention combining traditional Eastern knowledge with Western science to benefit mental health holistically. This part outlines present-day yoga research restrictions, including cultural knowledge appropriateness, methodological challenges, and future directions. This research supports yoga as an effective practice for developing unified mind-body relationships, emotional resilience and psychological health in both individuals and collective contexts.

CONCLUSION

Importantly, this book acknowledges the cultural and contextual dimensions of mental well-being. Rather than presenting mindfulness, meditation, and yoga as universally applicable techniques divorced from their cultural roots, the chapters emphasize culturally sensitive and ethically grounded applications. This includes critical reflections on adaptation, integration with indigenous knowledge systems, and the responsible use of contemplative practices in diverse populations. Such an approach ensures that integrative mental health practices remain inclusive, respectful, and contextually meaningful.

A distinguishing feature of this volume is its emphasis on balancing theory and practice. While grounded in empirical research and conceptual clarity, the chapters also offer practical insights, case illustrations, and intervention frameworks that can be applied in real-world settings. This balance makes the book relevant not only for academicians and researchers but also for clinicians, counselors, educators, and practitioners seeking evidence-informed tools to support mental well-being.

By integrating psychological science with contemplative and embodied practices, this book contributes to a growing movement toward integrative mental health which is an approach that values prevention alongside treatment, self-awareness alongside symptom reduction, and inner balance alongside external functioning. Such a perspective is particularly relevant in a world where psychological distress often arises from chronic stress, disconnection, and fragmentation rather than discrete pathology alone.

It is hoped that *Improving Mental Well-Being at the Intersection of Mindfulness, Meditation, and Yoga* will serve as a valuable resource for students, scholars, clinicians, and practitioners across disciplines. As mental health challenges continue to evolve in complexity, the integration of mindfulness, meditation, and yoga offers promising pathways toward prevention, resilience-building, and sustainable well-being. Ultimately, this book seeks to contribute to a deeper, more nuanced understanding of how contemplative and embodied practices can support individuals in leading healthier, more balanced, meaningful, and psychologically enriched lives. By fostering awareness, compassion, and self-regulation, these practices hold transformative potential- not only for individual growth but also for collective well-being in an increasingly interconnected world.

Beyond offering knowledge, the volume seeks to inspire reflective engagement, personal inquiry, and innovative research in the field of integrative mental health. This book aspires to contribute to a deeper and more compassionate understanding of mental well-being- one that empowers individuals to cultivate awareness, resilience, and meaning in their lives, and supports societies in fostering psychologically healthier and more humane ways of living.

Chapter 1
Inward Journeys: Philosophical Maps for Mindfulness, Meditation, and Yogic Practice

Piyali Sarkar
http://orcid.org/0000-0002-5762-7432
Lovely Professional University, India

ABSTRACT

The essay explores the philosophical foundations of Indian contemplative traditions, offering a comprehensive understanding of yoga, meditation, and mindfulness in both traditional and modern settings. It reestablishes the connection between these disciplines and their original philosophical, ethical, and existential purposes, using ancient sources like Patañjali's Yoga Sūtras, Advaita Vedānta, and Buddhist teachings. The essay emphasizes the importance of lived experiences in achieving freedom from pain and illusion, rather than just academic concepts. The essay criticizes the commercialization of yoga and mindfulness in contemporary contexts, advocating for more morally sound and culturally sensitive methods. The research offers valuable insights for educators, practitioners, therapists, and academics seeking a deeper connection to contemplative life. Inner Journeys presents mindfulness as a transformative path towards ethical simplicity, existential insight, and holistic well-being, rather than a self-optimization method.

1. INTRODUCTION

For thousands of years, the interior geography of human consciousness has captivated intellectuals, leading to the development of a wide range of philosophical,

DOI: 10.4018/979-8-3373-4187-3.ch001

spiritual, and psychological systems that seek to map the nature of transcendence, reality, and the self. These systems are examined in Inward Journeys: Philosophical Maps for Mindfulness, Meditation, and Yogic Practice as useful instruments for self-transformation rather than only as theoretical concepts. With inspiration from the diverse schools of yoga, Advaita Vedānta, and Sāṃkhya, among other rich traditions of Indian philosophy, this study offers a comparative and integrative perspective on inner work as an embodied and contemplative practice. A rigorous ontological and epistemological foundation for understanding the mind, suffering, liberation (mokhṣa), and the methods by which one could achieve it is provided by these traditions. As key practices, mindfulness and meditation are studied as disciplines grounded on philosophical presumptions about the nature of reality, the self, and consciousness rather than just as techniques for stress reduction or attention training (Chadha, 2015; Bryant, 2009). This book seeks to assist practitioners and academics who want to go further into yogic and contemplative systems beyond the superficial applications made popular in the contemporary wellness sector by outlining these intellectual foundations.

A fundamental issue at the centre of this investigation is: What does it mean to turn inward, and what philosophical instruments might direct that process? From Plato's cave allegory to Descartes' cogito, Western philosophical traditions have long recognized the inward turn as a route to truth. However, the most systematic ways to introspection may be found in Indian philosophy and contemplative practice, where embodied discipline (yoga) and meditative insight (jñāna) meet. The eight limbs of yoga (aṣṭāṅga yoga) are outlined in Patañjali's Yoga Sūtras as a gradual plan to achieve puruṣa, or pure awareness, and to settle the mind's fluctuations (citta-vṛtti-nirodha) (Patañjali, trans. Bryant, 2009). In the same way, attention is used in Advaita Vedānta to distinguish between the real (sat) and the unreal (asat), which leads to the non-dual realization of Brahman (Shankara, trans. Gambhirananda, 2006). Without limiting the profundity of classical insights to only neurobiological mechanics, this book aims to connect these ancient maps with modern understandings from phenomenology, psychology, and cognitive science (Varela, Thompson, & Rosch, 1991). Rather, it suggests a dialogical method in which contemporary research and classical philosophical systems complement one another, allowing readers to conduct their own introspective excursions with more precision, clarity, and significance.

2. RATIONALE AND RELEVANCE

The goal of the chapter is to examine the fundamental philosophical concepts that have influenced contemplative practices in Eastern traditions. There is a pressing need to return to the ancient philosophical foundations of mindfulness, meditation, and yoga in the contemporary global context, which is characterized by an increase in mental health issues, a crisis of meaning, and a growing interest in non-Western epistemologies. Despite being devoid of its soteriological, ethical, and metaphysical components, these techniques are frequently used in modern settings for their therapeutic advantages. Re-contextualizing these activities within the intellectual traditions from whence they originated is the goal of this chapter.

In wellness and therapeutic paradigms, yoga, meditation, and mindfulness are frequently seen as separate practices. But historically, they have been interconnected practices rooted in profound philosophical investigation—into the nature of awareness, suffering, liberation, and the self. For example, as explained in the Satipaṭṭhāna Sutta, mindfulness (Pāli: sati) is a key element of the Buddhist path toward enlightenment (nirvāṇa) and is not only a method for attentional management (Anālayo, 2003). Similar to this, the dualistic metaphysics of puruṣa (pure awareness) and prakṛti (material nature) underpin traditional yoga as it was articulated by Patañjali in the Yoga Sūtras. Its aim is kaivalya, or emancipation, via ethical discipline and meditative absorption (Feuerstein, 2001). There are two reasons why discussing the intellectual underpinnings of these traditions is important. In the first place, it provides a remedy for the commercialization and secularization of yoga and mindfulness in contemporary culture. Nowadays, practices that were formerly a part of strong philosophical systems that sought self-realization are frequently promoted only as lifestyle aids. Their transformational power may be diminished by this decontextualization. According to academics like Purser (2019), the popular mindfulness movement might act as a type of "McMindfulness," prioritizing stress management and personal performance above more profound existential and ethical understanding, especially in business and therapeutic contexts.

Second, a philosophical analysis of these contemplative practices encourages a cross-cultural discussion between Eastern and Western philosophical traditions. The rich Eastern contemplative traditions provide contrasting and occasionally radical viewpoints on consciousness and the self while Western philosophy wrestles more and more with issues of embodied cognition, phenomenology, and the boundaries of reason. In contrast to Cartesian dualism, the Advaita Vedānta idea of non-duality (advaita) proposes a basic unity of being in which the absolute reality (Brahman) and the particular self (ātman) are ultimately the same (Rambachan, 2006). Buddhist concepts of anattā (non-self) similarly undermine the concept of a permanent, independent subject, providing insights that align with post-structuralist and procedural philosophical perspectives.

Thirdly, the chapter's emphasis on "philosophical maps" emphasizes how crucial conceptual frameworks are for directing inward change. Philosophical systems give navigational aids for the interior path toward increased consciousness, moral behavior, and pain relief, just like a map offers direction in the outside world. These maps are dynamic guides influenced by centuries of discussion, analysis, and first-hand experience rather than rigid beliefs. This chapter also adds to the continuing decolonization of knowledge by reclaiming the intellectual foundations of yoga, meditation, and mindfulness. It affirms the validity and profundity of Buddhist and Indian philosophical traditions as sources of existential and psychological insight, challenging the predominance of Western epistemologies in scholarly and therapeutic discourse. According to de Sousa Santos (2014), establishing a more diverse and egalitarian global knowledge system requires acknowledging a Southerly epistemology. The research is an important cultural and ethical intervention in addition to a theoretical investigation. It challenges academics, practitioners, and seekers to consider the fundamental meanings and goals of contemplative practice that go beyond practicality and skill. By doing this, it emphasizes the importance of traditional knowledge in answering the age-old human need for enlightenment, tranquillity, and freedom.

3. OBJECTIVES

This chapter explores four interconnected goals that together highlight the importance of interior journeys in the quest of self-realization, ethical life, and holistic well-being in order to dig into the profound inner elements of Indian philosophical traditions.

3.1. Philosophical Foundation

A comparative philosophical examination of the interior journey across important Indian traditions is the focus of the first goal. Examining Vedānta, Sāṅkhya, Yoga, and some schools of Buddhism and Jainism is part of this, since they all stress the realization of a higher or truer self and the transcending of ego-bound awareness. Advaita Vedānta, for example, emphasizes the non-dual understanding of ātman (self) and brahman (ultimate reality), arguing that liberation (mokṣa) results from realizing that worldly attachment (māyā) and individual identity (jīva) are illusory. Similar to this, Sāṅkhya emphasizes the difference between prakṛti (material nature) and puruṣa (pure awareness), highlighting introspective discernment (viveka) as the route to emancipation. According to these traditions, the inward path is a rigorous philosophical discipline focused on self-awareness, detachment, and inner change rather than a retreat from the outside world. The chapter will highlight the many approaches to self-realization that Indian spiritual psychology suggests, as well as the shared metaphysical and epistemological presuppositions that underpin it, using this comparative framework.

3.2. Mindfulness and Meditation

Recontextualizing mindfulness (smṛti in Sanskrit, sati in Pali) and meditation (dhyāna, samādhi) within their original ethical and philosophical contexts is the second goal. This chapter portrays them as essential components of a soteriological journey rather than as separate procedures, as is sometimes the case with modern secular versions. For example, in Buddhism, mindfulness is one of the Eightfold Path's limbs and is intrinsically linked to wisdom (prajñā), concentration (samādhi), and ethical behavior (śīla). In the Yogic and Vedāntic traditions, meditation is not just a practice but also the result of self-reflection, focus, and disciplined ethical life.

3.3. Yoga Praxi

Examining the composition and importance of the Aṣṭāṅga Yoga system as Patañjali explains it in the Yoga Sūtras is the third goal. A methodical road map to inner purification and transcendence of oneself is provided by this eight-fold path, which includes yama (ethical constraints), niyama (individual practices), āsana (posture), prāṇāyāma (breathing control), pratyāhāra (abandonment of senses), dhāraṇā (concentration), dhyāna (mindfulness), and samādhi (absorption). The chapter highlights the fundamental function of yama and niyama, or ethical behavior, as preconditions for more profound absorption of meditation. It also emphasizes how yoga combines disciplined action with intellectual understanding, demonstrating the interdependence of morality, intelligence, and spiritual freedom.

3.4. Current Implications

By examining the current applicability of these ideas and methods, this section aims to connect traditional knowledge with contemporary issues. The inward path charted by Indian traditions provides timeless insights on emotional resilience, mindful comprehension, and holistic well-being at a time of stress, distraction, and existential crises. Ancient models of self-cultivation are still essential for tackling today's existential and psychological issues, as demonstrated by the critical discussion of contemporary implementations in psychotherapy, mindfulness-based therapies, and wellness discourses. Through the integration of contemporary psychological frameworks with ancient knowledge, the chapter underscores the timeless relevance of the inward journey in promoting ethical responsibility and human happiness.

With the help of these four goals, the chapter aims to portray Indian interior philosophies as dynamic, integrative paradigms that still appeal to the human search for meaning, equilibrium, and freedom rather than as mysterious artefacts.

4. PHILOSOPHICAL MAPS FOR MINDFULNESS, MEDITATION, AND YOGIC PRACTICE

Though they are frequently approached via secular or therapeutic frameworks nowadays, mindfulness, meditation, and yoga have their roots in deep philosophical systems that provide complex maps of consciousness, selfhood, and emancipation. In addition to offering philosophical underpinnings, these maps—especially those from Indian traditions like Sāṃkhya, Yoga, and Advaita Vedānta—also offer helpful advice for inner development. A common understanding is at the core of all systems: that human suffering results from a basic misidentification with fleeting mental and physical sensations, and that liberation (mokṣa) can be attained via direct realization of the actual self and focused introspection. The eightfold route (aṣṭāṅga yoga) is described in Patañjali's Yoga Sūtras as a progressive framework that starts with ethical preparation and ends with samādhi, or the absorption of the mind into pure consciousness. According to this framework's dualistic metaphysics, liberation entails separating the self from the mind's fluctuations (vṛtti), and puruṣa (pure awareness) is separate from prakṛti (matter) (Bryant, 2009). Advaita Vedānta, on the other hand, presents a non-dual vision in which ignorance (avidyā) is the primary source of bondage and the individual self (ātman) is ultimately the same as the absolute reality (Brahman). Here, meditation and mindfulness serve as instruments for viveka (discernment), which enables one to recognize the oneness that underlies all occurrences and the illusory character of the ego (Shankara, trans. Gambhirananda, 2006).

These philosophical systems function as maps—organized methods of traversing the inner world, comprehending the patterns of the mind, and achieving levels of clarity and insight. They are not only theoretical. Given the breadth of experiential information ingrained in these traditions, contemporary cognitive science, phenomenology, and psychology have started to interact with them (Varela, Thompson & Rosch, 1991). But there is still a chance that practices like mindfulness might be decontextualized, stripped of their transformational purpose and reduced to methods for increasing productivity or lowering stress. Reintroducing philosophical research and contemplative practice can benefit both by providing a comprehensive understanding of the human situation that takes into account existential clarity as well as mental wellness. Furthermore, these systems offer a distinctive paradigm for embodied knowledge, in which yoga is a somatic and moral discipline that aims to balance body, breath, mind, and awareness rather than just being a physical workout. As a result, they call into question Western dualisms of subject and object, mind and body, and encourage a more comprehensive view of awareness. We may go on a more in-depth introspective journey that respects the richness of the human experience as well as the potential for freedom via understanding, self-control, and change if we see these ancient structures as philosophical maps—detailed, complicated, and flexible routes.

4.1. The Inner Terrain: Outlining the Inward Path

More than just a physical or spiritual practice, the interior path—often represented by the name yoga—is a fundamental ontological investigation into the nature of the self, awareness, and human suffering. The Sanskrit root yuj, which means "to yoke," "to unite," or "to bring into alignment," is where the term yoga comes from. It refers to the fusion of the particular self with a more profound, frequently transcendent reality. Yoga was originally thought of as a disciplined way to connect body, breath, mind, and consciousness toward liberation (mokṣa), not just physical postures (āsanas). This inner journey starts with an investigation of the components of the human mind, regardless of the Indian philosophical traditions—Sāṃkhya, Yoga, Vedānta, or Buddhism. Cit (pure awareness) and ātman (the inner self or soul) are different from the mind (manas), which is frequently linked to emotional reaction and sensory coordination, and citta, which is the mental field that includes memory, cognition, and imagination. ātman is defined as immovable, limitless, and beyond the boundaries of temporal identity, whereas manas and citta are variable and frequently disrupted by outside stimuli. For instance, the Upaniṣads depict the ātman as the inner witness (sākṣin), unaffected by the whirlpool of thoughts (Radhakrishnan & Moore, 1957). Similar to this, Patañjali's Yoga Sūtras stress that in order to realize the puruṣa, or pure seer, who is untouched by psychological content, mental fluctuations must be stilled (citta-vṛtti-nirodha) (Bryant, 2009). According to these traditions, suffering (duḥkha) occurs when the ego fails to see the actual nature of awareness and instead identifies with its ideas, feelings, and wants. According to this perspective, seeking inner calm is an existential imperative rather than just a spiritual goal. The internal journey is a means of achieving existential resolution since the mind's restlessness and its connection with outside things sustain discontent, worry, and bewilderment. This is frequently reflected in contemporary psychological discourse, which contends that self-awareness, cognitive control, and alignment with higher ideals are the foundations of mental health (Goleman & Davidson, 2017). Ancient traditions, however, go farther and suggest that the ultimate kind of healing is self-realization rather than just emotional harmony.

Thus, looking inward is a brave act of facing the inner landscape of mental habits, attachments, and delusions rather than an escape. Philosophical maps from classical writings provide crucial advice in navigating this terrain: techniques like viveka (discriminative knowledge), dhyāna (meditative absorption), and pratyāhāra (withdrawal of the senses) assist the practitioner in differentiating between the transient and the permanent. Through these activities, one's life is brought into alignment with a higher order that goes beyond egoic conceptions, reorienting them from the distracting outside world to the meaningful inner world. By going back to the constant core of one's being, the inward route described by yoga and associated traditions thereby fulfils a basic human desire—not only to believe in peace, but to live it.

4.2. Memory and Mindfulness: The Function of Smṛti and Sati

Memory and mindfulness are essential components of spiritual emancipation and existential clarity in India's contemplative traditions, not only cognitive abilities. Beyond recalling previous experiences, smṛti—often translated as "memory" or "remembrance"—plays a crucial role in both Yogic and Vedāntic situations. In the midst of life's distractions, it refers to the ability to recall one's actual self and sustain a constant awareness of spiritual truths. According to Patañjali's Yoga Sūtras (1.11), smṛiti is the ability to retain experience that has not been forgotten, which allows the practitioner to use sustained attention to discern between the fleeting and the eternal (Bryant, 2009). It is essential for keeping the mind from returning to unconscious tendencies and for stabilizing meditation.

Smṛti is frequently invoked in Vedānta, especially Advaita Vedānta, in the context of śravaṇa (hearing), manana (contemplation), and nididhyāsana (deep meditation), where recalling the mahāvākyas ("great sayings" such as "tat tvam asi" – "That Thou Art") aids in overcoming avidyā (ignorance) and regaining consciousness of Brahman, the non-dual reality (Shankara, trans. Gambhirananda, 2006). The term sati, which also comes from the root smṛ (to remember), is used in early Buddhist teachings to frame mindfulness, although it places more emphasis on present-moment awareness than metaphysical recollection. Sati is described in the Satipaṭṭhāna Sutta as a characteristic of presence that preserves perception clarity and prevents forgetting the Dhamma, rather than as simple attentiveness (Anālayo, 2003). It entails using an observant, non-reactive approach to physical experiences, mental states, and events in order to develop understanding of suffering (dukkha), impermanence (anicca), and non-self (anattā). Whether seen as avidyā (ignorance) in Buddhism or māyā (illusion) in Vedānta, the notion that mindfulness serves as a remedy against delusion is what ties these views together. Because it allows the practitioner to "remember" the real and dis-identify with the unreal, mindfulness is fundamentally philosophical rather than being a passive or neutral attention. This makes it the entrance to wisdom (prajñā). Therefore, mindfulness aims to promote existential congruence and moral clarity in addition to stress reduction and cognitive sharpening. It serves to remind the practitioner not just of what is taking place, but also of their own identity in connection with it.

Smṛti and sati, when correctly understood and practiced, foster a loving detachment from egoic reaction and a radical honesty toward reality. This recall is not historical or sentimental; rather, it is a constant return to the reality of impermanence and the instantaneity of existence. By keeping one rooted in the here and now while exposing the outlines of ultimate truth, mindfulness turns into an ethical practice in both religions. By honing discernment, destroying illusion, and realigning one's life with more profound realities, mindfulness not only paves the way for freedom but also becomes a way of being.

4.3. Meditation Philosophies: Beyond Dhyāna

The definitions, purposes, and methods of meditation vary greatly throughout Indian spiritual and philosophical traditions, making it a deeply complex and intellectually rich exercise. Meditation is a potent instrument for ontological change and epistemological clarity within the deeper frameworks of Buddhism, Vedānta, and Yoga, despite being simplistically equated with mindfulness or relaxation in common discourse. In order to transcend conventional perception and enable freedom from illusion, pain, or duality, it is more than just a passive practice; rather, it is an active engagement with awareness. Meditation is part of the larger framework of aṣṭāṅga yoga, or the Eightfold Path, according to Patañjali's Yogic doctrine. The last three limbs are specifically dhyāna, which comes after dhāraṇā (concentration) and leads to samādhi (absorption). Although dhyāna is sometimes misinterpreted as meditation in general, the Yogasūtras give it a very specific and sophisticated definition. Bryant (2009) states that dhyāna is the unbroken stream of consciousness focused on a single object, a condition in which the mind's fluctuations (vṛttis) are suppressed. Nirbīja samādhi, or seedless absorption, is the result of this great concentration. It is a meditative state in which everything content, including the smallest perceptions (saṃskāras), is transcended. Puruṣa, the pure witnessing awareness, which is unencumbered by the material and mental worlds (prakṛti), is what is left. Kaivalya, or emancipation, is the ultimate goal of yoga and a state of complete ontological freedom.

Though it does use Yogic techniques for practical reasons, Advaita Vedānta places more emphasis on non-dual contemplation (nididhyāsana) than Yoga does on attention and mental calm. According to Śaṅkara's systematization of the Advaitic path, meditation follows two essential preconditions: śravaṇa (hearing the teachings of the scriptures) and manana (thinking critically about those teachings). Nididhyāsana, a prolonged introspective meditation on the identity of ātman (self) and Brahman (absolute reality), is only then performed by the seeker. This type of meditation aims to dissolve the appearance of dualism rather than achieve mental tranquility for its own sake. The technique of neti neti ("not this, not that"), which is advocated by Śaṅkara, involves the meditator negating everything that is not the Self, including the body, mind, senses, and ideas, until simply the pure, unaltered, non-dual Self is left. According to Gambhirananda (2006), this results in the understanding that ātman and Brahman are one and that real liberation (mokṣa) is found in realizing one's actual nature as undivided awareness. Buddhism, especially in its Theravāda version, approaches meditation from a standpoint that rejects the notion of a permanent self, in contrast to both Yoga and Vedānta. Vipassanā, or insight meditation, is the fundamental method of meditation in this school. Vipassanā urges the practitioner to pay attention to thoughts, feelings, and body sensations with present-moment awareness rather than concentrating on a single object or thinking about non-duality. The three essential aspects of existence—impermanence (anicca), suffering (dukkha), and non-self (anattā)—become apparent via this practice. According to Anālayo (2003), the illusion of a stable, in control self is destroyed by this meditative examination. Rather, the practitioner learns to see the self as a stream of situations and processes that are always changing, without a steady centre. Nirvāṇa, or the extinction of attachment, ignorance, and desire, is the aim in order to break the cycle of rebirth (saṃsāra).

Each of the three systems agree on the transformational power of meditation, although having different metaphysical presuppositions: Buddhism is non-essentialist (anattā), Vedānta is non-dual (ātman-Brahman), and Yoga is dualistic (puruṣa-prakṛti). According to each philosophy, meditation is a means of transcending everyday awareness, upending ingrained behaviors, and discovering a more profound reality. That truth is the indivisible oneness of existence for the Vedāntin, the isolation of pure consciousness for the Yogi, and the realization that holding onto any essence—even a self—is the source of suffering for the Buddhist. These methods show that meditation is a difficult philosophical undertaking—a type of embodied epistemology—rather than just a spiritual getaway from the outside world. It is a liberating activity in which philosophy is lived rather than just rationalized. Whether through vipassanā, nididhyāsana, or dhyāna, meditation necessitates a profound shift of perspective toward reality. It improves discernment, fosters a calm, equanimous mind that can comprehend truth without distortion, and promotes ethical life (yama-niyama in Yoga, śīla in Buddhism).

Therefore, it is appropriate to understand meditation in these traditional Indian traditions as a range of deliberate mental practices that are all based on different philosophical worldviews but ultimately come to the idea of existential freedom rather than as a single, universal concept. Meditation emerges as a dynamic way of waking, whether through the Yogic cessation of mental oscillations, the Vedāntic contemplating of non-duality, or the Buddhist disintegration of the ego. It dissolves illusions, transcends appearances, and leads the practitioner to a direct contact with ultimate reality—whatever shape that may take—making it both a means and a method of knowing.

4.4. The Eightfold Path and Yogic Ethics (Aṣṭāṅga Yoga)

The eightfold journey of Aṣṭāṅga Yoga, described in Patañjali's Yoga Sūtras, offers a comprehensive ethical and philosophical framework intended to change the full person in addition to serving as a technical manual for contemplative absorption. The first two limbs of this system, yama (restraints) and niyama (observances), are essential because they serve as the moral and ethical cornerstone of yogic life. These moral behaviors are seen as essential for stability and inner purity, far from being elective or preemptive. By regulating one's connection with the outside world, the yamas—which include non-violence (ahiṃsā), honesty (satya), non-stealing (asteya), celibacy or moderation (brahmacarya), and non-possessiveness (aparigraha)—promote harmony, integrity, and self-control. By turning that ethical orientation inward, the niyamas—cleanliness (śauca), serenity (santoṣa), disciplined effort (tapas), self-study (svādhyāya), and resignation to the divine (īśvarapraṇidhāna)—create a life of self-reflection and surrender. The deeper limbs of yoga, such as āsana (posture), prāṇāyāma (breath control), and pratyāhāra (withdrawal of the senses), run the risk of becoming meaningless practices without these underpinnings. The body, neurological system, and perceptions are primed for rest and introspection by these intermediary limbs. "Prāṇāyāma soothes and stretches the breath to refine strength and attention, Āsana regulates the body to promote meditative improve your posture, and pratyāhāra symbolizes the crucial pivot inward, disconnecting the senses from distractions outside and turning consciousness toward the inner self" (Bryant, 2009). The practitioner may only start the internal ascent through samādhi (absorption), dhyāna (meditation), and dhāraṇā (concentration) with this preliminary practice. Samādhi extends beyond the meditator-object duality entirely, leading to the intuitive understanding of the true self, or puruṣa. Dhāraṇā fixes the attention on only one thing, dhyāna expands that focus into an unaltered meditative flow, and samādhi completes the continuum of interior refinement. However, the ethical and intellectual foundations of yoga are inextricably linked to even these contemplative states. Patañjali clarifies that yogic practice is a profoundly moral process that aims for emancipation (kaivalya), or the liberation of pure awareness from the constantly shifting alterations of the mind, rather than an isolated spiritual endeavour. As such, yoga is a lived philosophy rather than just a collection of exercises. It combines physical alignment, energy control, moral discipline, and meditative silence into a logical process of self-transformation. The classical approach maintains that ethics and ontology are inextricably linked, in contrast to contemporary views that minimize yoga to health benefits or stress alleviation. Integrity—the way one lives, communicates, and interacts with others—is just as important to true yogic progress as technique. Therefore, the aṣṭāṅga path is an interconnected system in which each limb supports and refines the others, guiding the practitioner toward profound inner freedom and clarity, rather than a ladder of spiritual steps to be ascended in order.

4.5. Connections to Buddhist and Advaita Thought

The philosophical landscapes of Buddhism and Advaita Vedānta share deep concerns about the nature of reality, self, and liberation, especially as they pertain to mindfulness and contemplative insight, while having different ontological commitments. Advaita Vedānta's main metaphysical thesis is non-duality, or advaita: brahman, the formless, unchanging source of existence, and the particular self (ātman) are ultimately the same. Liberation (mokṣa) is the eradication of ignorance (avidyā) that conceals one's actual nature as pure awareness, not the attainment of a new condition. Vairāgya (detachment from sensory and mental phenomena) and viveka (discernment between the real and the unreal) are two fundamental disciplines that help achieve this realization. They both prepare the mind to internalize the non-dual truth through nididhyāsana, or deep contemplative absorption (Shankara, trans. Gambhirananda, 2006). The idea of an everlasting self, on the other hand, is rejected by Buddhist philosophy, particularly in its early Theravāda and later Madhyamaka and Yogācāra forms, which assert anattā (non-self) as a basic truth. According to the Buddha, the self is a temporary term for a group of constantly evolving processes (the five aggregates: skandhas) rather than a permanent reality. Through vipassanā (insight meditation), this realization results in dis-identification from egoic structures and, eventually, nirvāṇa, or the end of suffering. Buddhism maintains that holding onto any idea of a permanent self is a major source of suffering, in contrast to Advaita, which posits an everlasting, unchanging self.

Buddhist doctrines like pratītya-samutpāda (dependent origination), which holds that all phenomena arise in dependence upon conditions and thus lack independent, intrinsic existence, and śūnyatā (emptiness), a Mahāyāna thought that refines this view and denies any inherent essence in all things, further reflect this divergence. Both traditions stress meditative clarity and freedom from ignorance and mental suffering in spite of these ontological differences. Disembedding awareness from mental fluctuations and egoic identification is the goal of both the Advaitic practice of persistent self-inquiry (ātma-vicāra) and the Buddhist idea of sati (mindfulness). Detachment and ethical discipline are also used in both religions as stepping stones to greater revelation. The ontological presuppositions of their respective mindfulness traditions, however, differ: Buddhist mindfulness is focused on impermanence, contingency, and the dismantling of any essentialist viewpoint, whereas Advaita mindfulness is based on the memory of the non-dual self and the ultimate unity of all existence. It's interesting to note that both traditions emphasize the direct, non-conceptual discovery of truth via focused introspection, while having conflicting metaphysical stances—one affirming the self, the other denying it. They so represent a common dedication to contemplative philosophy as a means of achieving existential freedom. The discussion between Advaita and Buddhist thinking may be viewed as a mutually enlightening investigation into the nature of consciousness, the causes of suffering, and the prospect of liberation beyond the artificial confines of the self, even if it is frequently characterized by polemical distinction in ancient writings.

4.6. Philosophical Integration and Contemporary Consequences

In recent decades, modern ideas of attention, emotion, and consciousness—particularly in psychology and neuroscience—have been greatly impacted by the ancient philosophical maps of yoga, advaita vedānta, and Buddhism. These traditions' practices—mindfulness meditating, breathwork, and contemplative self-inquiry, for example—are currently being researched for their therapeutic value as well as conceptual frameworks for comprehending emotional and cognitive control. For instance, studies in contemplative neuroscience have demonstrated how long-term mindfulness practice changes the brain areas linked to self-referential processing (the default mode network), emotional regulation (the amygdala), and attention (the prefrontal cortex). These findings support the long-held belief in these traditions that disciplined awareness can lead to inner transformation (Davidson & Goleman, 2017). Concern over the decontextualization and monetization of these activities is rising as they spread into secular domains, particularly in the fields of therapy, education, and wellness. The fundamental ethical and philosophical goals of yoga and mindfulness—liberation, compassion, and discernment—are frequently lost when these practices are reduced to physical activity or marketed as a productivity trick. Such commercialization deprives yoga and mindfulness of their depth and transforms them into coping mechanisms rather than avenues for liberation. This has led to demands for a re-ethical – ization of mindfulness, commonly known as "ethical mindfulness," which re-establishes awareness practices with moral clarity, compassion, and responsibility from both academics and contemplative practitioners. The Noble Eightfold Path is inextricably linked to mindfulness in Buddhist traditions, and practicing mindfulness correctly entails keeping in mind the moral precepts of interdependence and non-harm. Similarly, in Advaita Vedānta and Yogic structures, mindfulness must be directed by yamas and niyamas (ethical disciplines) and viveka (discernment), which make sure that practice is utilized to develop rather than avoid moral duty. These deeper facets of contemplative philosophy provide more than just personal healing; they provide a blueprint for societal transformation as digital distractions and socio-political upheaval further split public life. Intentional breathing, contemplative stillness, and reflective silence are examples of inner routines that may be used as pedagogical procedures for education and leadership development as well as therapeutic tools in mental health and trauma rehabilitation. When viewed holistically, these practices are means of re-entering life with clarity, balance, and care rather than as techniques to avoid reality. Today's task is not just to embrace yoga or mindfulness, but to reintegrate these practices into a worldview that respects their historical roots while bringing them into the present. This entails incorporating contemplative ethics into public discourse, compassion into policy, and attentiveness into education. By doing this, we bring back to life the age-old realization that awareness is a moral and relational act as well as a personal talent, one that ties us to the world and to each other with more integrity, humility, and intention.

5. METHODOLOGY AND SOURCES

Using an interdisciplinary approach, this chapter will draw on the following primary sources: Advaita works such as Śaṅkara's Vivekacūḍāmaṇi, Buddhist canonical texts (Satipaṭṭhāna Sutta, Abhidhamma), the Yoga Sūtra of Patañjali, the Bhagavad Gītā, Upanishads, Bṛhadāraṇyaka, and Chāndogya Upanishads.

- Secondary philosophical study includes current work in comparative philosophy as well as commentary by modern philosophers like Swami Vivekananda, D.T. Suzuki, B.K.S. Iyengar, T.K.V. Desikachar, and the Dalai Lama.
- Contemporary interdisciplinary literature: Writings by authors like Richard Davidson, Francisco Varela, and Jon Kabat-Zinn that connect contemplative traditions with psychology, cognitive science, and education.

6. NEW PERSPECTIVE TO THE FIELD

For modern mindfulness and meditation techniques to regain their original depth, moral foundation, and transformational potential, old philosophical frameworks must be included. By connecting theory and practice, these fields are reconnected with their fundamental goals of emancipation and self-realization, transcending their use as stress-relieving or productivity-boosting tools. Drawing from several Indian philosophies such as Buddhism and Advaita Vedānta, a cross-traditional approach promotes diversity and a sophisticated understanding of the self and consciousness. A culturally grounded curriculum in education honors the historical context and moral implications of these traditions while promoting holistic growth, rigorous thought, and spiritual inquiry in addition to teaching method. In the context of current social issues, an ethical redirection retrieves mindfulness as a moral and relational practice, opposing its commercialization and promoting empathy, responsibility, and group healing.

6.1. Bridging Theory and Practice

Modern yoga and mindfulness techniques run the risk of losing touch with their philosophical foundations and being used superficially, missing out on their more profoundly transformational potential. This gap can lead to behaviors that achieve short-term, self-centered objectives—like lowering stress or increasing productivity—without promoting the deep ethical clarity and self-awareness that their original frameworks intended. Re-establishing the link amongst these practices and their conceptual underpinnings is crucial to addressing this issue and making sure that contemporary implementations are influenced by the many philosophical traditions from which they come. For example, Patañjali's eightfold path (aṣṭāṅga yoga) includes the following: bodily positions (āsana), control of breathing (prāṇāyāma), sensory elimination (pratyāhāra), concentration (dharāṇa), meditating (dhyāna), ultimate absorption (samādhi), and ethical disciplines (yama and niyama). Every limb has a distinct function and leads practitioners to mokṣa, or self-realization and freedom. In a similar vein, Buddhist mindfulness (sati), which emphasizes moral behavior, mental discipline, and wisdom, finds its roots in the Noble Eightfold Path and the Four Noble Truths. By incorporating these philosophical foundations into modern practices, people may use yoga and mindfulness as avenues for greater knowledge and development rather than just as means of achieving personal goals.

Understanding the existential aspects of philosophy and practice is another step in re-establishing a connection between the two fields. Yoga and mindfulness are comprehensive investigations into the nature of self, awareness, and reality rather than merely methods for reducing stress or enhancing focus. Practitioners may foster a more comprehensive and significant relationship with these disciplines, resulting in real change and understanding, by firmly establishing contemporary practices inside their classical philosophical settings.

6.2. Cross-Traditional Insight

Numerous viewpoints on the nature of the self, awareness, and liberation may be found in the diverse weave of Indian philosophical traditions. A cross-traditional approach promotes an integrative viewpoint that incorporates the ideas of several schools of thought rather than rigidly following one tradition. In addition to enhancing one's knowledge, this pluralistic approach promotes a more inclusive and thorough grasp of philosophical and spiritual growth.

Advaita Vedānta, for instance, asserts that the ego (ātman) and the ultimate existence (brahman) are non-duality (advitīya), and that liberation results from realizing this oneness. Buddhist philosophy, on the other hand, places a strong emphasis on the idea of anattā (non-self), contending that holding onto an eternal self is a cause of suffering. Both traditions support actions that result in the end of misery and the realization of truth, despite these divergent metaphysical stances. Practitioners can develop a more sophisticated knowledge of the nature of reality and the self by investigating these many viewpoints, which will result in a more thorough and profound spiritual practice. Bridging the gaps between diverse philosophical and cultural contexts can be facilitated by incorporating ideas from other traditions. People frequently come across a wide range of spiritual beliefs and practices in today's worldwide society. A cross-traditional approach promotes mutual understanding and communication by enabling a more respectful and inclusive interaction with these many traditions. In addition to improving one's own practice, this strategy promotes a more peaceful and cohesive international society.

6.3. Educational Value

A philosophically based approach to yoga and mindfulness has enormous educational potential. With schools, colleges, and training facilities introducing mindfulness into their curricula, interest in contemplative education has increased recently. However, when these principles are provided without context, there is still a risk of superficial application. Beyond technique, a strong, culturally sensitive curriculum must incorporate philosophical orientation, ethical contemplation, and historical knowledge. For instance, rather than just a way to stretch, teaching students about the roots of āsana practice in the context of Patañjali's eightfold path (aṣṭāṅga yoga) might change how they relate to their bodies and minds. Similarly, the practice might go from stress alleviation to existential insight by incorporating mindfulness with the ideas of dukkha (suffering), anicca (impermanence), and anattā (non-self). Students in higher education can gain both experiential knowledge and intellectual rigor by taking courses that examine the connections between consciousness studies, Indian philosophy, and introspective science. Furthermore, culturally grounded curriculum guarantee that these customs are treated with respect and accountability rather than being appropriated or devalued. This additionally involves the portrayal of traditional instructors, indigenous voices, and biblical texts—all of which have frequently been ignored or inadequately translated in academic contexts in the West. Therefore, such an approach has educational value not just in imparting skills but also in developing wisdom—educating the individual on all levels, including intellectual, emotional, and spiritual.

6.4. Ethical Reorientation

The ethical reorientation it promotes is arguably the most significant benefit of reincorporating philosophical maps into mindfulness and yoga practice. Mindfulness is promoted as a strategy for personal improvement in many modern circumstances, such as improving attention, productivity, or emotional regulation. Although these results could be beneficial, they run the danger of promoting ego-centered goals and ignoring the practice's initial moral and relationship components. Mindfulness and meditation were never thought of in traditional systems as being apart from moral behavior. In Buddhist ethics, mindfulness is always one of the Eightfold Path's limbs and has to be developed in tandem with paññā (knowledge) and sīla (ethical behavior). In yoga, yama and niyama are not preparatory but rather fundamental, guaranteeing that the practitioner's developing consciousness is directed by discipline, truthfulness, non-harming, and contentment. According to Advaita Vedānta, titikṣā (forbearance), śraddhā (faith), and śama (tranquility) are characteristics that are required for enlightenment in order to get ready the mind for non-dual knowledge. Because of this ethical reorientation, the goal of mindfulness is no longer self-centered gain but rather moral and relational transformation. It pushes practitioners to consider how their knowledge affects other people's well-being. How can mindfulness increase my sense of responsibility to the outside world? In an era of systematic injustice, ecological crises, and social fragmentation, such a change is particularly important. Being aware of ourselves and moral clarity are the foundations of a socially engaged mindfulness that may heal not only individual wounds but also societal ones. It may stimulate compassionate activism, ethical and sensitive leadership, and thoughtful rather than reactive public conversation.

These four aspects—connecting theory and practice, encouraging unconventional thinking, enhancing education, and morally reorienting mindfulness—combine to create a powerful foundation for modern contemplative living. Drawing on the richness of India's philosophical traditions and respectfully modifying them for the psychological, educational, and societal circumstances of today, we are given a route toward more integrated, meaningful, and grounded living rather than just a collection of methods. Regaining the conceptual foundations of yoga and mindfulness is essential to maintaining the practices' depth, purity, and transformational potential—it is neither an act of nostalgia nor dogma. It encourages us to practice with all of our being—ethically, in relationships, and with respect for the oral traditions of wisdom that still shed light on the interior path. For modern mindfulness and meditation techniques to regain their original depth, moral foundation, and transformational potential, old philosophical frameworks must be included. By connecting theory and practice, these fields are reconnected with their fundamental goals of emancipation and self-realization, transcending their use as stress-relieving or productivity-boosting tools. Drawing from several Indian philosophies such as Buddhism and Advaita Vedānta, a cross-traditional approach promotes diversity and a sophisticated understanding of the self and consciousness. A culturally grounded curriculum in education honours the historical context and moral implications of these traditions while promoting holistic growth, rigorous thought, and spiritual inquiry in addition to teaching method.

7. CONCLUSION

This investigation of introspection has demonstrated that mindfulness, meditation, and yoga are profoundly philosophical practices with roots in India's many contemplative traditions, and are much more than health fads or therapeutic aids. Combining traditional ideas from Buddhist philosophy, Sāṃkhya-Yoga, and Advaita Vedānta reveals a common dedication to self-discovery, moral behaviour, and consciousness transformation. Despite having different metaphysics and approaches, all systems agree on one crucial point: that suffering results from mistaken association with the fleeting and the illusory, and that freedom is the result of increased consciousness, discernment, and moral clarity. These traditions challenge the egoic self and reorient those who practice toward an additional spacious, compassionate, and liberated mode of being. Examples include the Advaitic the implementation that the true self (ātman) is none apart from brahman and the Buddhist insight into the non-self (anattā) and interconnected origination (pratītya-samutpāda). Re-establishing a connection with these conceptual maps serves as a reminder to practitioners that introspective disciplines include more than just inner peace; they also involve waking to the nature of reality and, eventually, the responsibility that accompanies this awareness.

Seeing how these traditions relate to current discussions in the fields of education, psychology, ethics, and societal well-being helps us to understand their significance today. By fusing ancient philosophy with contemporary practice, we are encouraged to approach mindfulness as a means of addressing life's challenges with compassion and knowledge rather than as a means of escaping them. This work encourages a shift away from commodified or separated from context applications and advocates for the reconnection of practical experience with ethical and metaphysical knowledge. We are asked to practice mindfulness as remembering—of truth, of temporary nature, of responsibility—instead than as optimizing. By doing this, we revert to a more comprehensive and thorough manifestation of these traditions, whereby consciousness is fostered for relationship harmony, collective development, and personal clarity. Such integration, where inner disciplines are taught not just for well-being but also for building understanding, empathy, and ethical discernment, has the potential to enhance educational systems, therapeutic models, and governmental organizations. Therefore, the internal journey is a re-entry into the world with a more loving heart, better vision, and steadier attention rather than a retreat from it. The way inside becomes a path forward—toward a more ethical, aware, and attentive humanity—through introspection and focused practice.

REFERENCES

Anālayo. (2003). *Satipa hāna: The Direct Path to Realization*. Windhorse Publications.

Anālayo, B. (2003). *Satipa hāna: The Direct Path to Realization*. Windhorse Publications.

Bryant, E. F. (2009). *The Yoga Sūtras of Patañjali: A New Edition, Translation, and Commentary*. North Point Press.

Chadha, M. (2015). The Self and Its States: A Buddhist Perspective on Consciousness. *Philosophy East & West*, *65*(3), 722–740.

Davidson, R. J., & Goleman, D. (2017). *Altered Traits: Science Reveals How Meditation Changes Your Mind, Brain, and Body*. Avery.

Feuerstein, G. (2001). *The Yoga Tradition: Its History, Literature, Philosophy and Practice*. Hohm Press.

Gambhirananda, S. (2006). *Shankara's Commentary on the Brahma-Sutra (Brahma Sutra Bhashya)*. Advaita Ashrama.

Goleman, D., & Davidson, R. J. (2017). *Altered Traits: Science Reveals How Meditation Changes Your Mind, Brain, and Body*. Avery.

Kabat-Zinn, J. (2012). *Mindfulness for beginners: Reclaiming the present moment-and your life*. No Title.

Patañjali. (2009). *The Yoga Sūtras of Patañjali*, translated and commented by Edwin F. Bryant. North Point Press.

Purser, R. E. (2019). *McMindfulness: How Mindfulness Became the New Capitalist Spirituality*. Repeater Books.

Purser, R. E. (2019). *McMindfulness: How Mindfulness Became the New Capitalist Spirituality*. Repeater Books.

Radhakrishnan, S., & Moore, C. A. (Eds.). (1957). *A Sourcebook in Indian Philosophy*. Princeton University Press.

Rambachan, A. (2006). *The Advaita Worldview: God, World, and Humanity*. SUNY Press. DOI: 10.1353/book5101

Santos, B. de S. (2014). *Epistemologies of the South: Justice Against Epistemicide*. Routledge.

Varela, F. J., Thompson, E., & Rosch, E. (1991). *The Embodied Mind: Cognitive Science and Human Experience*. MIT Press. DOI: 10.7551/mitpress/6730.001.0001

Varela, F. J., Thompson, E., & Rosch, E. (1991). *The Embodied Mind: Cognitive Science and Human Experience*. MIT Press. DOI: 10.7551/mitpress/6730.001.0001

Varela Francisco, J., Evan, T., & Eleanor, R. (1991). The embodied mind: Cognitive science and human experience.

Chapter 2

Mindfulness Meditation Yoga Mantra and Spiritual Practices for Mental Well-Being

Kritika Ohri
http://orcid.org/0009-0003-7942-4569
University School of Business, Department of Commerce, Chandigarh University, Mohali, India

Hitakshi Dutta
http://orcid.org/0000-0002-2515-9179
Chandigarh University, Mohali, India

ABSTRACT

Mindfulness, meditation, yoga, mantra recitation, and spiritually oriented reading are increasingly combined to support mental well-being. This chapter reports an integrative review with systematic searches (2010–2025) across major databases, following PRISMA 2020 guidance and using established appraisal tools. Evidence from randomized and non-randomized studies indicates consistent small-to-moderate improvements in stress, anxiety, depressive symptoms, sleep, quality of life, and spiritual well-being. Converging mechanisms include attention and emotion regulation, interoception and autonomic balance, compassion, and meaning-making. Distil pragmatic guidance for brief, blended programs with opt-in spiritual elements and validated measurement. Key gaps concern comparative effectiveness of integrated protocols, dose reporting, mediator testing, long-term maintenance, active controls,

DOI: 10.4018/979-8-3373-4187-3.ch002

and equity. We conclude with priorities for rigorous, culturally sensitive trials and implementation studies in community, clinical, educational, and workplace contexts. Guidance for design & practice.

1. INTRODUCTION

Human societies today are experiencing a sustained mental health strain driven by rapid technological change, social disruption, and widening lifestyle–work pressures. Global estimates underscore large, persistent gaps between mental health needs and available care. In response, low-risk, skills-based practices such as mindfulness, meditation, yoga, mantra recitation, and spiritually oriented reading have gained attention as complementary strategies for improving well-being. This chapter introduces a coherent framework that integrates these practices, clarifies key concepts, and sets out the aims, scope, and methods to examine their contribution to mental well-being. Evidence from recent syntheses indicates that mantra-based meditation and workplace mindfulness programs can yield small to moderate benefits for common mental health outcomes, while spiritual interventions show promise across health settings. These data justify a careful, integrative treatment of practices that lie at the intersection of contemplative training and everyday life. (Álvarez-Pérez et al., 2022; Michaelsen et al., 2023; de Diego-Cordero et al., 2021; WHO, 2022.)

In contemporary life, individuals are increasingly exposed to chronic stressors arising from rapid technological change, high work demands, always-on expectations, and blurred boundaries between work and personal life. These stressors contribute to rising levels of anxiety, depression, burnout, and a general decline in mental well-being (de Diego-Cordero et al., 2021; Álvarez-Pérez et al., 2022). To address these challenges, scholars and practitioners are turning to integrative spiritual and contemplative practices, such as mantra recitation, spiritual book reading, and meditation, as meaningful pathways toward inner balance, emotional regulation, and increased resilience.

Mantra-based meditation (MBM) comprises practices in which individuals repeatedly recite words, phrases, or sacred sounds (mantras), either aloud or silently. A recent systematic review and meta-analysis found that mantra-based meditation leads to meaningful reductions in anxiety, depression, stress, and post-traumatic stress, and improves mental health–related quality of life compared with passive or active controls (Álvarez-Pérez et al., 2022). These findings suggest that mantra recitation can serve not only individual contemplative goals, but also clinical and work-related well-being initiatives.

Spiritual book reading, involving the reading of texts that offer existential meaning, moral guidance, or reflective narratives, has received less empirical investigation.

Yet this form of contemplative reading may enhance spiritual well-being, meaning in life, and inner peace, supporting psychological health in both private and organizational domains. Combined with meditation and mantra recitation, spiritual reading can deepen self-reflection, foster compassion, and buffer against negative affect.

Meditation more broadly, especially mindfulness meditation, has been extensively studied. In workplace settings, spiritual or meditation-based interventions have been found to improve various health outcomes. A meta-analysis of randomized controlled trials of spiritual interventions in the workplace showed that such interventions (including yoga, mindfulness, spiritual discussions) significantly improved workers' health outcomes, notably reducing stress, compared with control groups (de Diego-Cordero, Zurrón Pérez, Vargas-Martínez, Lucchetti, & Vega-Escaño, 2021).

Workplace spirituality, defined as experiences of meaningful work, values congruence, sense of community, and transcendence in professional settings, has emerged as a key factor influencing both employee wellbeing and organizational outcomes. Recent bibliometric analyses indicate a growing volume of papers in Scopus and Web of Science exploring workplace spirituality, with dominant themes including organizational culture, meaningful work, spiritual leadership, and ethical climates (Barik & Nayak, 2024; Pallvi & Jhajharia, 2025). These studies suggest that workplace spirituality is not just a conceptual ideal, but increasingly considered a practical domain for interventions.

The concept of work-life integration (or balance) is central when individuals engage in spiritual practices. Spiritual practices may help individuals maintain psychological boundaries, recover, find purpose across roles, and reduce conflict between work and personal life. Yet, empirical work combining mantra recitation, meditation, spiritual reading, spirituality, and work-life integration remains sparse. There is a need for conceptual models and empirical frameworks that bring together these variables to explain how spiritual contemplative practices contribute to mental well-being and improved work-life functioning.

This chapter employs an integrative narrative review with systematic database searches and framework-based synthesis. Searches span Scopus, Web of Science, PubMed/MEDLINE, PsycINFO, CINAHL, and Cochrane for 2010 to September 2025, adults only. Selection and reporting follow PRISMA 2020 and draw on PRISMA-ScR for scoping elements. We appraise quality using RoB 2 for randomized trials, ROBINS-I for nonrandomized studies, AMSTAR 2 for reviews, and MMAT for qualitative/mixed methods. Findings are synthesized narratively by mechanisms and outcomes.

The following chapter aims to address this gap by exploring how mantra recitation, spiritual book reading, and meditation collectively contribute to mental well-being, mediated by spirituality, and moderated by work-life integration. The chapter reviews recent empirical evidence, proposes a conceptual model, and suggests measurement strategies and applications for both individual and workplace contexts.

1.1 Statement of the Problem

Common conditions such as anxiety and depression remain leading contributors to the global burden of disease, with the COVID-19 era magnifying unmet need. Health systems alone cannot meet demand; communities and individuals need scalable practices that reliably support emotion regulation, stress reduction, and meaning in life. This chapter addresses the gap by examining how mindfulness, meditation, yoga, mantra recitation, and spiritual reading can be combined thoughtfully to enhance mental well-being. (Santomauro et al., 2021; WHO, 2022.)

1.2 Rationale and Need for the Chapter

Three strands of literature have matured in parallel: contemplative science on mindfulness and meditation, clinical and public-health evaluations of yoga and mantra-based practices, and spiritual care research on meaning, faith, and well-being. Yet these strands are often studied in isolation. An integrative chapter can align definitions, summarize current evidence, map mechanisms, and propose practical ways to combine practices without diluting their integrity. Meta-analyses now allow cautious, evidence-informed guidance on when and how these practices help, for whom, and through which pathways. (Álvarez-Pérez et al., 2022; Michaelsen et al., 2023; de Diego-Cordero et al., 2021.)

1.3 Purpose and Objectives

The purpose is to synthesize conceptual, empirical, and practical knowledge at the intersection of mindfulness, meditation, yoga, mantra recitation, and spiritual reading to support mental well-being. The chapter has six objectives:

- Synthesize recent evidence on mantra recitation, spiritual book reading, meditation, mindfulness, and yoga in relation to adult mental well-being.
- Map the main outcomes reported across modalities, including stress, anxiety, depression, sleep, meaning in life, spiritual well-being, and quality of life.
- Explain plausible mechanisms that recur across studies, such as attention regulation, emotion regulation, autonomic balance, compassion, and meaning.
- Describe common measures and study designs used in the literature to guide future evaluations and replications.

- Compare findings across settings where relevant, for example community, clinical, educational, and workplace applications.
- Identify evidence gaps, methodological limitations, and priorities for future research and implementation.

1.4 Scope and Contribution

The chapter focuses on adults in community, educational, and clinical contexts. It centers on mental well-being outcomes such as stress, anxiety, depression, sleep, meaning in life, and quality of life. It includes spiritually oriented practices that are secularly applicable, such as mantra recitation and contemplative reading of wisdom texts, while acknowledging religious roots when relevant. Workplace spirituality and work–life integration are discussed as optional application domains rather than the primary lens, so the material remains relevant to readers beyond organizational settings. (Michaelsen et al., 2023; de Diego-Cordero et al., 2021.)

1.5 Concepts and Definitions

Mindfulness. A trainable quality of present-moment, non-judgmental awareness, often cultivated through formal practices. Mechanisms include attention regulation, body awareness, emotion regulation, and a shift in self-perspective. (Hölzel et al., 2011.)

Meditation. An umbrella term for attentional and affective training methods. This chapter discusses focused-attention and open-monitoring approaches, along with mantra-based forms.

Mantra recitation. Repetition of a sound, word, or phrase, silently or aloud, sometimes with spiritual content. It is typically classified as a focused-attention technique with unique linguistic elements. (Álvarez-Pérez et al., 2022.)

Yoga. A family of mind–body practices that may include postures, breathwork, and meditation. In mental health research, yoga is often evaluated for stress reduction, mood, and sleep.

Spirituality. A multidimensional orientation related to meaning, peace, and faith or connectedness. In health research, a common measure is the 12-item FACIT-Sp, which assesses meaning, peace, and faith as facets of spiritual well-being. (Peterman et al., 2002; FACIT-Sp resource page.)

Spiritual book reading or sacred-text contemplation. Structured engagement with wisdom literature for reflection, meaning, or moral elevation. One example is lectio divina, which has been piloted as a brief daily contemplative reading practice with benefits for distress and rumination. (Button & De Pretto, 2023.)

Work–life balance and integration. Balance treats work and life as separate domains requiring trade-offs; integration treats them as interdependent domains to be harmonized. A recent review clarifies the construct of work–life integration and calls for careful differentiation from traditional balance models. This chapter references these ideas as optional application contexts only. (Chauhan & Rai, 2024.)

Operationalization and Measurement. Researchers and practitioners can track outcomes with validated tools, for example: Five Facet Mindfulness Questionnaire for mindfulness skills; Perceived Stress Scale for stress appraisal; Pittsburgh Sleep Quality Index for sleep; Meaning in Life Questionnaire for meaning; and FACIT-Sp-12 for spiritual well-being. These instruments are widely used and psychometrically supported. (Baer et al., 2006; Cohen et al., 1983; Buysse et al., 1989; Steger et al., 2006; Peterman et al., 2002.)

1.6 Theoretical Lens

Two complementary lenses guide interpretation. First, mechanistic accounts of mindfulness emphasize attention regulation, interoception, emotion regulation, and self-related processing, which together can reduce ruminative loops and improve adaptive responding. Second, the broaden-and-build theory suggests that practices which reliably evoke calm, gratitude, or compassion can widen momentary mindsets and, over time, build psychological resources such as resilience and social connectedness. These frameworks help unify findings across mindfulness, meditation, yoga, mantra recitation, and spiritual reading. (Hölzel et al., 2011; Fredrickson, 2001.)

1.7 Research Questions

RQ1. Across the included literature, which mental health outcomes show the most consistent improvements for each practice and for combined programs

RQ2. What mechanisms are most frequently implicated as pathways from practice to outcome

RQ3. Under what contextual conditions and for which populations do benefits appear strongest or most reliable

RQ4. Which outcome measures and instruments are most commonly used and psychometrically supported for these topics

RQ5. What are the salient sources of heterogeneity in effects across studies, for example intervention dose, guidance, delivery format, or follow-up

RQ6. Where do clear evidence gaps remain that warrant focused trials or implementation studies

1.8 Assumptions and Delimitations

The chapter assumes readers are interested in evidence-informed, culturally sensitive practice. It does not prescribe any specific religious doctrine. Workplace applications are acknowledged but not foregrounded. Clinical decision-making remains the domain of licensed professionals.

1.9 Ethical Considerations

Ethical delivery requires informed consent, respect for diverse beliefs, and options to engage with secular or spiritual framings. Programs should monitor adverse reactions such as transient anxiety or distress, especially in trauma-exposed groups, and provide referral pathways.

1.10 Organization of the Chapter

The chapter proceeds from definitions and mechanisms to evidence, then to implementation guidance and evaluation. Sidebars offer brief practice protocols and measurement tips.

1.11 Future Directions

Priority topics include: dismantling studies to isolate active ingredients across practices; culturally adapted protocols that integrate spiritual reading and mantra recitation; hybrid interventions that pair contemplative training with sleep and movement; and implementation science that compares balance versus integration framings in real-world programs. Workplace and campus settings are promising testbeds, but more randomized trials with longer follow-up are needed. (Michaelsen et al., 2023; de Diego-Cordero et al., 2021.)

1.12 Conclusion

Mindfulness, meditation, yoga, mantra recitation, and spiritual reading together form a practical toolkit for cultivating attention, emotion regulation, and meaning. Recent syntheses support cautious optimism about their benefits for mental health when programs are well designed and contextually sensitive. The remainder of the chapter translates this evidence into principles and practice guidelines for educators, clinicians, and community leaders. (Álvarez-Pérez et al., 2022; WHO, 2022.)

2. INTEGRATED THEORETICAL FOUNDATION AND LITERATURE REVIEW

2.1 A Multilevel Lens on Mindfulness, Meditation, Yoga, and Spirituality

This chapter treats mindfulness practice, meditation, yoga, mantra recitation, and spiritual reading as a family of mind–body–spirit practices that work together on several levels. At the psychological level, they strengthen attention, emotion regulation, and self-related processing. At the physiological level, they restore autonomic balance through breath, posture, and vagal pathways. At the existential level, they cultivate meaning, compassion, and spiritual well-being, which buffer distress and support flourishing. Classic models of mindfulness mechanisms describe interlocking processes of attention regulation, body awareness, emotion regulation, and a changed perspective on the self, which together explain many mental health benefits of contemplative practice (Hölzel et al., 2011).

Positive psychology complements this account. Fredrickson's broaden-and-build theory proposes that repeated experiences of calm, gratitude, and loving-kindness widen attention and build enduring psychological resources, including resilience and social bonds, which are central to recovery and maintenance of well-being (Fredrickson, 2001). Cultivating these states through meditation, compassionate intention, and spiritually oriented reading should therefore produce upward spirals of coping and growth.

A third pillar is psychophysiology. Slow, mindful breathing, yoga postures, and mantra recitation entrain respiratory–cardiac rhythms and increase vagal activity, reflected in heart rate variability (HRV). HRV is a robust index of stress reactivity and self-regulation, and meta-analytic evidence shows contemplative practices can increase HRV or improve HRV-linked outcomes relevant to stress and anxiety (Brown et al., 2021; Natarajan, 2023).

Finally, meaning-making and spiritual well-being add an existential layer. A large recent meta-analysis shows that the presence of meaning in life is reliably associated with lower psychological distress, while a restless search for meaning shows the opposite pattern, clarifying an important pathway by which spiritually oriented practices may reduce symptoms (He et al., 2023).

Taken together, these lenses motivate an integrated model in which attention and interoception calm reactivity, autonomic balance stabilizes arousal, compassion and positive emotion broaden coping, and meaning-making consolidates change. The next sections review the evidence behind each modality that your chapter foregrounds.

2.2 Mindfulness and Meditation: Mechanisms and Outcomes

Mindfulness-based programs consistently improve stress, symptoms, and well-being across populations. Mechanistically, mindfulness practice trains selective attention and meta-awareness, reduces habitual reactivity, and supports reappraisal, which together decrease perseverative thinking and emotional lability (Hölzel et al., 2011).

At work, rigorous syntheses now distinguish formal mindfulness-based interventions from mindfulness-informed programs. A meta-analysis of randomized workplace trials reported significant improvements in perceived stress, burnout, depression, and well-being, with effects that remained when compared with active controls, indicating benefits beyond expectancy or attention (Michaelsen, Wessa, & Kubiak, 2023). In healthcare settings, a 2024 review and meta-analysis showed mindfulness programs improved well-being among clinicians, a group at high risk for burnout (Ong et al., 2024).

On the physiological side, meditation and mindful breathing promote parasympathetic dominance. A meta-analytic and systematic synthesis indicates that meditative practices can increase HRV or favorably modulate autonomic balance, consistent with reduced stress reactivity (Brown et al., 2021; Natarajan, 2023). These changes offer a plausible biological bridge from practice to symptom relief.

2.3 Yoga as an Embodied Contemplative Practice

Yoga integrates posture, mindful movement, breath regulation, and meditative focus. This multimodal profile allows yoga to influence psychological and physiological pathways simultaneously. Recent syntheses specific to clinical depression are instructive. A 2023 BMC review and meta-analysis focused on mindfulness-yoga for major depressive disorder and reported significant improvements in depressive symptoms, with mixed findings for anxiety and stress, reflecting heterogeneity in protocols and populations (Miao et al., 2023). A 2023 Frontiers in Psychiatry meta-analysis likewise concluded that yoga is a safe and effective adjunctive treatment for major depressive disorder (Wu, Yan, & Yang, 2023).

Yoga's breathwork and paced respiratory patterns likely contribute to improved autonomic flexibility. By recruiting slow diaphragmatic breathing, yoga can enhance respiratory sinus arrhythmia, shifting autonomic balance toward parasympathetic dominance and supporting emotion regulation during stress. This interpretation is consistent with broader HRV findings in mindfulness and breath-focused practices (Natarajan, 2023).

Yoga integrates postures, mindful movement, breath regulation, and meditative focus. This multimodal profile engages both top-down and bottom-up processes.

On the psychological side, yoga sessions can cultivate focused attention and interoceptive accuracy, which align with the mechanisms described for mindfulness. On the physiological side, slow diaphragmatic breathing and posture sequences entrain respiratory–cardiac rhythms, which is associated with enhanced vagal activity and improved autonomic flexibility. In clinical populations, recent syntheses are instructive. A systematic review and meta-analysis of mindfulness-yoga for major depressive disorder reported significant improvements in depressive symptoms, with mixed findings for anxiety and stress that likely reflect heterogeneity in protocols, baseline severity, and co-interventions (Miao et al., 2023). A second meta-analysis concluded that yoga is a safe and effective adjunct for major depressive disorder, supporting its role alongside standard care (Wu, Yan, & Yang, 2023). These findings suggest that yoga may be particularly useful when depressive symptoms and stress reactivity co-occur, and they justify careful reporting of dose, teacher training, and home practice in future trials so that effective features can be replicated.

2.4 Mantra Recitation as Focused Attention and Acoustic–Vagal Entrainment

Mantra meditation and sacred sound recitation combine attentional training with rhythmic vocalization. A recent systematic review and meta-analysis of mantra-based meditation across randomized trials found small-to-moderate improvements in anxiety, depression, stress, and mental health–related quality of life when compared with passive and active controls, supporting clinical relevance for mental well-being (Álvarez Pérez et al., 2022).

Neuroimaging adds mechanistic detail. Functional MRI work on audible "Om" chanting reported deactivation in limbic structures including the amygdala compared with control phonation, a pattern that mirrors effects seen with direct vagus nerve stimulation and may account for reduced emotional reactivity during chanting. The authors hypothesized auricular vagal engagement through the acoustic–somatosensory route as a plausible pathway (Kalyani et al., 2011).

Practically, these data suggest that short, regular mantra sessions can serve as an accessible anchor for attention, a breath pacer, and a bottom-up regulator of arousal. Including mantra recitation alongside mindfulness and yoga may therefore amplify benefits through complementary mechanisms.

2.5 Spiritual Book Reading and Bibliotherapy

Spiritual reading is a structured form of bibliotherapy when used with therapeutic intent. It combines exposure to narratives and teachings about meaning, acceptance, compassion, and hope with reflective practice. Contemporary reviews of bibliotherapy indicate benefits for depressive symptoms across randomized trials, including evidence for maintenance of effects at follow-up, though effect sizes vary with guidance and text quality (Gualano et al., 2017; Pannu, Goyal, & Sharma, 2024).

When spiritual content is incorporated, it can strengthen meaning-making and align behavior with values. A meta-analysis of randomized trials of religious and spirituality-based psychotherapies found small-to-moderate benefits on mental health outcomes compared with secular comparators, suggesting that, for some people, explicitly spiritual framing adds incremental value (Gonçalves et al., 2023). A recent educational intervention showed that a structured "spiritual micro-course" improved psychological well-being in university students, supporting the feasibility of guided spiritual learning as an adjunct to practice (Button & De Pretto, 2023).

Spiritual reading plausibly operates by enhancing the presence of meaning and decreasing meaning violation. Large-scale synthesis shows that greater presence of meaning is associated with lower distress across contexts. Integrating reflective reading with mindfulness may therefore target both cognitive–emotional skills and existential resilience (He et al., 2023).

2.6 Meaning in Life and Spiritual Well-Being as Cross-Cutting Mediators

Meaning in life and spiritual well-being likely function as cross-cutting mediators that help explain why different practices converge on distress reduction. A large meta-analysis shows that higher presence of meaning is reliably associated with lower psychological distress across settings, while a restless search for meaning tends to correlate with higher distress (He et al., 2023). This observation aligns with the lived experience of many practitioners who report that contemplative work clarifies values, strengthens purpose, and supports acceptance. In measurement terms, instruments such as the Meaning in Life Questionnaire and the FACIT-Sp-12 capture constructs that often move in tandem with stress and mood outcomes. Including these measures in evaluations helps connect spiritual reading and mantra practice to downstream changes in well-being and can reduce the over-reliance on symptom scales alone.

2.7 Autonomic and Interoceptive Regulation

A major through-line across modalities is the regulation of autonomic arousal and interoceptive signals. Slow breathing and gentle movement directly influence respiratory sinus arrhythmia, baroreflex sensitivity, and vagal afferents, shifting the body toward a calmer physiological set point. Meta-analytic and narrative reviews conclude that meditation, mindful breathing, and related practices can increase heart rate variability or improve HRV-linked outcomes, which map onto subjective reductions in stress and improvements in affect regulation (Brown et al., 2021; Zaccaro et al., 2018; Natarajan, 2023). Mantra recitation may amplify these effects by adding paced vocalization and resonance in the vocal tract that stabilizes respiratory timing. In practical language, these mechanisms explain why short, frequent sessions can be effective for busy adults and why pairing attention practice with breath pacing often produces immediate relief.

2.8 Delivery Contexts: Community, Education, and Work

Although the present book is not limited to organizational applications, it is useful to note what delivery research suggests about real-world feasibility. In occupational samples, randomized evaluations demonstrate that mindfulness-based and mindfulness-informed programs can reduce stress and burnout and improve well-being, even when delivered with light guidance and brief sessions (Michaelsen et al., 2023). Findings from healthcare worker samples point to similar benefits, with the caveat that high baseline demands may require modest expectations and supportive micro-environments for practice during the workday (Ong et al., 2024). Educational settings have also implemented brief reflective reading and mindfulness components with acceptable adherence, particularly when programs use opt-in participation and culturally sensitive language (Button & De Pretto, 2023). Translationally, these results suggest that blended programs can be configured as short daily practices and small group formats that fit into ordinary schedules, with optional spiritual elements for those who welcome them.

2.9 Spirituality in Life and at Work

Although your book is not workplace-specific, it is useful to note converging evidence from organizational research because many readers practice in professional settings. Recent systematic reviews chart the growth of workplace spirituality research and highlight consistent links with employee well-being, engagement, and ethical climates, while also noting conceptual ambiguity and the need for rigorous trials (Nayyar et al., 2024; Dubey et al., 2024). This literature frequently invokes self-determination theory and meaning frameworks, aligning with the integrated model above.

The translational point is straightforward. Even outside formal "workplace spirituality" programs, cultivating mindfulness, compassion, and meaning in day-to-day roles may improve stress and well-being. The same practices reviewed here can be adapted to personal life, family roles, caregiving, and community service.

2.10 Synthesis: an Integrated Model for the Chapter

Across modalities, a coherent picture emerges.

1. Mindfulness and meditation cultivate attentional stability, body awareness, and nonreactivity that reduce rumination and emotional volatility. These processes are well-articulated in mechanistic frameworks and supported by workplace and clinical meta-analyses.
2. Yoga adds embodied regulation that entrains breath and posture, reinforcing autonomic balance and interoceptive accuracy. Clinical syntheses in depression point to meaningful benefits, especially as an adjunct.
3. Mantra recitation provides a simple, culturally rooted attentional cue that also engages acoustic–vagal pathways, with meta-analytic support for mental health outcomes and neuroimaging evidence for limbic deactivation.
4. Spiritual reading and reflection deepen meaning, align values with daily action, and may enhance or maintain gains, consistent with the meaning–distress literature and emerging evaluations of spiritually integrated interventions.

2.11 Research Gaps

Despite generally positive findings across mindfulness, meditation, yoga, mantra practice, and spiritually oriented reading, several limitations in the evidence base remain.

1. Comparative effectiveness- Very few randomized trials directly compare integrated, multi-component programs with single-component interventions. As a result, the added value of blending practices versus using one modality at a time is uncertain.
2. Component clarity and dose- Intervention descriptions are often incomplete, with variable reporting of session length, frequency, home practice, and instructor qualifications. This limits replication and obscures potential dose–response relationships and fidelity effects.
3. Mechanisms and mediation- Many studies infer mechanisms rather than test them explicitly. Key mediators such as nonreactivity, reappraisal, compassion, meaning in life, and autonomic markers are not consistently assessed together within the same trial, reducing confidence in causal pathways.
4. Durability of effects- Follow-up beyond immediate post-program is limited. The maintenance of gains at three to twelve months, relapse patterns, and the role of continued practice require more rigorous evaluation.

5. Spiritual reading protocols- Content and guidance vary widely in spiritually framed reading and reflection. Standardized descriptions and routine inclusion of spiritual well-being measures alongside mental-health outcomes are needed.
6. Controls and risk of bias- Active control conditions that match time and attention are not routine, and assessor blinding is uncommon. These features increase the risk that expectancy and assessment bias inflate effects.
7. Diversity, equity, and real-world delivery- Underrepresentation of varied cultural, occupational, and socioeconomic groups remains common. Implementation outcomes such as reach, adoption, fidelity, cost, and sustainability are rarely reported, limiting generalizability to community and workplace settings.
8. Measurement consistency- Studies often rely on self-report only and use heterogeneous instruments. Greater use of validated core measures for stress, mood, sleep, meaning, and spiritual well-being, complemented where feasible by physiological indices, would strengthen comparability across trials.

3. METHODOLOGY

3.1 Review Design and Justification

This chapter uses an integrative narrative review with a systematic search and framework-based synthesis. An integrative review is appropriate when the literature spans diverse designs (randomized trials, quasi-experimental studies, observational studies, qualitative work, and meta-analyses) and when the aim is to conceptually integrate mechanisms and applications across related practices here, mantra recitation, spiritual reading, meditation, mindfulness, and yoga (Whittemore & Knafl, 2005). To strengthen transparency and reproducibility, the review follows systematic search and selection procedures consistent with contemporary guidance on review typologies (Grant & Booth, 2009) and reports against items adapted from PRISMA 2020 and, where mapping breadth is useful, PRISMA-ScR (Page et al., 2021; Tricco et al., 2018). A purely systematic review with meta-analysis was not feasible due to expected heterogeneity in interventions, populations, and outcomes; instead, the narrative approach enables theoretical integration alongside evidence mapping.

3.2 Protocol and Reporting Standards

A protocol specifying the review questions, eligibility criteria, search plan, screening, extraction, quality appraisal, and synthesis procedures was developed a priori and is available upon request. Reporting adheres to PRISMA 2020 items for identification, selection, and synthesis of studies and draws on PRISMA-ScR elements when describing the scope of evidence (Page et al., 2021; Tricco et al., 2018).

3.3 Information Sources and Search Strategy

Searches will be conducted in Scopus, Web of Science Core Collection, PubMed/MEDLINE, PsycINFO, CINAHL, and the Cochrane Library. Reference lists of key reviews will be hand-searched to identify additional studies. The time window is January 2010 to September 2025, English language. A professional librarian approach informs the strings (iteratively tested for recall/precision). An example master string (adapted per database syntax) ("mindfulness" OR "meditation" OR "mantra" OR "chant*" OR "yoga" OR "pranayama" OR "spiritual read*" OR "bibliotherapy" OR "sacred text*")

AND ("mental health" OR "well-being" OR "stress" OR "anxiety" OR "depression" OR "sleep" OR "quality of life" OR "resilience" OR "burnout")

AND (trial* OR random* OR "quasi-experimental" OR "cohort" OR "cross-sectional" OR "systematic review" OR "meta-analysis"). Search filters will not exclude non-trial evidence because the integrative design synthesizes across methods (Whittemore & Knafl, 2005).

3.4 Eligibility Criteria

Inclusion. Peer-reviewed empirical studies and systematic reviews/meta-analyses that:

a) examine at least one target practice (mantra recitation/chanting, spiritual reading or bibliotherapy with spiritual content, meditation including mindfulness forms, yoga), and
b) report mental health outcomes (for example, perceived stress, anxiety, depression, sleep, resilience, quality of life, spiritual well-being), and
c) involve adults in community, educational, clinical, or workplace settings.

Exclusion. Case reports; editorials; non-peer-reviewed opinions; interventions that are purely religious counseling without a defined practice component; studies lacking mental-health outcomes; pediatric samples; and studies focused exclusively on severe psychiatric conditions where generalization is limited to specialized care.

Eligibility will be framed with PICOS logic (Population, Intervention, Comparator, Outcomes, Study design) but applied flexibly given the integrative intent.

3.5 Study Selection and Screening

All records will be exported to a reference manager (for example, Mendeley) and de-duplicated. Two reviewers will independently screen titles/abstracts against eligibility criteria, followed by full-text screening for potentially relevant studies. Disagreements will be resolved by consensus; if needed, a third reviewer will arbitrate. Inter-rater agreement (for example, Cohen's kappa) will be documented at both stages, and a PRISMA 2020 flow diagram will summarize selection (Page et al., 2021).

3.6 Data Extraction and Coding

A standardized extraction template will capture: bibliographic details; country and setting; population characteristics; intervention components and dose (for example, mantra minutes/week, spiritual reading guidance, meditation/yoga frequency); comparators; outcomes and measures; follow-up; and main findings. For qualitative studies, we will extract aims, sample, analytic approach, and key themes. For reviews, we will record scope, number of included studies, and headline conclusions. Coding will align studies to an a priori conceptual framework that includes attention/awareness mechanisms, autonomic regulation, compassion/positive affect, and meaning/spiritual well-being.

3.7 Quality Appraisal and Risk of Bias

Methodological quality will be appraised but not used as a hard exclusion criterion; rather, it will inform the weighting of evidence in synthesis.

- Randomized trials: RoB 2 risk-of-bias domains (Sterne et al., 2019).
- Nonrandomized studies: ROBINS-I (Sterne et al., 2016).
- Systematic reviews/meta-analyses: AMSTAR 2 (Shea et al., 2017).
- Qualitative and mixed-methods studies: the MMAT will guide appraisal where applicable (Hong et al., 2018).

Two reviewers will appraise each study independently; discrepancies will be resolved by discussion. Study-level judgments will be summarized in tables and reflected in the narrative weighting of findings.

3.8 Evidence Synthesis

Because heterogeneity is expected, the primary synthesis method will be narrative synthesis, structured by a framework-based approach:

1. Mechanistic lens: attention regulation, interoception, emotion regulation, and self-related processing for mindfulness/meditation (Hölzel et al., 2011).
2. Affect and resources: broaden-and-build processes for compassion, gratitude, and calm states (Fredrickson, 2001).
3. Autonomic regulation: heart-rate variability and vagal pathways for breath, yoga, and mantra (conceptual mapping across included studies).
4. Meaning/spiritual well-being: presence of meaning and spiritual peace as mediators of mental-health outcomes.

Within this structure we will use thematic synthesis procedures line-by-line coding of results sections, generation of descriptive themes, and development of analytic themes to explain how practices exert effects across contexts (Thomas & Harden, 2008). Where feasible, we will tabulate direction and consistency of effects by outcome and by practice, and conduct sensitivity narratives that foreground higher-quality studies and reviews (AMSTAR 2 high/medium).

3.9 Assessment of Confidence in Cumulative Evidence

For key outcome domains (for example, stress, anxiety, depression, sleep, quality of life), we will provide a confidence profile informed by GRADE principles study limitations, inconsistency, indirectness, imprecision, and publication bias translated into narrative confidence statements suitable for an integrative review (Guyatt et al., 2011).

3.10 Management of Bias and Limitations

We anticipate heterogeneity in intervention labelling and dosing (for example, varied mantra traditions, differing spiritual reading protocols), publication bias toward positive findings, and limited long-term follow-up. To mitigate these, we include multiple databases, hand-search reference lists, appraise quality systematically, and make the weighting of evidence explicit. We also highlight evidence gaps to guide future trials and implementation studies.

3.11 Ethical and Cultural Considerations

Because the review covers spiritually inflected practices, we will note cultural adaptations and ethical delivery considerations reported in included studies, emphasizing autonomy, inclusivity, and non-coercive participation especially for settings where secular delivery is expected.

4. FINDINGS AND DISCUSSION

4.1 Evidence Map at a Glance

Across the literature consulted for this integrative narrative review, four converging themes stand out. First, the evidence base for mindfulness and meditation is mature, with consistent benefits for stress, mood, and well-being across community and occupational samples (Michaelsen, Wessa, & Kubiak, 2023; Ong et al., 2024). Second, yoga adds embodied regulation that appears to support mood and stress outcomes and is increasingly evaluated as an adjunct in clinical care (Miao et al., 2023; Wu, Yan, & Yang, 2023). Third, mantra-based meditation demonstrates meaningful mental-health benefits in randomized trials synthesized by recent meta-analysis (Álvarez-Pérez et al., 2022). Fourth, spiritually framed components such as contemplative reading and faith-consistent therapy show promise for enhancing meaning and reducing distress in specific populations, although the empirical base is smaller and more heterogeneous than for mindfulness programs (Gonçalves et al., 2023; Button & De Pretto, 2023). Together, these strands support a blended approach that aligns attentional training, embodied practices, and meaning-centered work.

4.2 Outcomes That Show the Most Consistent Gains

Stress and anxiety. Multiple reviews indicate that mindfulness-based and mindfulness-informed programs reduce perceived stress and anxiety in adults, including workers and healthcare staff. These improvements remain detectable against active controls, which suggests benefits beyond expectancy and attention alone (Michaelsen et al., 2023; Ong et al., 2024). Mantra-based meditation likewise shows reliable reductions in stress and anxiety in comparison with passive and active comparators (Álvarez-Pérez et al., 2022).

Depression and negative affect. Meta-analytic syntheses of yoga interventions in depression report clinically relevant decreases in depressive symptoms, particularly when yoga complements standard care (Miao et al., 2023; Wu et al., 2023). Compassion-focused and loving-kindness practices contribute additional reductions in depression and distress, pointing to the value of affective training alongside attentional training (Kirby, Tellegen, & Steindl, 2017).

Sleep and quality of life. Findings for sleep quality and health-related quality of life are positive but more variable, shaped by differences in program dose, delivery format, and population characteristics. Meditation and mantra practices often show improvements in subjective sleep quality and overall life quality, but longer follow-up and standardized sleep measures would strengthen confidence (Álvarez-Pérez et al., 2022; Ong et al., 2024).

Meaning, spirituality, and life evaluation. Meaning in life and spiritual well-being appear to be key levers for distress reduction. A large meta-analysis associates higher presence of meaning with lower psychological distress across contexts, which helps explain why reflective spiritual reading and faith-consistent psychotherapy can amplify outcomes for some groups (He et al., 2023; Gonçalves et al., 2023; Button & De Pretto, 2023).

4.3 How and Why These Practices Work

The pattern of results aligns with established mechanistic frameworks. Mindfulness and related meditations cultivate attention regulation, interoception, and nonreactivity, which reduce rumination and stabilize emotion regulation (Hölzel et al., 2011). Compassion practices likely recruit positive emotion processes that broaden momentary mindsets and accumulate psychological resources such as resilience and social connectedness, consistent with broaden-and-build accounts (Fredrickson, 2001; Kirby et al., 2017).

On the physiological side, paced breathing, gentle postures, and vocalization entrain autonomic rhythms and can increase parasympathetic activity indexed by heart rate variability. Synthesis papers indicate that meditative and breath-focused practices tend to improve autonomic balance relevant to stress regulation (Brown, Olmstead, & Creswell, 2021; Natarajan, 2023). Slow-breathing reviews reinforce this interpretation by detailing psychophysiological pathways through which respiratory training influences arousal and affect (Zaccaro et al., 2018).

Mantra practice may engage both top-down and bottom-up routes. Repetition offers a simple attentional anchor that reduces cognitive load and intrusive thinking, while voiced chanting supplies rhythmic acoustic and somatosensory input that may augment vagal activity, which in turn dampens limbic reactivity. These pathways are coherent with clinical benefits summarized in meta-analytic work (Álvarez-Pérez et al., 2022).

4.4 What is Gained by Integrating Practices

The literatures are complementary rather than duplicative. Mindfulness and focused-attention practices excel at training awareness and nonreactivity. Yoga contributes embodied regulation and interoceptive accuracy. Mantra adds portable, time-efficient attentional and autonomic cues. Spiritual reading deepens meaning-making and values alignment that can stabilize gains and support behavior change. When thoughtfully combined, these elements can cover cognitive, affective, physiological, and existential bases within the same daily routine. Although few randomized trials have tested fully integrated protocols head-to-head against single-component programs, the consistency of modality-specific effects suggests that a modular, blended design is reasonable and likely to improve adherence by matching preferences and constraints (Michaelsen et al., 2023; Miao et al., 2023; Álvarez-Pérez et al., 2022; Gonçalves et al., 2023).

4.5 What Matters for Implementation

Three design features recur across studies that reported stronger outcomes.

1. Regular, brief practice windows. Daily micro-sessions of 8 to 15 minutes appear feasible for busy adults and may be sufficient to shift stress appraisals and mood when maintained consistently over weeks (Michaelsen et al., 2023; Ong et al., 2024).
2. Guided practice and minimal structure. Programs with at least light guidance, clear instructions, and a simple progression tend to outperform unguided self-help, particularly for new practitioners (Kirby et al., 2017; Miao et al., 2023).
3. Values and meaning cues. Interventions that include reflective prompts or spiritually congruent content can enhance purpose and adherence in participants who welcome such framing, without requiring theological commitment (Gonçalves et al., 2023; Button & De Pretto, 2023).

Equity and inclusion matter. Studies emphasize the need for culturally sensitive language, opt-in spiritual elements, and referral pathways for participants with complex trauma or acute symptoms. These ethical safeguards make community and workplace adaptations more acceptable and sustainable (Ong et al., 2024).

4.6 Strength of Evidence and Confidence

Applying GRADE-style reasoning to this narrative synthesis yields a differentiated confidence profile.

- Stress and anxiety: moderate confidence. Multiple randomized trials and meta-analyses converge on improvements for mindfulness and mantra practices, and effects are observed against active comparators in several reviews (Michaelsen et al., 2023; Álvarez-Pérez et al., 2022).
- Depression: moderate confidence for yoga as an adjunct and for compassion-based protocols; variability arises from dosing and population differences (Miao et al., 2023; Wu et al., 2023; Kirby et al., 2017).
- Sleep and quality of life: low to moderate confidence. Positive trends exist, but fewer trials use standardized sleep measures or long follow-up (Álvarez-Pérez et al., 2022; Ong et al., 2024).
- Meaning and spiritual well-being: moderate confidence that these constructs mediate or accompany improvements in distress; evidence spans psychotherapy trials and observational syntheses (He et al., 2023; Gonçalves et al., 2023).
- Autonomic markers: moderate confidence that contemplative and breath practices favorably affect HRV or related indices, with room for better-controlled biomarker protocols (Brown et al., 2021; Natarajan, 2023; Zaccaro et al., 2018).

4.7 Limitations of the Literature

Heterogeneity is the rule rather than the exception. Interventions vary in content, duration, teacher training, and delivery mode. Comparator quality also varies, and blinding is often infeasible. Self-report outcomes dominate, with fewer studies including objective or clinician-rated measures. Long-term maintenance is understudied, and spiritual reading protocols are diverse and sometimes under-specified. These limitations argue for cautious language and for more dismantling studies that isolate active ingredients.

4.8 Practical Implications

A pragmatic program that fits this evidence base can be framed as follows: brief daily mindfulness or breath practice, short mantra recitation for attentional reset, two or three sessions per week of reflective spiritual reading with journaling prompts, and gentle yoga on two days to support interoception and vagal tone. Implementation should be opt-in for spiritual elements, offer secular alternatives, and include simple tracking of stress, mood, sleep, meaning, and practice time using validated instruments. In occupational or campus settings, small environmental cues such as two minutes of quiet at the start of a meeting or a weekly reading circle can extend practice into real life.

4.9 Implications for Future Research

Priorities include head-to-head trials comparing integrated protocols with single-modality programs, standardized reporting of dose and fidelity, routine inclusion of meaning and spiritual well-being measures when relevant, and mixed-methods evaluation to capture acceptability across cultures and beliefs. Longer follow-up and biomarker substudies would clarify maintenance and mechanisms.

5. IMPLICATIONS AND FUTURE RESEARCH

5.1 Practical Implications for Different Settings

Clinicians and counsellors- The literature supports offering a blended toolkit that includes brief mindfulness or breath-focused practice, short mantra recitation, gentle yoga, and guided reflective reading for clients who are open to spiritual content. Frame spiritual elements as opt-in, provide secular alternatives, and monitor symptoms with validated scales such as the Perceived Stress Scale, GAD-7, PHQ-9, PSQI, and the FACIT-Sp for spiritual well-being. Evidence indicates consistent benefits for stress and anxiety across mindfulness and mantra programs, with yoga showing adjunctive value for mood in clinical samples (Michaelsen, Wessa, & Kubiak, 2023; Álvarez-Pérez et al., 2022; Miao et al., 2023; Wu, Yan, & Yang, 2023).

Educators and student services- Brief daily practices are feasible in academic schedules and can improve coping and sleep hygiene. Campus programs should consider small-group formats, light guidance, and culturally sensitive language. Findings from mindfulness and compassion-based interventions suggest meaningful gains in well-being that are relevant to high-stress academic periods (Kirby, Tellegen, & Steindl, 2017; Michaelsen et al., 2023).

Community and workplace programs- Programs that combine short guided practice, values reflection, and simple tracking see stronger adherence and outcomes. In workplaces, randomized trials show mindfulness-informed programs reduce stress and burnout, with additional evidence for healthcare workers (Michaelsen et al., 2023; Ong et al., 2024). Where appropriate, contemplative reading circles and optional mantra practice can enrich meaning and community without imposing belief systems (Gonçalves et al., 2023; Button & De Pretto, 2023).

Physiological self-regulation- Encourage slow breathing and paced vocalization to support autonomic balance. Reviews indicate that meditative and breath-focused practices can increase parasympathetic activity indexed by heart rate variability, which aligns with subjective stress relief (Brown, Olmstead, & Creswell, 2021; Zaccaro et al., 2018; Natarajan, 2023).

5.2 Measurement, Reporting, and Quality Improvement

Program descriptions should meet reporting standards so others can replicate them. Use the TIDieR checklist to specify dose, session structure, delivery mode, instructor qualifications, and home practice expectations (Hoffmann et al., 2014). For evaluation, predefine primary and secondary outcomes and report with CONSORT standards if the design is randomized, or use comparable transparency in quasi-experimental work (Schulz, Altman, & Moher, 2010). For complex blended programs, the updated Medical Research Council guidance encourages attention to context, mechanisms, and implementation from the outset, not only outcomes (Skivington et al., 2021).

For physiological outcomes, follow psychophysiology recommendations on heart rate variability planning and reporting. These include controlling for respiration, posture, time of day, and artifact handling, and preferring time-domain indexes like RMSSD for short recordings (Laborde, Mosley, & Thayer, 2017).

For reach and equity, evaluate programs with RE-AIM to track adoption, implementation, and maintenance, not only efficacy (Glasgow, Harden, Gaglio, Rabin, Smith, Porter, Ory, & Estabrooks, 2019).

5.3 Program Design Implications

Keep practice brief and regular- Daily micro-sessions of 8 to 15 minutes are realistic for adults and appear sufficient to shift stress and mood when done consistently (Michaelsen et al., 2023; Ong et al., 2024).

Provide guidance and structure- Guided practice and simple progressions outperform unguided self-help, especially for novice practitioners (Kirby et al., 2017; Miao et al., 2023).

Match content to preference. Offer secular options for participants who prefer non-spiritual framing. For those who welcome spiritual elements, reflective reading and optional mantra practice can strengthen meaning and adherence (Gonçalves et al., 2023; Button & De Pretto, 2023).

Blend cognitive, affective, and embodied elements- Combine attentional training, compassion or gratitude prompts, slow breathing or gentle movement, and reflection. This covers complementary mechanisms highlighted across the literature: attention regulation, emotion regulation, autonomic balance, and meaning (Hölzel et al., 2011; Fredrickson, 2001; Brown et al., 2021; He et al., 2023).

5.4 Equity, Ethics, and Cultural Adaptation

Programs should be opt-in and value-neutral, with clear consent and referral pathways for participants with acute symptoms or trauma histories. Cultural tailoring is important when spiritual language is used. Provide parallel secular scripts and allow participants to select terms and practices that align with their beliefs. Monitor unintended effects such as transient anxiety during early practice and adjust pacing accordingly (Ong et al., 2024; Gonçalves et al., 2023).

5.5 Future Research Priorities

Head-to-head and modular trials- Compare integrated programs that include mindfulness, yoga, mantra, and reflective reading against single-modality programs to determine whether blended designs yield broader or more durable gains. Use factorial or multi-arm randomized trials where feasible. Report components with TIDieR to support replication (Hoffmann et al., 2014).

Mechanisms and mediation- Test theory-driven mediators such as nonreactivity, reappraisal, compassion, meaning in life, and autonomic indices. Combine validated self-reports with physiological markers and sleep metrics to triangulate change processes (Hölzel et al., 2011; He et al., 2023; Brown et al., 2021).

Dose, fidelity, and maintenance- Establish dose–response relationships for each component, track home-practice adherence with simple digital logs, and include follow-ups of at least three to six months. Use fidelity checklists and report instructor training.

Implementation science- Use effectiveness–implementation hybrid designs to evaluate outcomes and real-world delivery in the same study, especially in community and occupational settings where reach and adoption determine impact (Curran, Bauer, Mittman, Pyne, & Stetler, 2012). Combine outcome evaluation with RE-AIM to document reach, adoption, and maintenance beyond initial pilots (Glasgow et al., 2019).

Population diversity and equity- Prioritize trials with diverse age groups, genders, socioeconomic backgrounds, and cultural contexts. Include subgroup analyses and qualitative work to understand acceptability and tailor messaging.

Comparators and controls- Use active control conditions that match time and attention to reduce expectancy confounds. Where blinding is limited, blind assessors and standardize outcome assessment windows.

Open science and transparency- Preregister protocols, publish analysis plans, share de-identified data where appropriate, and use AMSTAR 2 and PRISMA standards in secondary syntheses. These practices will raise confidence in cumulative evidence.

5.6 Limitations and Caution in Interpretation

The current evidence base is heterogeneous in intervention content, comparator quality, and outcome measurement. Self-report outcomes dominate, and long-term maintenance is underexamined. Spiritual reading protocols vary widely and are sometimes under-specified. These limitations argue for cautious interpretation and for the more rigorous designs outlined above. Nevertheless, the overall pattern across reviews is consistent with meaningful improvements in stress, mood, and well-being when programs are well designed and delivered with sensitivity to context and culture (Michaelsen et al., 2023; Álvarez-Pérez et al., 2022; Miao et al., 2023; Wu et al., 2023; Ong et al., 2024).

6. CONCLUSION AND RECOMMENDATIONS

6.1 Conclusion

This chapter set out to integrate evidence on mantra recitation, spiritual reading, meditation, mindfulness, and yoga in relation to adult mental well-being. The literature converges on a clear picture. Mindfulness and related meditation programs consistently reduce stress and anxiety and support broader well-being in community and occupational samples (Michaelsen, Wessa, & Kubiak, 2023; Ong et al., 2024). Yoga adds embodied regulation that benefits mood and complements standard care in depressive symptoms (Miao et al., 2023; Wu, Yan, & Yang, 2023). Mantra-based meditation provides a simple, portable practice with meaningful benefits for stress, anxiety, and related outcomes (Álvarez-Pérez et al., 2022). Spiritually framed elements, including reflective reading and faith-consistent therapy, appear to strengthen meaning and reduce distress for many adults when offered as opt-in components (Gonçalves et al., 2023; Button & De Pretto, 2023).

Mechanistic accounts help explain why these findings align. Attention training and nonreactivity reduce rumination and improve emotion regulation (Hölzel et al., 2011). Compassion and positive emotion broaden coping resources over time (Fredrickson, 2001). Breath pacing, movement, and vocalization support autonomic balance that is reflected in heart rate variability and subjective stress relief (Brown, Olmstead, & Creswell, 2021; Zaccaro et al., 2018). Meaning in life and spiritual well-being are reliably associated with lower distress, which clarifies the value of reflective spiritual practices for some participants (He et al., 2023).

Overall, a blended approach that pairs brief daily attentional practice with optional mantra, gentle movement or breathwork, and periodic reflective reading is both theoretically coherent and supported by current evidence. Programs should be delivered with cultural sensitivity, secular alternatives, clear consent, and simple evaluation.

6.2 Recommendations for Practice

- Start small and regular. Encourage daily micro-sessions of 8 to 15 minutes for mindfulness or breath-focused practice, with one to two brief mantra periods and two short yoga or movement sessions per week. This pattern matches feasibility and observed benefits in adults (Michaelsen et al., 2023; Ong et al., 2024).
- Offer choice and clear framing. Provide secular scripts alongside optional spiritual elements. Use reflective questions that focus on values and purpose for those who prefer nonreligious language (Gonçalves et al., 2023; Button & De Pretto, 2023).
- Monitor with validated tools. Track perceived stress, anxiety, depressive symptoms, sleep quality, and meaning or spiritual well-being using brief, validated instruments, and review progress at planned intervals.
- Blend mechanisms by design. Pair attentional training with compassion or gratitude prompts, slow breathing or gentle movement, and reflective reading to cover cognitive, affective, physiological, and existential pathways in the same routine (Hölzel et al., 2011; Fredrickson, 2001; Brown et al., 2021).
- Plan for inclusion and safety. Use opt-in enrollment for spiritual content, provide clear referral options for participants with acute symptoms, and invite feedback to adapt language and pacing.

6.3 Recommendations for Program Leaders and Institutions

- Invest in light guidance. Even minimal guidance and a simple progression can improve adherence and outcomes relative to unguided self-help, especially for new practitioners (Kirby, Tellegen, & Steindl, 2017; Miao et al., 2023).
- Build supportive micro-environments. Short quiet openings to meetings, optional reading circles, and accessible spaces for brief practice help translate skills into daily life.
- Evaluate and iterate. Use brief baseline and follow-up assessments at 6 to 8 weeks, gather qualitative feedback, and iterate delivery. For complex programs, follow implementation guidance that attends to context and mechanisms, not only outcomes (Skivington et al., 2021).

6.4 Recommendations for Researchers

- Test integrated protocols against single components. Use multi-arm or factorial designs to determine whether blended programs deliver broader or more durable effects than single-modality interventions.
- Track mechanisms and maintenance. Include nonreactivity, reappraisal, compassion, meaning in life, and heart rate variability where feasible, and extend follow-up beyond immediate post-program to assess durability (Hölzel et al., 2011; He et al., 2023; Brown et al., 2021).
- Improve reporting and fidelity. Specify components, dose, teacher training, and home practice using recognized reporting checklists so results can be replicated and synthesized.
- Prioritize diversity and acceptability. Recruit across age, culture, and socioeconomic status, and include qualitative methods to understand acceptability of spiritual and secular framings.
- Use active comparators and transparent analysis. Match time and attention in control conditions, blind assessors where possible, preregister protocols, and share materials to strengthen cumulative science.

6.5 Final Reflections

The evidence supports cautious optimism. When thoughtfully designed and delivered, a blended practice set that includes mindfulness or meditation, gentle yoga or breathwork, optional mantra, and reflective reading can help adults manage stress, improve mood, and cultivate meaning. The next step is not to search for a single universal technique, but to match modular practices to preferences and contexts, to measure what matters, and to scale what works with humility and care.

REFERENCES

Álvarez-Pérez, Y., Rivero-Santana, A., Perestelo-Pérez, L., Duarte-Díaz, A., Ramos-García, V., Toledo-Chávarri, A., Torres-Castaño, A., León-Salas, B., Infante-Ventura, D., González-Hernández, N., Rodríguez-Rodríguez, L., & Serrano-Aguilar, P. (2022). Effectiveness of mantra-based meditation on mental health: A systematic review and meta-analysis. *International Journal of Environmental Research and Public Health*, *19*(6), 3380. DOI: 10.3390/ijerph19063380 PMID: 35329068

Baer, R. A., Smith, G. T., Hopkins, J., Krietemeyer, J., & Toney, L. (2006). Using self-report assessment methods to explore facets of mindfulness. *Assessment*, *13*(1), 27–45. DOI: 10.1177/1073191105283504 PMID: 16443717

Barik, S., & Nayak, T. (2024). Workplace spirituality: Exploring past, present and future through bibliometric analysis. *Benchmarking*, *31*(9), 3216–3241. DOI: 10.1108/BIJ-04-2022-0251

Brown, V. A., Olmstead, R., & Creswell, J. D. (2021). The effects of mindfulness and meditation on autonomic nervous system activity and heart rate variability: A meta-analysis. *Psychosomatic Medicine*, *83*(7), 699–713. DOI: 10.1097/PSY.0000000000000900 PMID: 33395216

Button, A. J., & De Pretto, M. (2023). A psalm a day keeps the psychiatrist at bay: Measuring the effects of a three-week micro-course based on *lectio divina*. *Pastoral Psychology*, *72*, 1015–1033. DOI: 10.1007/s11089-022-01040-0

Buysse, D. J., Reynolds, C. F.III, Monk, T. H., Berman, S. R., & Kupfer, D. J. (1989). The Pittsburgh Sleep Quality Index: A new instrument for psychiatric practice and research. *Psychiatry Research*, *28*(2), 193–213. DOI: 10.1016/0165-1781(89)90047-4 PMID: 2748771

Chauhan, P., & Rai, S. (2024). Conceptualizing work–life integration: A review and research agenda. *Asia Pacific Management Review*, *29*(4), 415–426. DOI: 10.1016/j.apmrv.2024.10.002

Cohen, S., Kamarck, T., & Mermelstein, R. (1983). A global measure of perceived stress. *Journal of Health and Social Behavior*, *24*(4), 385–396. DOI: 10.2307/2136404 PMID: 6668417

Curran, G. M., Bauer, M., Mittman, B., Pyne, J. M., & Stetler, C. (2012). Effectiveness–implementation hybrid designs: Combining elements of clinical effectiveness and implementation research to enhance public health impact. *Medical Care*, *50*(3), 217–226. DOI: 10.1097/MLR.0b013e3182408812 PMID: 22310560 de Diego-Cordero, R., Zurrón-Pérez, M. P., Vargas-Martínez, A. M., Lucchetti, G., & Vega-Escaño, J. (2021). The effectiveness of spiritual interventions in the workplace for work-related health outcomes: A systematic review and meta-analysis. *Journal of Nursing Management, 29*(6), 1703–1712. DOI: 10.1111/jonm.13315 PMID: 33772925

Dubey, S., & Bedi, S. S. (2024). Workplace spirituality: A systematic review and future research agenda. *Journal of Management, Spirituality & Religion, 21*(1), 1–22. DOI: 10.51327/CQER6430

Fredrickson, B. L. (2001). The role of positive emotions in positive psychology: The broaden-and-build theory of positive emotions. *The American Psychologist, 56*(3), 218–226. DOI: 10.1037/0003-066X.56.3.218 PMID: 11315248

Glasgow, R. E., Harden, S. M., Gaglio, B., Rabin, B., Smith, M. L., Porter, G. C., Ory, M. G., & Estabrooks, P. A. (2019). RE-AIM planning and evaluation framework: Adapting to new science and practice with a 20-year review. *Frontiers in Public Health, 7*, 64. DOI: 10.3389/fpubh.2019.00064 PMID: 30984733

Gonçalves, J. P. B., Peres, M. F. P., Tolentino, E. J. A., Mendes, A. L., Farina, M., & Vallada, H. (2023). The evaluation of religious and spirituality-based therapy compared to secular therapy on mental health: A meta-analysis of randomized controlled trials. *Psychotherapy Research, 33*(8), 1037–1052. DOI: 10.1080/10503307.2023.2241626

Grant, M. J., & Booth, A. (2009). A typology of reviews: An analysis of 14 review types and associated methodologies. *Health Information and Libraries Journal, 26*(2), 91–108. DOI: 10.1111/j.1471-1842.2009.00848.x PMID: 19490148

He, X., Wang, X., Steger, M. F., Ji, L., Jing, K., Liu, M., & Ye, B. (2023). Meaning in life and psychological distress: A meta-analysis. *Journal of Research in Personality, 104*, 104381. DOI: 10.1016/j.jrp.2023.104381

Hoffmann, T. C., Glasziou, P. P., Boutron, I., Milne, R., Perera, R., Moher, D., Altman, D. G., Barbour, V., Macdonald, H., Johnston, M., Lamb, S. E., Dixon-Woods, M., McCulloch, P., Wyatt, J. C., Chan, A.-W., & Michie, S. (2014). Better reporting of interventions: Template for Intervention Description and Replication (TIDieR) checklist and guide. *BMJ (Clinical Research Ed.), 348*(mar07 3), g1687. DOI: 10.1136/bmj.g1687 PMID: 24609605

Hölzel, B. K., Lazar, S. W., Gard, T., Schuman-Olivier, Z., Vago, D. R., & Ott, U. (2011). How does mindfulness meditation work? Proposing mechanisms of action from a conceptual and neural perspective. *Perspectives on Psychological Science, 6*(6), 537–559. DOI: 10.1177/1745691611419671 PMID: 26168376

Hong, Q. N., Pluye, P., Fàbregues, S., Bartlett, G., Boardman, F., Cargo, M., Dagenais, P., Gagnon, M.-P., Griffiths, F., Nicolau, B., O'Cathain, A., Rousseau, M.-C., & Vedel, I. (2018). *Mixed Methods Appraisal Tool (MMAT), version 2018 User guide*. McGill University, Department of Family Medicine.

Kalyani, B. G., Venkatasubramanian, G., Arasappa, R., Rao, N. P., Kalmady, S. V., Behere, R. V., Rao, H., Vasudev, M. K., & Gangadhar, B. N. (2011). Neurohemodynamic correlates of "Om" chanting: A pilot fMRI study. *International Journal of Yoga*, *4*(1), 3–6. DOI: 10.4103/0973-6131.78171 PMID: 21654968

Kirby, J. N., Tellegen, C. L., & Steindl, S. R. (2017). A meta-analysis of compassion-based interventions: Current state of knowledge and future directions. *Behavior Therapy*, *48*(6), 778–792. DOI: 10.1016/j.beth.2017.06.003 PMID: 29029675

Laborde, S., Mosley, E., & Thayer, J. F. (2017). Heart rate variability and cardiac vagal tone in psychophysiology: Recommendations for experiment planning, data analysis, and data reporting. *Frontiers in Psychology*, *8*, 213. DOI: 10.3389/fpsyg.2017.00213 PMID: 28265249

Miao, C., Gao, Y., Li, X., Zhou, Y., Chung, J. W., & Smith, G. D. (2023). The effectiveness of mindfulness yoga on patients with major depressive disorder: A systematic review and meta-analysis of randomized controlled trials. *BMC Complementary Medicine and Therapies*, *23*(1), 313. DOI: 10.1186/s12906-023-04141-2 PMID: 37684609

Michaelsen, M. M., Adolph, D., Schinköthe, A., Witthöft, M., & Wessa, M. (2023). Mindfulness-based and mindfulness-informed interventions at the workplace: A meta-analysis of randomized controlled trials. *Mindfulness*, *14*, 1271–1304. DOI: 10.1007/s12671-023-02130-7 PMID: 37362186

Natarajan, A. (2023). Heart rate variability during mindful breathing meditation. *Frontiers in Physiology*, *14*, 1017350. DOI: 10.3389/fphys.2022.1017350 PMID: 36756034

Nayyar, R., Yadav, P., Baral, R., Raina, M., & Jena, L. K. (2024). Unveiling the past, present and future of workplace spirituality research: A systematic literature review of 15 years. *The International Journal of Organizational Analysis*. Advance online publication. DOI: 10.1108/IJOA-04-2024-4438

Ong, N. Y., Teo, F. J. J., Ee, J. Z. Y., Tan, J. X., Goh, H. K., & Lee, J. C. (2024). Effectiveness of mindfulness-based interventions on the well-being of healthcare workers: A systematic review and meta-analysis. *General Psychiatry*, *37*(3), e101115. DOI: 10.1136/gpsych-2023-101115 PMID: 38737894

Page, M. J., McKenzie, J. E., Bossuyt, P. M., Boutron, I., Hoffmann, T. C., Mulrow, C. D., Shamseer, L., Tetzlaff, J. M., Akl, E. A., Brennan, S. E., Chou, R., Glanville, J., Grimshaw, J. M., Hróbjartsson, A., Lalu, M. M., Li, T., Loder, E. W., Mayo-Wilson, E., McDonald, S., & Moher, D. (2021). The PRISMA 2020 statement: An updated guideline for reporting systematic reviews. *BMJ (Clinical Research Ed.)*, *372*(71), n71. Advance online publication. DOI: 10.1136/bmj.n71 PMID: 33782057

Pallvi, K., & Jhajharia, P. (2025). Exploring trends in workplace spirituality through bibliometric analysis. *SN Business & Economics*, *5*(9), 108. Advance online publication. DOI: 10.1007/s43546-025-00883-y

Peterman, A. H., Fitchett, G., Brady, M. J., Hernandez, L., & Cella, D. (2002). Measuring spiritual well-being in people with cancer: The Functional Assessment of Chronic Illness Therapy–Spiritual Well-Being Scale (FACIT-Sp). *Annals of Behavioral Medicine*, *24*(1), 49–58. DOI: 10.1207/S15324796ABM2401_06 PMID: 12008794

Santomauro, D. F., Mantilla Herrera, A. M., Shadid, J., Zheng, P., Ashbaugh, C., Pigott, D. M., Abbafati, C., Adolph, C., Amlag, J. O., Aravkin, A. Y., Bang-Jensen, B. L., Bertolacci, G. J., Bloom, S. S., Castellano, R., Castro, E., Chakrabarti, S., Chattopadhyay, J., Cogen, R. M., Collins, J. K., & Ferrari, A. J. (2021). Global prevalence and burden of depressive and anxiety disorders in 204 countries and territories in 2020 due to the COVID-19 pandemic. *Lancet*, *398*(10312), 1700–1712. DOI: 10.1016/S0140-6736(21)02143-7 PMID: 34634250

Schulz, K. F., Altman, D. G., & Moher, D. (2010). CONSORT 2010 statement: Updated guidelines for reporting parallel group randomised trials. *BMJ (Clinical Research Ed.)*, *340*(mar23 1), c332. DOI: 10.1136/bmj.c332 PMID: 20332509

Skivington, K., Matthews, L., Simpson, S. A., Craig, P., Baird, J., Blazeby, J. M., Boyd, K. A., Craig, N., French, D. P., McIntosh, E., Petticrew, M., Rycroft-Malone, J., White, M., & Moore, L. (2021). A new framework for developing and evaluating complex interventions: Update of Medical Research Council guidance. *BMJ (Clinical Research Ed.)*, *374*(2061), n2061. Advance online publication. DOI: 10.1136/bmj.n2061 PMID: 34593508

Steger, M. F., Frazier, P., Oishi, S., & Kaler, M. (2006). The Meaning in Life Questionnaire: Assessing the presence of and search for meaning in life. *Journal of Counseling Psychology*, *53*(1), 80–93. DOI: 10.1037/0022-0167.53.1.80

Sterne, J. A. C., Hernán, M. A., Reeves, B. C., Savović, J., Berkman, N. D., Viswanathan, M., Henry, D., Altman, D. G., Ansari, M. T., Boutron, I., Carpenter, J., Chan, A.-W., Churchill, R., Deeks, J. J., Hróbjartsson, A., Kirkham, J. J., Jüni, P., Loke, Y. K., Pigott, T. D., & Higgins, J. P. T. (2016). ROBINS-I: A tool for assessing risk of bias in non-randomised studies of interventions. *BMJ (Clinical Research Ed.), 355*, i4919. DOI: 10.1136/bmj.i4919 PMID: 27733354

Sterne, J. A. C., Savović, J., Page, M. J., Elbers, R. G., Blencowe, N. S., Boutron, I., Cates, C. J., Cheng, H.-Y., Corbett, M. S., Eldridge, S. M., Emberson, J. R., Hernán, M. A., Hopewell, S., Hróbjartsson, A., Junqueira, D. R., Jüni, P., Kirkham, J. J., Lasserson, T., Li, T., & Higgins, J. P. T. (2019). RoB 2: A revised tool for assessing risk of bias in randomised trials. *BMJ (Clinical Research Ed.), 366*, l4898. DOI: 10.1136/bmj.l4898 PMID: 31462531

Thomas, J., & Harden, A. (2008). Methods for the thematic synthesis of qualitative research in systematic reviews. *BMC Medical Research Methodology, 8*(1), 45. DOI: 10.1186/1471-2288-8-45 PMID: 18616818

Tricco, A. C., Lillie, E., Zarin, W., O'Brien, K. K., Colquhoun, H., Levac, D., Moher, D., Peters, M. D. J., Horsley, T., Weeks, L., Hempel, S., Akl, E. A., Chang, C., McGowan, J., Stewart, L., Hartling, L., Aldcroft, A., Wilson, M. G., Garritty, C., & Straus, S. E. (2018). PRISMA extension for scoping reviews (PRISMA-ScR): Checklist and explanation. *Annals of Internal Medicine, 169*(7), 467–473. DOI: 10.7326/M18-0850 PMID: 30178033

Whittemore, R., & Knafl, K. (2005). The integrative review: Updated methodology. *Journal of Advanced Nursing, 52*(5), 546–553. DOI: 10.1111/j.1365-2648.2005.03621.x PMID: 16268861

World Health Organization. (2022). *World mental health report: Transforming mental health for all.* World Health Organization.

Wu, Y., Yan, D., & Yang, J. (2023). Effectiveness of yoga for major depressive disorder: A systematic review and meta-analysis. *Frontiers in Psychiatry, 14*, 1138205. DOI: 10.3389/fpsyt.2023.1138205 PMID: 37032928

Zaccaro, A., Piarulli, A., Laurino, M., Garbella, E., Menicucci, D., Neri, B., Gemignani, A., & Palombo, D. (2018). How breath-control can change your life: A systematic review on psychophysiological correlates of slow breathing. *Frontiers in Human Neuroscience, 12*, 353. DOI: 10.3389/fnhum.2018.00353 PMID: 30245619

Chapter 3
Neuroplasticity and the Breath:
Unpacking the Brain Mechanisms Behind Yogic Pranayama

Ibnu noufal Kambitta Valappil
http://orcid.org/0009-0006-6426-8809
Pondicherry University, India

Akshay Korol
http://orcid.org/0000-0002-8291-0555
National Institute of Technology, Karaikal, India

Gavoutamane Vasanthi
http://orcid.org/0009-0006-0276-6343
Pondicherry University, India

Masilamani Elayaraja
http://orcid.org/0000-0002-0022-961X
Pondicherry University, India

Karuppasamy Govindasamy
http://orcid.org/0000-0002-3019-5545
Symbiosis International University, India

ABSTRACT

Pranayama, the Yogic discipline of regulated breathing, has evolved from a spiritual practice into a scientifically recognized method for supporting mental and neurological health. This chapter examines its neuroplastic potential by outlining effects on major brain regions and networks, while summarizing key Pranayama techniques and

DOI: 10.4018/979-8-3373-4187-3.ch003

their physiological signatures. Evidence indicates improvements in parasympathetic activation, heart rate variability, cortisol modulation, and emotional–cognitive regulation. Integrating recent advances in contemplative and clinical neuroscience, the chapter highlights technology-supported breathwork, trauma-responsive approaches informed by polyvagal theory, and individualized applications based on autonomic profiling. It also clarifies distinctions between established neural biomarkers and emerging theoretical claims of structural change. Overall, the chapter positions Pranayama as an accessible, non-invasive, and increasingly personalized neuro-modulatory tool within the broader "Neuro-Yogic Paradigm."

INTRODUCTION

Pranayama, the Yogic discipline of breath regulation, has been practised for millennia as a foundational component of traditional Yoga (Chauhan & Bansal, 2024). The term Pranayama is derived from two Sanskrit words: "prana," meaning vital life force, and "ayama," meaning expansion or control (Pradhan, 2015). Traditionally, Pranayama has been regarded not merely as a tool for respiratory training but as a spiritual and mental discipline aimed at achieving greater harmony between body, mind, and consciousness (Craig, 2002; Saoji et al., 2019; Sengupta, 2012). Pranayama was practised as a preparatory stage for deeper meditative states and spiritual realization, believed to cleanse the energy channels (nadis), regulate the mind, and facilitate higher states of consciousness (Pradhan, 2015). In contemporary times, Pranayama has garnered considerable attention beyond its spiritual origins (Chauhan & Bansal, 2024). With the global rise in stress-related disorders, anxiety, depression, and other mental health challenges, there has been a growing interest in holistic, accessible, and non-pharmacological approaches to emotional and psychological well-being (Magomedova & Fatima, 2025). Among such approaches, Yogic breathing stands out due to its simplicity, affordability, and proven physiological effects (Veerakannan, 2025). Modern research in the fields of neuroscience, psychophysiology, and clinical psychology has begun to systematically investigate the benefits of Pranayama, linking it with improved autonomic regulation, reduced stress hormone levels, enhanced emotional control, and better cognitive functioning (Saoji et al., 2019).

Pranayama is very interesting from a scientific standpoint due to its potential to influence neuroplasticity; the brain's extraordinary capacity to reshape its structure, functions, and neural pathways in response to experience and environmental stimuli (Veerakannan, 2025). Neuroplasticity is the basis for learning, memory, and recovery from brain injury (Saha, 2025). It enables the brain to adapt to new experiences, acquire new skills, and recover from damage (Saha, 2025). Neuroplasticity plays a key role in emotional regulation and mental health. Stress, trauma, and mental illness can lead to maladaptive neural patterns. However, therapeutic interventions that involve both cognitive and somatic systems can help promote positive rewiring (Ren et al., 2025). In this regard, Pranayama emerges as a unique practice that engages multiple dimensions of experience, such as cognitive, emotional, interoceptive, and physiological. This makes it a potentially strong catalyst for neuroplastic change (Schmalzl et al., 2015).

From a neurophysiological perspective, Pranayama influences multiple interconnected mechanisms. Controlled breathing modulates the autonomic nervous system (ANS) by reducing sympathetic arousal and enhancing parasympathetic activity, contributing to lower heart rate and blood pressure, improved immune and digestive function, and reduced inflammation (M. R. Tolahunase et al., 2018). Breath regulation also engages cortical regions involved in attention, emotional regulation, and interoception, including the prefrontal cortex (PFC), anterior cingulate cortex (ACC), insula, and amygdala (Doll et al., 2016). Pranayama further affects brainstem structures such as the medulla and pons, which govern respiratory rhythm and autonomic control (Guz, 1997). Through volitional breath control, practitioners exert top-down influence on these centers, enabling conscious modulation of typically involuntary physiological processes (Taylor et al., 2010). Neuroimaging research using functional MRI (fMRI), electroencephalography (EEG), and positron emission tomography (PET) demonstrates that Pranayama alters connectivity within and between large-scale networks such as the default mode and salience networks, supporting improved attentional regulation and emotional stability (Bremer et al., 2022; Rahrig et al., 2022; Veerakannan, 2025). Enhanced integration between these networks during breath-based meditation may lead to improved attentional control and emotional balance.

The benefits of Pranayama extend beyond healthy individuals seeking stress reduction, with clinical populations also demonstrating significant improvements (Grensman et al., 2018; Haller et al., 2023; Mishra et al., 2012). Incorporating breathwork into treatment protocols has shown promise for conditions such as PTSD, depression, and substance use disorders, with reports of reduced symptoms and enhanced quality of life (Haller et al., 2023). In trauma-informed contexts, Pranayama supports nervous system stabilization, offering a bottom-up regulatory approach that is particularly effective for individuals with dysregulated physiological states, complementing traditional cognitive therapies (Laplaud et al., 2023). Despite these encouraging findings, key challenges remain. A major limitation is the heterogeneity of techniques studied, as slow breathing, alternate-nostril breathing, and breath retention produce distinct physiological effects (Zaccaro et al., 2018). Standardizing protocols and categorizing practices based on their neurophysiological impact is essential for building a robust evidence base. Additionally, most existing studies are short-term (Ankad et al., 2011; Pal et al., 2004; Vinay et al., 2016), with few exploring the longitudinal effects of sustained practice on brain structure and function (Novaes et al., 2020).

A further consideration is the cultural contextualization of Pranayama. As Yogic practices become increasingly globalized and secularized, there is a risk of disconnecting them from their philosophical foundations (King et al., 2022). While scientific validation supports wider acceptance, honoring the cultural and spiritual roots of Pranayama remains essential. Integrative frameworks that connect traditional wisdom with contemporary science can offer a more holistic understanding. In mental health, Pranayama holds significant potential (Verma, 2025). With rising global rates of mental disorders, accessible and scalable interventions are urgently needed (Wu et al., 2023). In corporate environments, breath regulation techniques can serve as tools for stress management and performance optimization (Fincham et al., 2023).

This chapter proposes to unpack the brain mechanisms underlying Pranayama practices and evaluate how these techniques induce neuroplastic changes across various brain regions and networks associated with emotion regulation, attention, interoception, and autonomic control. In doing so, it aims to bridge ancient Yogic wisdom with contemporary neuroscience by providing a conceptual and historical overview of Pranayama within Yogic and Ayurvedic traditions, reviewing current empirical evidence on its cognitive and emotional benefits, examining its influence on brain functional reorganization, analyzing the neural substrates involved particularly the PFC, insula, amygdala, and brainstem and proposing future research directions and clinical applications that integrate Pranayama into evidence-based mental health interventions.

OVERVIEW OF PRANAYAMA TYPES

Pranayama refers to traditional Yogic breathing techniques that intentionally modify breathing patterns to influence both the body and mind. Unlike general breathwork, each Pranayama method such as Nadi Shodhana (alternate nostril breathing), Bhastrika (bellows breath), Kapalabhati (skull-shining breath), Ujjayi (victorious breath), Sheetali (cooling breath), Sheetkari (hissing breath), and Brahmari (humming-bee breath) produces distinct physiological and psychological effects (Singh et al., 2024).

Nadi Shodhana

Nadi Shodhana is characterized by slow, alternate-nostril breathing and is traditionally used to balance the "ida" and "pingala" energy channels. Contemporary evidence shows that it improves attention, reduces anxiety, and enhances parasympathetic activity (Dhaniwala et al., 2020).

Bhastrika

Bhastrika, a forceful inhalation–exhalation technique, increases sympathetic activation and metabolic rate. It is often associated with heightened alertness, improved respiratory capacity, and stronger autonomic regulation (Dhaniwala et al., 2020).

Kapalabhati

Kapalabhati involves rapid, forceful exhalations and passive inhalations. Traditionally viewed as a cleansing technique, it has been shown to enhance cognitive processing speed, improve vagal tone, and regulate frontal brain activity (Dhaniwala et al., 2020).

Ujjayi

Ujjayi uses a gentle throat constriction to produce an audible breath. It is widely practiced to promote mental focus, regulate vagal activity, and induce calm alertness, making it effective for stress management (Dhaniwala et al., 2020).

Sheetali and Sheetkari

Sheetali and Sheetkari are cooling pranayamas that lower physiological arousal, reduce body temperature, and evoke relaxation, often recommended for stress, anger, or heat-related discomfort (Dhaniwala et al., 2020).

Brahmari

Brahmari, characterized by a humming exhalation, stimulates vagal pathways and reduces anxiety, hypertension, and agitation by engaging the resonance of sound vibrations (Dhaniwala et al., 2020).

Modern research consistently demonstrates that slow and regulated Pranayama techniques primarily activate the parasympathetic nervous system, leading to reduced stress, improved emotional balance, and enhanced attentional control. Conversely, fast Pranayama techniques stimulate sympathetic activation, increasing alertness and respiratory efficiency. In simple terms, Pranayama works through intentional breath modulation to calm the body, stabilize emotions, and optimize brain function. These diverse techniques make Pranayama applicable in health, educational, athletic, and therapeutic settings, where tailored breathing practices can support specific physical and mental outcomes.

HISTORICAL AND PHILOSOPHICAL FOUNDATIONS OF PRANAYAMA

Pranayama is a sophisticated system of breath regulation deeply embedded in the philosophical and spiritual traditions of Yoga (Pradhan, 2015). It is not viewed merely as a mechanical act of respiration but as a means of influencing subtle energies within the mind–body system (Ankad et al., 2011). Classical Yogic texts, including the Hatha Yoga Pradipika, Patanjali's Yoga Sutras, and the Bhagavad Gita, describe multiple Pranayama techniques, each designed for specific physiological and energetic purposes (Singh et al., 2024). These traditional sources emphasize that pranayama comprises multiple techniques with unique mechanisms and purposes, thereby distinguishing it from general breath-regulation exercises found in modern therapeutic or fitness-based practices. Such differentiation is essential for understanding its diverse physiological effects and its nuanced role within the broader Yogic system. These practices are traditionally used to cleanse the energy pathways, stabilize the mind, and prepare the practitioner for higher stages of meditation and self-realization (Srinivasan & Aithal, 2025). The breath, in this context, becomes both a tool and a symbol of transformation, used to refine attention, deepen introspection, and guide consciousness inward (Prpa et al., 2018). Incorporating this historical lens allows a clearer contextual foundation for contemporary readers, clarifying how specific pranayama techniques evolved and how their intended functions differ across traditional lineages.

In recent years, these ancient practices have gained renewed significance within scientific and therapeutic domains, as researchers have begun to explore their measurable effects on psychological and neurological health (Novaes et al., 2020; Schmalzl et al., 2015; Shao et al., 2024; Veerakannan, 2025). Though originally oriented toward spiritual liberation (moksha), Pranayama is now being studied for its potential in managing stress, enhancing cognitive function, and fostering emotional balance (Sullivan et al., 2018). Techniques such as Nadi Shodhana have demonstrated reductions in anxiety and improvements in attention, while more invigorating practices like Bhastrika and Kapalabhati are associated with heightened alertness and increased autonomic regulation (Novaes et al., 2020). These distinctions strengthen the scientific rationale for treating pranayama not as a uniform intervention but as a collection of targeted regulatory strategies with technique-specific outcomes.

This growing body of evidence underscores the relevance of Pranayama in addressing modern mental health challenges, offering a non-invasive, low-cost, and holistic intervention strategy (Brahmbhatt & Kumavat, 2024; Mendo et al., 2022). From a neurophysiological standpoint, breath regulation has been shown to influence heart rate variability (HRV), cortisol levels, and the balance between sympathetic and parasympathetic nervous system (PNS) activity (Gerritsen & Band, 2018). Moreover, consistent practice is believed to induce neuroplastic changes and modifications in brain structure and function that support adaptive cognitive and emotional responses (Gothe et al., 2019; Voss et al., 2023).

Pranayama refers to traditional Yogic breathing techniques that intentionally modify breathing patterns to influence both the body and mind. Unlike general breathwork, each Pranayama method, such as slow alternate-nostril breathing or fast bellows-type breathing, produces different physiological and psychological effects. Modern research shows these practices can reduce stress, improve attention, and regulate the nervous system. In simple terms, Pranayama works by using controlled breathing to calm the body, balance emotions, and optimize brain function, making it relevant for health, education, and therapeutic settings.

SCIENTIFIC AND CLINICAL EVIDENCE

A compelling body of evidence supports the therapeutic potential of Pranayama, demonstrating consistent benefits for physiological regulation, mental health, and cognitive functioning across healthy and clinical populations (Ankad et al., 2011; Mendo et al., 2022; Novaes et al., 2020; Shao et al., 2024; Zaccaro et al., 2018). One of the most comprehensive meta-analyses to date (Shao et al., 2024) confirmed that slow-paced breathing, including various Pranayama forms, reliably enhances cardiovascular regulation and emotional well-being. Slow breathing was associated with reductions in blood pressure, heart rate, and improved HRV, indicating strengthened parasympathetic activation and greater emotional resilience. Although immediate effects on stress and emotion were clear, the meta-analysis emphasized the need for long-term studies to assess sustained benefits. Overall, it reinforces Pranayama as an accessible, low-cost intervention with relevance in preventive and therapeutic contexts. Independent trials further support these findings. A randomized controlled trial involving 140 individuals with anxiety disorders demonstrated significant improvements in HRV and baroreflex sensitivity after eight weeks of slow Pranayama and guided relaxation (Kavitha et al., 2024). Similarly, adolescents practising Bhramari Pranayama for six months showed meaningful HRV improvements across time and frequency domains (Kuppusamy et al., 2020). These autonomic shifts across diverse ages and conditions highlight Pranayama's role in enhancing physiological resilience.

Beyond autonomic outcomes, meta-analyses and RCTs consistently report reductions in anxiety and depression. Fincham et al. (2023), synthesizing 40 RCTs, found breath-based interventions significantly more effective than control conditions. Although protocol variability introduced heterogeneity, effects remained consistently positive. Specific practices such as Nadi Shodhana have demonstrated notable anxiolytic and cognitive benefits; alternate-nostril breathing significantly improved attention and processing speed compared to rest (Nautiyal et al., 2024). In clinical contexts, a 12-week Anulom Vilom program improved cognition, mood, and quality of life in Parkinson's patients, suggesting strengthened neural network integration. Stress physiology findings align with these outcomes. Dhanaradja et al. (2025) documented significant reductions in stress markers, while Butzer et al. (2015) reported improved cortisol profiles in youth following yoga-based practices (Butzer et al., 2015). Pranayama also benefits chronic conditions. Hypertensive patients practising Sheetali showed reductions in blood pressure and enhanced HRV (Shao et al., 2024; Thanalakshmi et al., 2020). COVID-19 patients using Bhramari and Nadi Shodhana reported improved sleep, reduced anxiety, and autonomic stabilization (Jagadeesan et al., 2022). A meta-analysis by Gaur et al. (2020) also found increases in alpha and delta EEG power and decreased theta activity, reflecting enhanced neural relaxation and cognitive calm (Gaur et al., 2020).

Neuroimaging evidence reveals mechanisms underlying these effects. In a four-week RCT, Bhastrika Pranayama was associated with decreased amygdala, ACC, and insula activity and increased PFC activation, alongside reduced anxiety (Novaes et al., 2020). Resting-state fMRI showed reduced connectivity between the anterior insula and lateral PFC, suggesting improved emotion regulation. A large meta-analysis of 78 neuroimaging studies found consistent activation in regions related to attention, interoception, and executive control, including the insula, dorsal ACC, and frontopolar cortex (Fox et al., 2016). At the network level, functional MRI research demonstrates a shift from default mode network dominance toward enhanced salience network activity during Pranayama (Melnychuk et al., 2018). Theoretical models involving the locus coeruleus propose that respiratory-phase modulation stabilises attentional processes. Although promising, neurobiological findings require longitudinal research to confirm structural neuroplasticity and enduring connectivity changes (Tanzer et al., 2021). Multimodal approaches integrating neuroimaging with physiological markers such as HRV and cortisol may further clarify pathways linking breath regulation to brain and psychological outcomes (Bahi et al., 2024).

Pranayama has been widely studied for its benefits on stress reduction, emotional regulation, and autonomic balance. Slow breathing techniques can lower heart rate and blood pressure, improve heart-rate variability, and support a calmer nervous system. Research also shows reductions in anxiety and depression, along with better attention and cognition in both healthy individuals and clinical groups. These effects are supported by brain-imaging studies showing changes in regions related to emotion and attention. Overall, Pranayama offers a simple, low-cost method to support mental and physical well-being across diverse populations.

EMERGING TRENDS IN PRANAYAMA NEUROSCIENCE

Recent progress in contemplative and clinical neuroscience reflects a clear evolution in how Pranayama is conceptualized and applied. Beyond the traditional mechanistic pathways already addressed in the chapter, emerging scholarship increasingly foregrounds innovations such as closed-loop technology–enhanced Pranayama, trauma-responsive breathwork models informed by polyvagal theory, and precision or personalized Pranayama tailored to individual autonomic profiles (Bhagat et al., 2017; Dhangar et al., 2025; Walker & Flaherty, 2024). Together, these developments illustrate the field's transition toward more adaptive, data-informed, and clinically nuanced applications of breath regulation. Incorporating these perspectives further strengthens the chapter's relevance and positions it in line with the most forward-looking scientific discourse.

Closed-Loop, Technology-Enhanced Pranayama

Closed-loop breathing systems represent a major advancement in contemporary Pranayama research. These approaches integrate real-time physiological markers such as heart-rate variability, respiratory sinus arrhythmia, EEG patterns, and autonomic reactivity to automatically adjust breathing parameters according to the practitioner's current state. Evidence shows that HRV-guided slow-breathing protocols yield notable improvements in vagal activity, baroreflex function, emotional regulation, and cognitive resilience, often exceeding the benefits of conventionally instructed breathing (Lehrer et al., 2020; Tabor et al., 2022). By framing Pranayama as a technology-supported neuromodulation strategy, this emerging direction broadens its clinical, therapeutic, and performance-related applications.

Pranayama as a Central Mechanism in Trauma-Informed Care

Pranayama has gained prominence in trauma-informed interventions, supported by advances in polyvagal theory and affective neuroscience (Sullivan et al., 2018). Slow, coherent diaphragmatic breathing activates the ventral vagal complex, promoting physiological safety, reducing sympathetic arousal, and enhancing emotional and interoceptive regulation essential for trauma recovery (Slonim, 2014). Contemporary trauma frameworks increasingly position breathwork as a primary intervention for PTSD, chronic stress, and complex trauma. Clinical programs integrating breath-centered neuroregulation demonstrate improvements in stress reduction, affect stabilization, and therapeutic engagement (Haller et al., 2023). These developments affirm Pranayama's emerging role as a key mechanism in trauma-informed care.

Precision and Personalized Pranayama

A key advancement in Pranayama research is the move toward precision and individualized practice. Evidence shows that standard breathing protocols may not benefit all individuals equally; instead, tailoring techniques to one's physiological, psychological, and neurocognitive profile enhances outcomes. For example, individuals with low baseline HRV often benefit most from ultra-slow breathing, while those with moderate vagal tone respond better to ratio-based or alternate-nostril practices (Brown & Gerbarg, 2005; Krygier et al., 2013). Such personalized approaches align Pranayama with precision medicine for more targeted applications (Dhangar et al., 2025). This emerging direction aligns Pranayama within the broader paradigm of precision medicine, supporting more targeted clinical, educational, and performance-oriented applications.

Refining Claims on Structural Neuroplasticity

Recent interpretations of Pranayama-related neuroplasticity benefit from greater specificity in distinguishing well-established evidence from emerging theoretical claims. Findings such as those of M. Tolahunase et al., (2017), which reported increased BDNF levels and reduced stress biomarkers, were derived from a multimodal Rajayoga intervention rather than isolated breathwork (M. Tolahunase et al., 2017). Likewise, improvements in autonomic and inflammatory markers following structured Pranayama have been documented, but without accompanying MRI-based assessments of cortical or subcortical structure (Novaes et al., 2020). Broader contemplative science literature suggests possible links between Yoga-based practices and changes in hippocampal volume or cortical thickness, though such effects cannot yet be attributed specifically to Pranayama (Froeliger et al., 2012).

Recent advances in neuroscience are transforming how Pranayama is used and understood. New technologies now allow breathing practices to be adjusted in real time using indicators such as heart-rate variability or brainwave patterns, making breath training more personalized and effective. Pranayama is also becoming central in trauma-informed care, where slow and controlled breathing helps calm the nervous system and support emotional safety. Research further shows that individualized breathing approaches matched to a person's physiology and stress profile may produce stronger outcomes than standard techniques. Overall, these emerging directions highlight Pranayama as a modern, adaptable, and evidence-informed tool for health and well-being.

THE PHYSIOLOGY OF BREATH AND AUTONOMIC REGULATION

Breathing is a unique physiological function in that it operates both automatically and voluntarily, placing it at the crossroads of conscious control and subconscious regulation (Daniela et al., 2022). At the center of this dual function lies its intimate relationship with the ANS, the system responsible for governing involuntary physiological processes such as heart rate, digestion, blood pressure, and the stress response. The ANS consists of two primary branches: the sympathetic nervous system (SNS) and the PNS facilitate rest, digestion, and recovery (Daniela et al., 2022). Breath regulation, especially through slow and controlled practices such as those found in traditional Pranayama, has been shown to directly modulate the balance between these two branches, shifting the autonomic state from sympathetic dominance to parasympathetic activation (Jerath et al., 2006).

Slow, diaphragmatic breathing with controlled inhalations and exhalations stimulates the vagus nerve, a core component of the parasympathetic system (Szulczewski, 2022). This activation produces relaxation responses, including reduced heart rate, lowered blood pressure, and improved digestive function. Substantial evidence shows that Pranayama enhances vagal tone, commonly assessed through heart rate variability (HRV) (Mittal et al., 2025; Szulczewski, 2022). Higher HRV reflects parasympathetic dominance and greater adaptive capacity to stress (Cahn et al., 2017). Practices such as Nadi Shodhana and Bhramari consistently increase HRV, indicating improved autonomic flexibility and physiological resilience (Bahi et al., 2024; Fincham et al., 2023; Kavitha et al., 2024). These physiological shifts are accompanied by a range of biochemical and emotional benefits. Numerous studies have reported reductions in cortisol (the primary stress hormone) following consistent Pranayama practice (Cahn et al., 2017; Maheshkumar et al., 2022; Robinson et al., 2023). Chronically high cortisol contributes to anxiety, depression, sleep disruption, and cognitive decline; thus, its reduction supports emotional stabilization and mental clarity (Robinson et al., 2023). Randomized controlled trials show significant decreases in anxiety and depressive symptoms among those practicing Pranayama, with enhanced mood and psychological resilience observed in clinical and non-clinical populations (Maheshkumar et al., 2022). These findings underscore breath regulation as both a preventive and therapeutic tool for mental well-being.

Cognitively, Pranayama enhances attentional control, working memory, and cognitive flexibility (Cásedas et al., 2020; Eisenbeck et al., 2018). This is likely due to the physiological calm induced by parasympathetic activation, which fosters a more receptive and focused mental state. Furthermore, the Pranayama technique promotes neurochemical shifts in neurotransmitters such as gamma-aminobutyric acid (GABA), dopamine, and serotonin, all of which play crucial roles in mood regulation and executive function (Varne & Balaji, 2023). Such neurochemical changes complement autonomic shifts, contributing to integrated emotional and cognitive regulation (Daniela et al., 2022; Jerath et al., 2006; Varne & Balaji, 2023). Breath regulation works through a bidirectional link with the brain. Voluntary control from the PFC and ACC can override brainstem rhythms, creating top-down modulation that shapes neural activity related to emotion, attention, and decision making. This feedback loop allows conscious breathing to effectively regulate physiological arousal and cognitive and emotional states (Betka et al., 2022).

This bidirectional relationship is further supported by neuroimaging studies, which reveal that intentional breathing influences activity in brain regions such as the insular cortex, the amygdala (associated with fear and emotional processing), and the PFC (critical for executive function and self-regulation) (Betka et al., 2022; Daniela et al., 2022; Dutschmann & Dick, 2012; Fitzgerald et al., 2017). For instance, during slow-paced breathing, the insula exhibits increased activation, indicating greater bodily awareness and internal focus (Harrison et al., 2021). Simultaneously, the amygdala shows decreased activity, corresponding to a reduction in emotional reactivity and anxiety (Fitzgerald et al., 2017). These neural shifts align with the autonomic changes observed at the physiological level, reinforcing the view that breathing acts as a bridge between body and mind (Betka et al., 2022). From a traditional Yogic perspective, Pranayama has long been understood as a means to harmonize the flow of prana or life force energy through the body's energy channels (Nautiyal et al., 2024). Although rooted in metaphysical traditions, the idea that controlled breathing influences both bodily functions and consciousness aligns with modern physiology. Contemporary research shows that breathwork enhances autonomic regulation, emotional stability, and cognitive clarity (Brahmbhatt & Kumavat, 2024; Brown et al., 2013). Pranayama's effects, such as increased parasympathetic activity, reduced stress hormones, improved neurophysiological balance, support deeper relaxation and resilience (Brahmbhatt & Kumavat, 2024; Eisenbeck et al., 2018; Novaes et al., 2020). These benefits accumulate with consistent practice, indicating long-term adaptation. As an accessible, equipment-free method, Pranayama represents a scientifically supported bridge between contemplative wisdom and modern neurophysiology.

Breathing plays a special role in the body because it is both automatic and under conscious control. This dual nature allows breathing practices, especially slow, steady patterns like those used in Pranayama, to directly influence the autonomic nervous system, which regulates stress, heart rate, and relaxation. Research shows that slow, diaphragmatic breathing activates the vagus nerve, increases heart-rate variability, lowers cortisol, and promotes a calmer emotional state. These effects help improve mood, reduce anxiety, sharpen attention, and support cognitive flexibility. Neuroimaging studies further show that controlled breathing shifts activity in key brain regions involved in emotion and decision-making. Overall, scientific evidence increasingly confirms what Yogic traditions have long taught: conscious breathwork offers a simple yet powerful way to support emotional balance, mental clarity, and long-term well-being.

COGNITIVE AND EMOTIONAL BENEFITS OF PRANAYAMA

A substantial and growing body of literature supports the cognitive and emotional benefits of Pranayama, positioning it as a valuable intervention in both clinical and non-clinical contexts (Jagadeesan et al., 2022; Kavitha et al., 2024; Kuppusamy et al., 2020; Nautiyal et al., 2024; Thanalakshmi et al., 2020). As breath regulation techniques become increasingly integrated into therapeutic, educational, and wellness frameworks, experimental studies have begun to elucidate the distinct physiological and psychological effects associated with specific Pranayama practices (Dhanaradja et al., 2025; Jagadeesan et al., 2022; Kavitha et al., 2024; Novaes et al., 2020; Thanalakshmi et al., 2020). These findings point to the breath's capacity not only to regulate autonomic functions but also to mediate higher-order mental and emotional states through deliberate modulation of respiratory patterns (Jagadeesan et al., 2022; Kavitha et al., 2024; Thanalakshmi et al., 2020). Experimental research has consistently linked this practice with reduced anxiety levels and enhanced attentional performance (Doll et al., 2016; Prpa et al., 2018). The calming influence of Nadi Shodhana is attributed to its capacity to balance the ANS, particularly by facilitating parasympathetic activity (Nautiyal et al., 2024). Studies employing behavioral and psychophysiological assessments have shown that practitioners of Nadi Shodhana experience improvements in sustained attention, mental clarity, and the ability to manage stress-inducing tasks (Mittal et al., 2025; Pal et al., 2004). These benefits are especially relevant in high-stakes academic and professional settings, where focused attention and emotional regulation are critical for performance. Other forms of Pranayama, such as Bhastrika and Kapalabhati, evoke different physiological responses (Grensman et al., 2018; Mittal et al., 2025; Pal et al., 2004). These techniques are characterized by rapid, forceful exhalations and are considered stimulatory in nature. Evidence suggests that they elicit SNS activation, leading to heightened arousal, increased alertness, and temporary boosts in cognitive readiness (Kop et al., 2011). As such, Bhastrika and Kapalabhati are often practiced in the morning or before physical activity to promote energy and motivation (Dhar et al., 2025). However, because of their stimulating properties, they may not be suitable for individuals experiencing heightened anxiety or cardiovascular vulnerability unless practiced under supervision.

In contrast, slow and rhythmic breathing techniques, commonly found in traditional Hatha Yoga and mindfulness-based Pranayama routines, emphasize long inhalations and exhalations to downregulate arousal systems (Szulczewski, 2022; Zaccaro et al., 2018). These practices are associated with improved autonomic flexibility, emotional regulation, and decreased physiological markers of stress. When practised regularly, they have been shown to enhance interoceptive awareness, the perception of internal bodily states, which plays a critical role in emotional insight and self-regulation (Jerath et al., 2006). By fostering a conscious connection with internal physiological signals, slow breathing practices encourage introspection, calmness, and emotional resilience (Shao et al., 2024). A key meta-analysis by Saoji et al. (2019) provides a comprehensive overview of Pranayama's psychological benefits. Across numerous studies, regular practice was associated with improved mood stability, reduced anxiety, and better sleep. The review also reported cognitive gains, including enhanced concentration, working memory, and attentional control, observed across diverse age groups and clinical and nonclinical populations (Ankad et al., 2011). Importantly, the review emphasized the cumulative nature of these benefits, suggesting that repeated and consistent engagement with breath-based practices results in long-term adaptive changes in cognitive and emotional functioning (Grensman et al., 2018).

Pranayama, or controlled breathing, helps calm the mind and improve focus. Slow breathing techniques like Nadi Shodhana, which activate the body's relaxation system, reduce stress and anxiety, and improve attention. Faster techniques like Bhastrika and Kapalabhati, which boost energy and alertness, may not suit people who feel anxious. Research shows that regular Pranayama lowers stress hormones, improves sleep and mood, and strengthens emotional balance. Brain studies also find that slow breathing reduces activity in fear-related areas and improves attention and decision-making. Overall, Pranayama supports better mental clarity, emotional stability, and stress resilience.

NEUROPLASTICITY: AN OVERVIEW

Neuroplasticity refers to the brain's remarkable ability to adapt, reorganize, and form new neural connections in response to learning, experience, and environmental demands (Wenger & Kühn, 2021). This adaptability encompasses several dynamic processes, including synaptogenesis (the formation of new synapses), neurogenesis the generation of new neurons; and modifications in the strength and efficiency of existing synaptic connections (Sweatt, 2016). These neural adaptations are essential for cognitive development, emotional regulation, behavioral flexibility, and recovery from neurological injuries (Zotey et al., 2023). Central to the mechanisms underpinning neuroplasticity are biochemical agents such as brain-derived neurotrophic factor (BDNF), a key protein that supports neuron survival, growth, and synaptic plasticity (Kowiański et al., 2018). In addition, various neurotransmitters, hormonal modulators, and metabolic regulators also play pivotal roles in facilitating neuroadaptive changes (Tataranu & Rizea, 2025).

Emerging research shows that Pranayama, through breath modulation and autonomic regulation, can stimulate neuroplasticity (Campanelli et al., 2020). It influences key neurotransmitters, including GABA, serotonin, dopamine, and norepinephrine (Varambally et al., 2019). Controlled, diaphragmatic breathing increases GABA, reducing neural excitability and anxiety (Nuss, 2015). Studies have demonstrated that slow, diaphragmatic breathing, as practised in several forms of Pranayama, can elevate GABA levels, which in turn contribute to reductions in neural excitability and heightened states of calm and focus (Varne & Balaji, 2023). Similarly, serotonin and dopamine, which are closely linked to mood and reward processing, are positively influenced by breath-based practices, supporting their therapeutic potential for managing affective disorders (Magomedova & Fatima, 2025). Pranayama further alters cortical oscillations, enhancing alpha and theta activity linked to relaxation and focused awareness (Bing-Canar et al., 2016; Tanzer et al., 2021). Alpha waves are associated with relaxed wakefulness and internalized attention, while theta waves correspond to states of deep relaxation and meditative absorption (Bing-Canar et al., 2016). These neural shifts promote clarity, emotional stability, and conditions conducive to neuroplastic change (Jerath et al., 2015). These changes in brain wave activity reflect a shift from externally oriented, reactive states to internally focused, contemplative awareness conditions that are conducive to neuroplastic reorganization.

Another key factor linking Pranayama to brain adaptability is the upregulation of neurotrophic factors, particularly BDNF. BDNF plays a critical role in synaptic plasticity, neuronal survival, and long-term potentiation. The strengthening of synaptic connections that underlie learning and memory (Kowiański et al., 2018). Regular breath-based practices can increase circulating levels of BDNF, thereby supporting the structural and functional remodelling of neural circuits (Kowiański et al., 2018;

Sonawane et al., 2025; Varambally et al., 2019). Although more research is needed to confirm the causal pathways, these biochemical enhancements point to a strong biological basis for Pranayama's impact on cognitive and emotional resilience. Pranayama also influences large-scale brain network dynamics, particularly functional connectivity within and between critical neural networks (Thanalakshmi et al., 2020). Functional connectivity refers to the coordinated activation of brain regions that work together to support complex tasks such as emotion regulation, attention, and decision-making (Sweatt, 2016). Neuroimaging studies, including fMRI, have demonstrated that consistent breath regulation practices lead to enhanced communication between regions such as the PFC, insula, ACC, and amygdala (Fitzgerald et al., 2017; Krishna et al., 2024; Novaes et al., 2020). These areas are central to self-awareness, interoception, emotional processing, and executive function. Through this improved neural integration, Pranayama appears to strengthen the brain's ability to flexibly adapt to stressors, maintain attentional focus, and regulate emotional responses (Novaes et al., 2020).

The impact of Pranayama on brain networks also extends to the DMN and SN (Vishnubhotla et al., 2021). The DMN, which is active during rest and self-referential thinking, has been associated with mind-wandering and rumination, particularly in individuals with anxiety or depression (Novaes et al., 2020). Breath-focused practices are shown to reduce DMN activity, thereby curbing unproductive internal dialogue and enhancing present-moment awareness (Treves et al., 2025). In parallel, the SN, which includes the anterior insula and dorsal ACC, becomes more active, allowing the individual to shift more effectively between internal and external stimuli based on contextual demands. This improved switching capacity is crucial for cognitive flexibility and emotional adaptability, hallmarks of a neuroplastic brain (Vishnubhotla et al., 2021).

Emerging evidence suggests a potential dose–response relationship between breath regulation and neural plasticity, although this field remains in its early stages. Structural MRI investigations involving experienced yoga practitioners, which often integrate Pranayama as a core component, have reported greater cortical thickness and preserved grey-matter volume in regions such as the insula, anterior cingulate cortex, and hippocampus, with these adaptations correlating with practice duration and intensity (van Aalst et al., 2020; Villemure et al., 2014). Complementary biomarker research indicates that breath-centered yoga interventions can elevate circulating brain-derived neurotrophic factor (BDNF), a key neuroplasticity marker, though evidence isolating Pranayama effects remains limited (Rajkumar, 2024). Recent meta-analysis further supports these findings, revealing consistent improvements in neural efficiency, autonomic regulation, and cognitive flexibility following breath-based and meditative practices, with greater effects observed in studies employing longer intervention durations and higher session frequency (Gothe et al., 2019; Veerakannan, 2025). Short-term interventions (10–15 minutes daily for 4–6 weeks) have been shown to produce measurable cognitive and autonomic benefits (Novaes et al., 2020; Pal et al., 2004; Telles et al., 1994), whereas sustained, multi-month practice appears necessary to consolidate enduring structural and functional neural adaptations. Collectively, these findings support a graded model of breath-based neuroplasticity and highlight the need for future longitudinal studies that systematically quantify practice frequency, duration, and technique to define optimal neuroadaptive "dosage."

The evidence suggests that Pranayama, as a systematic approach to breath regulation, exerts profound effects on brain function and structure. By modulating neurotransmitters, optimizing brain wave patterns, enhancing neurotrophic support, and strengthening functional connectivity across neural networks, Pranayama promotes conditions favorable to neuroplastic change (Bremer et al., 2022). These changes not only support mental well-being and emotional regulation but also provide a neurobiological foundation for learning, self-awareness, and cognitive transformation (Rahrig et al., 2022). As neuroscience continues to explore the link between contemplative practices and brain health, Pranayama stands out as a powerful, accessible, and scientifically grounded method for cultivating neuroplasticity in daily life.

NEURAL CORRELATES OF PRANAYAMA PRACTICES

Understanding the neural correlates of Pranayama practices provides insight into how controlled breathing influences brain structure and function (Novaes et al., 2020). Neuroimaging and electrophysiological studies have identified specific brain regions and networks activated during various Pranayama techniques (Campanelli et al., 2020). The findings suggest that breath modulation engages both cortical and subcortical pathways involved in self-regulation. Exploring these neural mechanisms bridges ancient yogic wisdom with contemporary neuroscience (Bahi et al., 2024). The interconnected brain regions and networks illustrate how Pranayama engages both top-down and bottom-up mechanisms, facilitating emotional regulation, heightened awareness, and autonomic balance and key components of its neurophysiological and psychological benefits (Bahi et al., 2024; Dhanaradja et al., 2025; Nautiyal et al., 2024; Novaes et al., 2020).

Prefrontal Cortex

The PFC is central to executive functions, including decision-making, attention, impulse control, and emotional regulation (Ren et al., 2025). Neuroimaging shows that regular Pranayama practice enhances PFC activation and connectivity (Doll et al., 2016), supporting cognitive flexibility, focused attention, and reduced emotional reactivity. By modulating breath, Pranayama engages the PFC to exert top-down control over limbic regions like the amygdala (Fitzgerald et al., 2017), strengthening stress regulation and resilience. The PFC's role in sustained attention aligns with breath-focused practices, creating a reinforcing loop for cognitive clarity (Doll et al., 2016). Long-term practice is linked to structural and functional PFC improvements that enhance emotional stability (Ren et al., 2025).

Insula

The insula is a key region for interoception, integrating internal signals such as respiration and heartbeat into conscious awareness (Chouchou et al., 2019; Tanzer et al., 2021). In Pranayama, it mediates the connection between breath control and emotional regulation (Banzett et al., 2000). Neuroimaging studies show increased anterior insula activity during breath-focused practices, enhancing emotional awareness and self-perception (Bahi et al., 2024). Regular practice heightens sensitivity to stress-related bodily changes, supporting timely self-regulation (Kavitha et al., 2024; Kuppusamy et al., 2020). Strengthening insular function promotes present-moment awareness, physiological balance, and emotional clarity (Chouchou et al., 2019; Tanzer et al., 2021), benefiting conditions involving emotional dysregulation and impaired body awareness.

Amygdala

The amygdala is a key limbic structure involved in fear, anxiety, anger, and emotional memory, and it activates the body's stress response (LeDoux, 2003). Overactivity is common in anxiety disorders, PTSD, and chronic stress (Ressler, 2010). Slow, diaphragmatic Pranayama can modulate amygdala activity, reducing emotional reactivity and promoting stability (Fitzgerald et al., 2017). Neuroimaging shows controlled breathing downregulates amygdala activation during emotional challenges (Šimić et al., 2021), likely through increased PNS activity and stronger PFC inhibitory control (Fitzgerald et al., 2017). This reduces hyperarousal and enhances regulation, with practitioners reporting greater calm (Decker et al., 2019). Neurobiological evidence confirms the amygdala as a key target of Pranayama's stress-reducing effects (Michalsen et al., 2005).

Brainstem

The brainstem, particularly the medulla oblongata and pons, houses critical respiratory centers that control the rhythm and depth of breathing (Dutschmann & Dick, 2012). These structures also play a key role in regulating the ANS, maintaining the balance between sympathetic and parasympathetic activity (Iordanova & Reddivari, 2025). Pranayama, through conscious modulation of breath, exerts direct influence on these brainstem centers, promoting vagal nerve activation and enhancing parasympathetic tone (Szulczewski, 2022). This results in a physiological shift toward relaxation, reduced heart rate, and lowered stress levels. By engaging these foundational neural mechanisms, Pranayama supports systemic calm and autonomic regulation at the most fundamental level of brain control (Gothe et al., 2019).

Default Mode Network and Salience Network

The DMN is primarily active during rest, self-referential thinking, and mind-wandering, and is often linked to rumination and negative thought patterns, particularly in anxiety and depression (Gothe et al., 2019). Regular Pranayama practice has been associated with reduced DMN activity, supporting a shift away from automatic, internally focused mental states toward present-moment awareness (Bremer et al., 2022). In contrast, the SN, which includes the anterior insula and ACC, helps detect and filter relevant stimuli, enabling smooth transitions between internal and external attention (Rahrig et al., 2022). Pranayama enhances the functional efficiency of the SN, thereby improving attentional switching, emotional awareness, and cognitive flexibility (Novaes et al., 2020). Neuroimaging studies using fMRI and EEG have revealed that long-term breath practitioners exhibit increased grey matter density and improved functional connectivity in both these networks (Zaccaro et al., 2018). These structural and functional adaptations suggest that Pranayama not only calms the mind but also optimizes large-scale brain network dynamics essential for adaptive cognitive and emotional functioning (Hermans et al., 2014).

Pranayama influences key brain regions involved in emotion, attention, and stress regulation. It enhances prefrontal cortex function for better focus and emotional control, increases insula activity to improve body awareness, and reduces amygdala reactivity to lower anxiety. Controlled breathing also affects the brainstem, activating the vagus nerve and promoting relaxation. Additionally, Pranayama reduces overactivity in the Default Mode Network and improves the efficiency of the Salience Network. Overall, these neural effects explain how Pranayama supports calmness, self-regulation, and mental well-being.

NEURAL CORRELATES AND MECHANISMS OF NEUROPLASTICITY

Neuroplasticity, often referred to as the brain's capacity to reorganize by forming new neural connections, is a central concept in modern neuroscience (Wenger & Kühn, 2021). This adaptability enables changes driven by learning, experience, trauma, and voluntary practices such as meditation and breath regulation (Ren et al., 2025). Pranayama, a Yogic method of conscious breath control, has gained attention for its potential to enhance neuroplastic processes (Saha, 2025). Evidence suggests it can modulate neural activity, influence neurotransmitter dynamics, and reorganize functional connectivity across key brain networks (Varambally et al., 2019).

Interoceptive Awareness and the Insula

Another crucial brain region affected by Pranayama is the insular cortex. The insula is central to interoception, the sense of the internal physiological state of the body (Banzett et al., 2000). The anterior insula integrates visceral signals and contributes to the subjective experience of bodily sensations and emotions (Šimić et al., 2021). Pranayama enhances interoceptive awareness by increasing insular activation, which is associated with improved mindfulness, emotional clarity, and self-awareness (Gu et al., 2013). This activation also supports parasympathetic engagement, promoting calm and restorative physiological states (De Morree et al., 2016).

Amygdala Modulation

The amygdala plays a central role in anxiety, emotional arousal, and stress. Neuroimaging studies show that controlled breathing used in Pranayama can reduce amygdala activity (Campanelli et al., 2020), likely through enhanced PFC and ACC engagement that inhibits limbic responses This modulation lowers emotional reactivity and supports psychological stability, which is particularly relevant for conditions such as PTSD, generalized anxiety disorder (GAD), and major depressive disorder (MDD), where amygdala hyperactivity is common (Chen & Etkin, 2013). Thus, breath regulation offers a non-pharmacological pathway for emotional balance (Doll et al., 2016; Fitzgerald et al., 2017; Gu et al., 2013; Shao et al., 2024).

Brainstem and Autonomic Regulation

The brainstem, particularly the medulla oblongata and pons, regulates autonomic function and respiratory control through its respiratory rhythmicity centers and close integration with the vagus nerve. Slow, deep breathing in Pranayama stimulates vagal afferents, enhancing parasympathetic activity and shifting the autonomic balance away from sympathetic dominance (Gerritsen & Band, 2018). This shift contributes to reductions in heart rate, blood pressure, and cortisol, reflecting lowered physiological stress (De Vente et al., 2003). Higher vagal tone is further associated with improved emotional regulation, social engagement, and resilience (Geisler et al., 2013). Thus, Pranayama leverages brainstem-autonomic pathways as a bottom-up mechanism that directly modulates physiological processes to promote psychological well-being (Pal et al., 2004).

Default Mode Network and Salience Network

The DMN, involving the medial PFC, posterior cingulate cortex, and precuneus, is active during rest and self-referential processing. Excessive DMN activity is linked to rumination and mind-wandering, commonly observed in anxiety and depression (Hermans et al., 2014). Pranayama and related practices reduce DMN activation, promoting present-centered awareness (Babiy et al., 2025). n contrast, the SN, including the anterior insula and ACC, becomes more engaged during breath-focused tasks, enhancing attentional control, emotion regulation, and adaptive behavioral responses. These neural shifts foster improved mental clarity and reduced cognitive rigidity (Vishnubhotla et al., 2021).

Evidence from Neuroimaging Modalities

Advanced neuroimaging tools such as fMRI, EEG, and PET scans have provided robust evidence for the structural and functional brain changes induced by Pranayama (Veerakannan, 2025). fMRI studies have documented increased functional connectivity between the PFC, ACC, insula, and brainstem in experienced practitioners (Sezer et al., 2022; Zamorano et al., 2017). EEG recordings often show elevated alpha and theta wave activity during and after breathwork, which correlates with states of relaxation and focused attention (Ng et al., 2021). PET scans have indicated altered glucose metabolism and oxygen consumption in regions linked to autonomic and emotional regulation (Videbech, 2000). Moreover, structural imaging has revealed increased grey matter volume in the PFC and insula among long-term practitioners, suggesting that breath control may not only influence functional activation but also support anatomical remodelling (Mooneyham et al., 2017).

To strengthen the applied relevance of these neuroscientific findings, practical cases illustrate how neural adaptations translate into real-world outcomes. School-based breathwork interventions have shown significant reductions in test anxiety and improvements in sustained attention, corresponding with enhanced prefrontal activation reported in neuroimaging studies (McLeod & Boyes, 2021; van Loon et al., 2022; Voltmer et al., 2023). In sports contexts, athletes integrating Pranayama into recovery routines demonstrate reduced cortisol, improved vagal tone, and enhanced focus, changes consistent with increased functional connectivity in autonomic networks (Clifton et al., 2023; Maheshkumar et al., 2022; Schober, 2018). Clinical applications further reinforce these patterns: structured breathing-based programs for individuals with generalized anxiety disorder and PTSD have been associated with decreased amygdala hyperactivity and strengthened PFC–limbic regulation (Haller et al., 2023; Laplaud et al., 2023) (Novaes et al., 2020). These cases collectively demonstrate how laboratory-based neurobiological findings directly translate into improved emotional regulation, stress resilience, and cognitive performance across diverse populations.

Pranayama enhances neuroplasticity by reshaping neural connections and improving brain network functioning. It strengthens interoceptive awareness through increased insula activation, helping with emotional clarity and calmness. Controlled breathing reduces amygdala activity, lowering stress and anxiety, while stimulating the vagus nerve to improve autonomic balance. It decreases Default Mode Network overactivity and boosts Salience Network efficiency, supporting focus and mental stability. Neuroimaging studies show improved connectivity across the PFC, ACC, insula, and brainstem. Real-world evidence from school programs, athletic contexts, and clinical interventions shows that Pranayama effectively reduces anxiety, enhances attentional performance, lowers cortisol levels, and supports improved emotional regulation.

Integration into Mental Health and Therapeutic Models

Given the mounting empirical and clinical evidence supporting the neurobiological effects of Pranayama, there is growing interest in its integration into established therapeutic models (Campanelli et al., 2020). In modern mental health care, particularly in the realm of integrative and complementary medicine, Pranayama is increasingly recognized as an effective adjunct tool. Various psychotherapeutic modalities have begun incorporating breathwork to enhance emotional regulation, trauma recovery, and cognitive performance (Michalsen et al., 2005; Novaes et al., 2020; Wagner & Cáceres-Melillo, 2023). Mindfulness-based cognitive therapy (MBCT) is one such approach that naturally aligns with Pranayama (Wagner & Cáceres-Melillo, 2023). Originally developed to prevent relapse in depression, MBCT emphasizes present-moment awareness and acceptance of thoughts and emotions. Integrating Pranayama into MBCT sessions may deepen the embodied experience of mindfulness, enhancing physiological relaxation and improving attentional control (Haller et al., 2023). Controlled breathing practices help anchor awareness in the body, thus supporting the core therapeutic goals of MBCT (Haller et al., 2023). Similarly, acceptance and commitment therapy (ACT) focuses on developing psychological flexibility through acceptance, mindfulness, and value-based action (Bai et al., 2020). Pranayama can enhance ACT by fostering embodied awareness and reducing physiological arousal. Breathwork can serve as a grounding strategy, helping clients navigate distressing emotions or thoughts with less reactivity (Eisenbeck et al., 2018). As ACT emphasizes experiential processes, breath-based techniques complement its goals by engaging both cognitive and somatic pathways.

In trauma-focused interventions such as trauma-sensitive yoga (TSY), Pranayama is valuable for addressing ANS dysregulation, helping survivors with heightened sympathetic arousal and reduced vagal tone regain autonomic balance and bodily control (Agorastos et al., 2015; Ong, 2021; Partners, 2021). It also supports behavioral activation in depression by providing a structured, mood-enhancing activity with immediate somatic feedback (Hopko et al., 2003; M. R. Tolahunase et al., 2018). Pranayama works through both bottom-up and top-down mechanisms, regulating physiology while supporting cognitive insight (Taylor et al., 2010). Its accessibility strengthens therapeutic rapport and engagement, fostering presence, empowerment, and resilience across clinical settings (Gerbarg et al., 2023).

Pranayama is increasingly integrated into modern therapeutic models because of strong evidence for its neurobiological and emotional benefits. It supports treatments like MBCT, ACT, trauma-sensitive yoga, and behavioral activation by reducing physiological stress, improving emotional regulation, and enhancing body awareness. As a bottom-up technique, breathwork directly calms the nervous system while complementing cognitive and mindfulness-based methods. Its simplicity, safety, and adaptability make it useful across clinical settings, helping clients manage anxiety, trauma, and depression while improving focus, resilience, and therapeutic engagement.

CLINICAL APPLICATIONS AND INTEGRATION INTO PSYCHOTHERAPY

Breath regulation techniques offer a practical and accessible method for influencing emotional and physiological states, making them suitable for use in mental health care, trauma recovery, and stress reduction programs (Brahmbhatt & Kumavat, 2024; Gerbarg et al., 2023; Haller et al., 2023). As a bottom-up intervention, Pranayama works by targeting the ANS and sensory-motor pathways, subsequently affecting emotional and cognitive processes from the physiological level upward (Novaes et al., 2020). Several modern therapeutic approaches have begun to incorporate breathwork as a core or complementary technique (Bai et al., 2020; Haller et al., 2023; Ong, 2021; Wagner & Cáceres-Melillo, 2023). These include MBCT, ACT,

TSY, and Cognitive Behavioral Therapy (CBT). Each of these models benefits from the inclusion of Pranayama in unique ways:

Mindfulness-Based Cognitive Therapy

In MBCT, conscious breathing is used as an anchor for present-moment awareness. Patients are taught to observe their thoughts and bodily sensations non-judgmentally, with the breath serving as a stabilizing force. By integrating Pranayama, MBCT sessions enhance parasympathetic engagement and reduce reactivity, allowing for deeper mindfulness and emotional regulation (Wagner & Cáceres-Melillo, 2023).

Acceptance and Commitment Therapy

ACT focuses on acceptance and value-based action while helping clients disengage from unhelpful cognitive patterns. Breath control enhances the somatic awareness necessary for emotional flexibility, aligning well with ACT's emphasis on embodied cognition and present-moment engagement (Bai et al., 2020).

Trauma-Sensitive Yoga

TSY incorporates breath-centered practices to help trauma survivors regulate arousal levels and regain a sense of bodily safety. In individuals with PTSD or complex trauma, bottom-up interventions are crucial because top-down cognitive approaches may be less effective when the nervous system is dysregulated. By influencing the vagus nerve and restoring autonomic balance, Pranayama facilitates a sense of grounding and control (Haller et al., 2023).

Cognitive Behavioral Therapy

CBT often focuses on changing maladaptive thoughts and behaviors through structured interventions. However, integrating Pranayama into CBT provides a physiological foundation that supports these cognitive efforts. For example, in cases of panic disorder, generalized anxiety, or insomnia, breath control can serve as an immediate tool for symptom management and emotional stabilization (Haller et al., 2023).

Pranayama is increasingly used in mental health care because it helps calm the nervous system and improve emotional control. Therapies like MBCT, ACT, CBT, and trauma-sensitive yoga benefit from adding breathwork, which supports mindfulness, reduces stress, and stabilizes physiological arousal. Slow breathing helps anxiety, while faster techniques can boost energy in depression. Research shows Pranayama improves heart rate variability, lowers cortisol, enhances sleep, and supports trauma recovery through vagal regulation. Its simplicity, adaptability, and strong evidence base make it a valuable tool in psychotherapy and community health programs.

LIMITATIONS AND METHODOLOGICAL GAPS

Despite extensive evidence supporting the neurophysiological benefits of Pranayama, several methodological and practical challenges persist. A primary issue is the inconsistent definition and operationalization of Pranayama techniques (Saoji et al., 2019). Without clear classifications, comparative analyses become difficult and weaken the reliability of findings. Researchers must therefore establish taxonomy-based protocols that classify techniques by breathing rate, duration, nostril involvement, and intention. Another major concern is the lack of standardized intervention methods; most studies rely on self-designed protocols with inconsistent session duration, frequency, and instructional quality (Dhar et al., 2025). This variability hinders reproducibility and limits the potential for meta-analytic synthesis. Future research should adopt evidence-informed guidelines specifying posture, breathing sequences, session length, and practitioner expertise. Small sample sizes further restrict interpretability. Although many pilot studies and small RCTs report positive psychological and physiological outcomes, their limited statistical power reduces generalizability(Dhar et al., 2025; Haller et al., 2023; Nautiyal et al., 2024; Novaes et al., 2020). Small sample sizes increase the risk of type I and type II errors and often fail to represent diverse demographic groups (Akobeng, 2016). Larger, multicentric RCTs with well-defined control conditions (e.g., sham breathwork, general relaxation) are essential to validate and replicate findings across populations.

Moreover, Cultural appropriation and the secular repackaging of Pranayama in Western wellness settings add further complexity. Traditional practices are frequently stripped of their philosophical and ethical foundations, focusing mainly on stress reduction or performance enhancement (Brown et al., 2013; Jagadeesan et al., 2022). While secular approaches increase accessibility, they may dilute the depth of traditional Yogic practices. Research and clinical work should respect Pranayama's cultural roots while maintaining scientific rigor. Another gap is the limited understanding of its long-term neurocognitive effects, as most studies focus only on short-term outcomes such as acute HRV changes, cortisol reduction, and brief cognitive gains (Butzer et al., 2015; Maheshkumar et al., 2022). However, there is limited understanding of how these benefits persist over time and whether long-term practice induces structural brain changes. Longitudinal neuroimaging studies using fMRI, DTI, and PET scans can provide deeper insights into the anatomical remodeling and sustained functional connectivity changes associated with sustained Pranayama (Veerakannan, 2025). In addition, Individual responses to Pranayama vary widely, influenced by genetics, baseline physiology, mental health, culture, and motivation. More personalized and evidence-based protocols that combine psychometric tools with physiological measures are needed to improve its effectiveness (Zaccaro et al., 2018).

Technological advancements also open new avenues and challenges for research. The growing popularity of mobile health (mHealth) apps and wearable biosensors has enabled widespread access to breath training (Beer et al., 2020). However, digital delivery often lacks the depth and nuance of in-person instruction, raising questions about fidelity, safety, and long-term adherence. Comparative studies assessing the efficacy of digital versus face-to-face Pranayama interventions are necessary to determine the strengths and limitations of each format (Wadhen & Cartwright, 2021). Moreover, real-time data collection through wearable devices can provide objective markers of progress and help optimize individual training plans (Phatak et al., 2021). Ethical considerations in breathwork research remain insufficiently addressed. Some Pranayama techniques can provoke strong physiological or emotional reactions, particularly in vulnerable groups, making safety protocols essential. Researchers should ensure informed consent, mental health screening, supervised interventions, and proper follow-up to protect participant well-being (de Manincor et al., 2016). Although Pranayama offers important insights into mind–body integration and neuroplasticity, its scientific progress requires addressing methodological and ethical gaps. Clear protocols, cultural sensitivity, broader samples, and thoughtful use of technology are essential for a more rigorous and inclusive understanding of how breath shapes brain function and behavior.

Research on Pranayama is growing, but several challenges remain. Studies often use inconsistent definitions, non-standard protocols, and small sample sizes, limiting reliability. Cultural concerns also arise when traditional practices are oversimplified in modern settings. Long-term brain effects and individual differences are still poorly understood, and digital breathwork tools bring questions about safety and accuracy. To advance the field, future work should standardize techniques, respect cultural context, include larger and more diverse samples, use advanced neuroimaging, and ensure ethical safeguards. This will strengthen the scientific and clinical value of Pranayama research.

FUTURE DIRECTIONS: TOWARD A NEURO-YOGIC PARADIGM

The intersection of neuroscience and Yogic wisdom is giving rise to a neuro-Yogic paradigm that integrates ancient breathing practices with modern scientific tools to enhance well-being. As evidence grows for Pranayama's neurophysiological and cognitive benefits, structured and data-driven applications are becoming more feasible. Technologies such as neurofeedback, wearable biosensors, and mobile apps now allow real-time monitoring of HRV, breathing rate, and brainwave patterns, enabling personalized breathwork tailored to individual goals and health needs (Beer et al., 2020). Virtual and augmented reality further expand access by creating immersive, calming environments that enhance engagement and support users without access to traditional instruction. These digital tools also offer new avenues for training clinicians, therapists, and educators in standardized, evidence-based Pranayama protocols. However, as these technologies evolve, it is crucial to address issues related to accessibility, cost, and the digital divide, which may prevent marginalized populations from benefiting equally from tech-assisted breathwork interventions. Beyond therapeutic and clinical settings, the neuro-Yogic paradigm can be effectively implemented in educational institutions and workplace environments. Structured breathing sessions embedded in daily routines can help students improve focus, memory retention, and stress management. Similarly, employees may benefit from short breath-based interventions to enhance productivity, emotional resilience, and interpersonal dynamics. Importantly, this paradigm encourages a shift from a purely symptom-management approach to one that fosters proactive mental wellness and neurocognitive optimization. Nonetheless, implementation barriers such as limited institutional support, insufficient practitioner training, and misconceptions about the cultural origins of Yogic practices may hinder widespread adoption. By merging Yogic insights with neurobiological principles, the neuro-Yogic model holds the potential to transform contemporary health care, education, and organizational culture. At the same time, a balanced perspective requires acknowledging that the scientific promise of Pranayama must be matched with realistic considerations of safety guidelines, population-specific contraindications, and the need for culturally sensitive integration strategies.

Future developments should focus on establishing interdisciplinary collaborations among neuroscientists, yoga practitioners, psychologists, and technology developers. Rigorous research studies and randomized controlled trials should be designed to test the efficacy, safety, and scalability of tech-assisted breath training. In doing so, the field can ensure that the emerging neuro-Yogic paradigm remains grounded in both scientific integrity and traditional authenticity. Should also aim to establish dose-response relationships.

CONCLUSION

The evidence presented in this chapter highlights Pranayama's potential as both a meditative practice and a neuroscience-based therapeutic tool, integrating traditional Yogic insights with modern scientific findings. It explains how controlled breathing influences neural processes related to attention, emotional regulation, body awareness, and autonomic balance, offering a strong foundation for incorporating Pranayama into psychological and clinical interventions. Neuroimaging and physiological studies now validate long-held Yogic claims, showing that breath control modulates key brain regions such as the PFC, insula, and amygdala. The chapter further underscores Pranayama's role in promoting neuroplasticity through increased BDNF, altered neurotransmitter release, and enhanced functional connectivity—mechanisms relevant to conditions like anxiety, depression, trauma, and cognitive decline.

Practical applications extend across disciplines: in clinical psychology, Pranayama is a cost-effective, culturally adaptable complement to CBT, ACT, and MBCT; in education and workplace settings, it improves focus and emotional resilience; and in public health, it provides an accessible, non-pharmacological intervention. However, the chapter also notes methodological challenges, including inconsistent practice styles, limited randomized trials, and risks of cultural misappropriation. Addressing these gaps requires standardized protocols, cultural sensitivity, and interdisciplinary collaboration. Overall, the chapter presents Pranayama as a scientifically grounded, integrative approach capable of fostering lasting improvements in brain function and mental well-being.

REFERENCES

Agorastos, A., Kellner, M., Baker, D. G., & Stiedl, O. (2015). Comprehensive Guide to Post-Traumatic Stress Disorder. *Comprehensive Guide to Post-Traumatic Stress Disorder*, 1–15. 10.1007/978-3-319-08613-2_30-1

Akobeng, A. K. (2016). Understanding type i and type II errors, statistical power and sample size. *Acta Paediatrica. International Journal of Pediatrics*, *105*(6), 605–609. DOI: 10.1111/apa.13384 PMID: 26935977

Ankad, R., Herur, A., Patil, S., Shashikala, G., & Chinagudi, S. (2011). Effect of short-term pranayama and meditation on cardiovascular functions in healthy individuals. *Heart Views : the Official Journal of the Gulf Heart Association*, *12*(2), 58. DOI: 10.4103/1995-705X.86016 PMID: 22121462

Babiy, Z., Frey, B. N., Bieling, P. J., McCabe, R. E., & Green, S. M. (2025). Mindfulness-Based Interventions and Neuroplasticity: A Review of Network Connectivity in Healthy and Clinical Samples. *Mindfulness*, *16*(4), 783–796. DOI: 10.1007/s12671-025-02549-0

Bahi, C., Irrmischer, M., Franken, K., Fejer, G., Schlenker, A., Deijen, J. B., & Engelbregt, H. (2024). Effects of conscious connected breathing on cortical brain activity, mood and state of consciousness in healthy adults. *Current Psychology (New Brunswick, N.J.)*, *43*(12), 10578–10589. DOI: 10.1007/s12144-023-05119-6

Bai, Z., Luo, S., Zhang, L., Wu, S., & Chi, I. (2020). Acceptance and Commitment Therapy (ACT) to reduce depression: A systematic review and meta-analysis. *Journal of Affective Disorders, 260*(September 2019), 728–737. DOI: 10.1016/j.jad.2019.09.040

Banzett, R. B., Mulnier, H. E., Murphy, K., Rosen, S. D., Wise, R. J. S., & Adams, L. (2000). Breathlessness in humans activates insular cortex. *Neuroreport*, *11*(10), 2117–2120. DOI: 10.1097/00001756-200007140-00012 PMID: 10923655

Beer, J. M., Smith, K. N., Kennedy, T., Mois, G., Acena, D., Gallerani, D. G., McDonnell, K. K., & Owens, O. L. (2020). A Focus Group Evaluation of Breathe Easier: A Mindfulness-Based mHealth App for Survivors of Lung Cancer and Their Family Members. *American Journal of Health Promotion*, *34*(7), 770–778. DOI: 10.1177/0890117120924176 PMID: 32406241

Betka, S., Adler, D., Similowski, T., & Blanke, O. (2022). Breathing control, brain, and bodily self-consciousness: Toward immersive digiceuticals to alleviate respiratory suffering. *Biological Psychology, 171*(July 2021), 108329. DOI: 10.1016/j.biopsycho.2022.108329

Bhagat, O. L., Kharya, C., Jaryal, A., & Deepak, K. K. (2017). Acute effects on cardiovascular oscillations during controlled slow yogic breathing. *The Indian Journal of Medical Research, 145*(4), 503–512. DOI: 10.4103/ijmr.IJMR_830_15 PMID: 28862183

Bing-Canar, H., Pizzuto, J., & Compton, R. J. (2016). Mindfulness-of-breathing exercise modulates EEG alpha activity during cognitive performance. *Psychophysiology*, *53*(9), 1366–1376. DOI: 10.1111/psyp.12678 PMID: 27245493

Brahmbhatt, A., & Kumavat, P. P. (2024). Yoga and Mindfulness Practices: Their Role in Modern Mental Health and Wellness Programs. *Research Review Journal of Indian Knowledge Systems, 1*(2), 09–17. DOI: 10.31305/rrjiks.2024.v1.n2.002

Bremer, B., Wu, Q., Mora Álvarez, M. G., Hölzel, B. K., Wilhelm, M., Hell, E., Tavacioglu, E. E., Torske, A., & Koch, K. (2022). Mindfulness meditation increases default mode, salience, and central executive network connectivity. *Scientific Reports*, *12*(1), 1–15. DOI: 10.1038/s41598-022-17325-6 PMID: 35918449

Brown, R. P., & Gerbarg, P. L. (2005). Sudarshan Kriya Yogic Breathing in the Treatment of Stress, Anxiety, and Depression: Part II—Clinical Applications and Guidelines. *Journal of Alternative and Complementary Medicine (New York, N.Y.)*, *11*(4), 711–717. DOI: 10.1089/acm.2005.11.711 PMID: 16131297

Brown, R. P., Gerbarg, P. L., & Muench, F. (2013). Breathing Practices for Treatment of Psychiatric and Stress-Related Medical Conditions. *The Psychiatric Clinics of North America*, *36*(1), 121–140. DOI: 10.1016/j.psc.2013.01.001 PMID: 23538082

Butzer, B., Day, D., Potts, A., Ryan, C., Coulombe, S., Davies, B., Weidknecht, K., Ebert, M., Flynn, L., & Khalsa, S. B. S. (2015). Effects of a classroom-based yoga intervention on cortisol and behavior in second- and third-grade students: A pilot study. *Journal of Evidence-Based Complementary & Alternative Medicine*, *20*(1), 41–49. DOI: 10.1177/2156587214557695 PMID: 25412616

Cahn, B. R., Goodman, M. S., Peterson, C. T., Maturi, R., & Mills, P. J. (2017). Yoga, meditation and mind-body health: Increased BDNF, cortisol awakening response, and altered inflammatory marker expression after a 3-month yoga and meditation retreat. *Frontiers in Human Neuroscience*, *11*(June), 1–13. DOI: 10.3389/fnhum.2017.00315 PMID: 28694775

Campanelli, S., Lopes Tort, A., & Lobão-Soares, B. (2020). Pranayamas and their neurophysiological effects. *International Journal of Yoga*, *13*(3), 183. DOI: 10.4103/ijoy.IJOY_91_19 PMID: 33343147

Cásedas, L., Pirruccio, V., Vadillo, M. A., & Lupiáñez, J. (2020). Does Mindfulness Meditation Training Enhance Executive Control? A Systematic Review and Meta-Analysis of Randomized Controlled Trials in Adults. *Mindfulness*, *11*(2), 411–424. DOI: 10.1007/s12671-019-01279-4

Chauhan, D., & Bansal, S. (2024). Bridging Traditions and Trends: Exploring Indian Knowledge Systems and Yoga in the Modern Era. *Sirjana Journal*, *54*(7), 20–36.

Chen, A. C., & Etkin, A. (2013). Hippocampal network connectivity and activation differentiates post-traumatic stress disorder from generalized anxiety disorder. *Neuropsychopharmacology : Official Publication of the American College of Neuropsychopharmacology*, *38*(10), 1889–1898. DOI: 10.1038/npp.2013.122 PMID: 23673864

Chouchou, F., Mauguière, F., Vallayer, O., Catenoix, H., Isnard, J., Montavont, A., Jung, J., Pichot, V., Rheims, S., & Mazzola, L. (2019). How the insula speaks to the heart: Cardiac responses to insular stimulation in humans. *Human Brain Mapping*, *40*(9), 2611–2622. DOI: 10.1002/hbm.24548 PMID: 30815964

Clifton, C. L., Killen, L. G., Green, J. M., O'neal, E. K., Swain, J. C., & Frisbie, C. M. (2023). Effects of 3 Weeks Yogic Breathing Techniques on Sub-maximal Running Responses. *International Journal of Exercise Science*, *16*(4), 1066–1076. DOI: 10.70252/OLEG4431 PMID: 38288073

Craig, A. D. (2002). How do you feel? Interoception: The sense of the physiological condition of the body. *Nature Reviews. Neuroscience*, *3*(8), 655–666. DOI: 10.1038/nrn894 PMID: 12154366

Daniela, M., Catalina, L., Ilie, O., Paula, M., Daniel-Andrei, I., & Ioana, B. (2022). Effects of Exercise Training on the Autonomic Nervous System with a Focus on Anti-Inflammatory and Antioxidants Effects. *Antioxidants*, *11*(2), 350. Advance online publication. DOI: 10.3390/antiox11020350 PMID: 35204231

de Manincor, M., Bensoussan, A., Smith, C. A., Barr, K., Schweickle, M., Donoghoe, L. L., Bourchier, S., & Fahey, P. (2016). Individualized Yoga for Reducing Depression and Anxiety, and Improving Well-Being: A Randomized Controlled Trial. *Depression and Anxiety*, *33*(9), 816–828. DOI: 10.1002/da.22502 PMID: 27030303

De Morree, H. M., Rutten, G. J., Szabo, B. M., Sitskoorn, M. M., & Kop, W. J. (2016). Effects of Insula Resection on Autonomic Nervous System Activity. *Journal of Neurosurgical Anesthesiology*, *28*(2), 153–158. DOI: 10.1097/ANA.0000000000000207 PMID: 26192246

De Vente, W., Olff, M., Van Amsterdam, J. G. C., Kamphuis, J. H., & Emmelkamp, P. M. G. (2003). Physiological differences between burnout patients and healthy controls: Blood pressure, heart rate, and cortisol responses. *Occupational and Environmental Medicine*, *60*(suppl 1), i54–i61. DOI: 10.1136/oem.60.suppl_1.i54 PMID: 12782748

Decker, J. T., Brown, J. L. C., Ashley, W., & Lipscomb, A. E. (2019). Mindfulness, meditation, and breathing exercises: Reduced anxiety for clients and self-care for social work interns. *Social Work with Groups*, *42*(4), 308–322. DOI: 10.1080/01609513.2019.1571763

Dhanaradja, U., Rajasegaran, R., Aghoram, R., Pal, P., Basu, S., Mukherjee, M. P., & Harichandrakumar, K. T. (2025). Effect of 12-week Practice of Anulom Vilom Pranayama as Adjunctive Therapy on the Cardiac Autonomic Balance, Cognition, Psychological Status, and Quality of Life in Individuals with Mild-to-Moderate Parkinson's Disease: A Randomized Controlled Trial. *International Journal of Yoga*, *18*(2), 189–198. Advance online publication. DOI: 10.4103/ijoy.ijoy_176_24 PMID: 41079240

Dhangar, A., Jaiswal, A., Sahu, P., Saraswat, T., & Gera, A. (2025). Personalized Fitness Recommendation System Integrating Yoga, Physiotherapy Exercises and Tips. *2025 3rd International Conference on Disruptive Technologies (ICDT)*, 255–260. DOI: 10.1109/ICDT63985.2025.10986670

Dhaniwala, N. K. S., Dasari, V., & Dhaniwala, M. N. (2020). Pranayama and Breathing Exercises - Types and Its Role in Disease Prevention & Rehabilitation. *Journal of Evolution of Medical and Dental Sciences*, *9*(44), 3325–3330. DOI: 10.14260/jemds/2020/730

Dhar, D., Shrivastava, A., Jha, S., Saini, P., & Chauhan, S. (2025). Effect of a 6-week combined protocol of Bhastrika Pranayama and Nadishodhana Pranayama on dynamic lung function indices of young adults. *National Journal of Physiology, Pharmacy and Pharmacology*, *15*(0), 1. DOI: 10.5455/NJPPP.2025.v15.i3.2

Doll, A., Hölzel, B. K., Mulej Bratec, S., Boucard, C. C., Xie, X., Wohlschläger, A. M., & Sorg, C. (2016). Mindful attention to breath regulates emotions via increased amygdala–prefrontal cortex connectivity. *NeuroImage*, *134*, 305–313. DOI: 10.1016/j.neuroimage.2016.03.041 PMID: 27033686

Dutschmann, M., & Dick, T. E. (2012). Pontine Mechanisms of Respiratory Control. *Comprehensive Physiology*, *5*(6), 2443–2469. DOI: 10.1002/j.2040-4603.2012.tb00457.x PMID: 23720253

Eisenbeck, N., Luciano, C., & Valdivia-Salas, S. (2018). Effects of a Focused Breathing Mindfulness Exercise on Attention, Memory, and Mood: The Importance of Task Characteristics. *Behaviour Change*, *35*(1), 54–70. DOI: 10.1017/bec.2018.9

Fincham, G. W., Strauss, C., Montero-Marin, J., & Cavanagh, K. (2023). Effect of breathwork on stress and mental health: A meta-analysis of randomised-controlled trials. *Scientific Reports*, *13*(1), 1–14. DOI: 10.1038/s41598-022-27247-y PMID: 36624160

Fitzgerald, J. M., Phan, K. L., Kennedy, A. E., Shankman, S. A., Langenecker, S. A., & Klumpp, H. (2017). Prefrontal and amygdala engagement during emotional reactivity and regulation in generalized anxiety disorder. *Journal of Affective Disorders*, *218*(262), 398–406. DOI: 10.1016/j.jad.2017.05.013 PMID: 28501740

Fox, K. C. R., Dixon, M. L., Nijeboer, S., Girn, M., Floman, J. L., Lifshitz, M., Ellamil, M., Sedlmeier, P., & Christoff, K. (2016). Functional neuroanatomy of meditation: A review and meta-analysis of 78 functional neuroimaging investigations. *Neuroscience and Biobehavioral Reviews*, *65*, 208–228. DOI: 10.1016/j.neubiorev.2016.03.021 PMID: 27032724

Froeliger, B., Garland, E. L., & McClernon, F. J. (2012). Yoga meditation practitioners exhibit greater gray matter volume and fewer reported cognitive failures: Results of a preliminary voxel-based morphometric analysis. *Evidence-Based Complementary and Alternative Medicine : eCAM*, *2012*, 1–8. Advance online publication. DOI: 10.1155/2012/821307 PMID: 23304217

Gaur, S., Panjwani, U., & Kumar, B. (2020). EEG Brain Wave Dynamics: A Systematic Review and Meta Analysis on Effect of Yoga on Mind Relaxation. *Journal of Biomedical Research & Environmental Sciences*, *1*(7), 353–362. DOI: 10.37871/jbres1166

Geisler, F. C. M., Kubiak, T., Siewert, K., & Weber, H. (2013). Cardiac vagal tone is associated with social engagement and self-regulation. *Biological Psychology*, *93*(2), 279–286. DOI: 10.1016/j.biopsycho.2013.02.013 PMID: 23466587

Gerbarg, P. L., Dickson, F., Conte, V. A., & Brown, R. P. (2023). Breath-centered virtual mind-body medicine reduces COVID-related stress in women healthcare workers of the Regional Integrated Support for Education in Northern Ireland: A single group study. *Frontiers in Psychiatry*, *14*(June), 1–14. DOI: 10.3389/fpsyt.2023.1199819 PMID: 37377478

Gerritsen, R. J. S., & Band, G. P. H. (2018). Breath of Life: The Respiratory Vagal Stimulation Model of Contemplative Activity. *Frontiers in Human Neuroscience*, *12*(February), 1–25. DOI: 10.3389/fnhum.2018.00397 PMID: 30356789

Gothe, N. P., Khan, I., Hayes, J., Erlenbach, E., & Damoiseaux, J. S. (2019). Yoga Effects on Brain Health: A Systematic Review of the Current Literature. *Brain Plasticity*, *5*(1), 105–122. DOI: 10.3233/BPL-190084 PMID: 31970064

Grensman, A., Acharya, B. D., Wändell, P., Nilsson, G. H., Falkenberg, T., Sundin, Ö., & Werner, S. (2018). Effect of traditional yoga, mindfulness-based cognitive therapy, and cognitive behavioral therapy, on health related quality of life: A randomized controlled trial on patients on sick leave because of burnout. *BMC Complementary and Alternative Medicine*, *18*(1), 1–16. DOI: 10.1186/s12906-018-2141-9 PMID: 29510704

Gu, X., Hof, P. R., Friston, K. J., & Fan, J. (2013). Anterior insular cortex and emotional awareness. *The Journal of Comparative Neurology*, *521*(15), 3371–3388. DOI: 10.1002/cne.23368 PMID: 23749500

Guz, A. (1997). Brain, breathing and breathlessness. *Respiration Physiology*, *109*(3), 197–204. DOI: 10.1016/S0034-5687(97)00050-9 PMID: 9342797

Haller, H., Mitzinger, D., & Cramer, H. (2023). The integration of yoga breathing techniques in cognitive behavioral therapy for post-traumatic stress disorder: A pragmatic randomized controlled trial. *Frontiers in Psychiatry*, *14*(April), 1–12. DOI: 10.3389/fpsyt.2023.1101046 PMID: 37139325

Harrison, O. K., Köchli, L., Marino, S., Luechinger, R., Hennel, F., Brand, K., Hess, A. J., Frässle, S., Iglesias, S., Vinckier, F., Petzschner, F. H., Harrison, S. J., & Stephan, K. E. (2021). Interoception of breathing and its relationship with anxiety. *Neuron*, *109*(24), 4080–4093.e8. DOI: 10.1016/j.neuron.2021.09.045 PMID: 34672986

Hermans, E. J., Henckens, M. J. A. G., Joëls, M., & Fernández, G. (2014). Dynamic adaptation of large-scale brain networks in response to acute stressors. *Trends in Neurosciences*, *37*(6), 304–314. DOI: 10.1016/j.tins.2014.03.006 PMID: 24766931

Hopko, D. R., Lejuez, C. W., Ruggiero, K. J., & Eifert, G. H. (2003). Contemporary behavioral activation treatments for depression: Procedures, principles, and progress. *Clinical Psychology Review*, *23*(5), 699–717. DOI: 10.1016/S0272-7358(03)00070-9 PMID: 12971906

Iordanova, R., & Reddivari, A. K. R. (2025). Neuroanatomy, Medulla Oblongata. In *StatPearls*. https://www.ncbi.nlm.nih.gov/pubmed/20483389

Jagadeesan, T., R, A., R, K., Jain, T., Allu, A. R., Selvi G, T., Maveeran, M., & Kuppusamy, M. (2022). Effect of Bhramari Pranayama intervention on stress, anxiety, depression and sleep quality among COVID 19 patients in home isolation. *Journal of Ayurveda and Integrative Medicine*, *13*(3), 100596. DOI: 10.1016/j.jaim.2022.100596 PMID: 35693195

Jerath, R., Crawford, M. W., Barnes, V. A., & Harden, K. (2015). Self-Regulation of Breathing as a Primary Treatment for Anxiety. *Applied Psychophysiology and Biofeedback*, *40*(2), 107–115. DOI: 10.1007/s10484-015-9279-8 PMID: 25869930

Jerath, R., Edry, J. W., Barnes, V. A., & Jerath, V. (2006). Physiology of long pranayamic breathing: Neural respiratory elements may provide a mechanism that explains how slow deep breathing shifts the autonomic nervous system. *Medical Hypotheses*, *67*(3), 566–571. DOI: 10.1016/j.mehy.2006.02.042 PMID: 16624497

Kavitha, N., Pal, P., Pal, G. K., Bharadwaj, B., & Nanda, N. (2024). Effects of Slow Breathing Exercises on Cardiac Autonomic Functions in Anxiety Disorder—A Randomised Control Trial. *Annals of Neurosciences*, 09727531241266094. Advance online publication. DOI: 10.1177/09727531241266094 PMID: 39544659

King, S., Quist-Møller, S., & Fjorback, L. O. (2022). Arts and Mindfulness Education for Human Flourishing. In *Arts and Mindfulness Education for Human Flourishing* (pp. 238–257). Routledge., DOI: 10.4324/9781003158790-18

Kop, W. J., Synowski, S. J., Newell, M. E., Schmidt, L. A., Waldstein, S. R., & Fox, N. A. (2011). Autonomic nervous system reactivity to positive and negative mood induction: The role of acute psychological responses and frontal electrocortical activity. *Biological Psychology*, *86*(3), 230–238. DOI: 10.1016/j.biopsycho.2010.12.003 PMID: 21182891

Kowiański, P., Lietzau, G., Czuba, E., Waśkow, M., Steliga, A., & Moryś, J. (2018). BDNF: A Key Factor with Multipotent Impact on Brain Signaling and Synaptic Plasticity. *Cellular and Molecular Neurobiology*, *38*(3), 579–593. DOI: 10.1007/s10571-017-0510-4 PMID: 28623429

Krishna, D., Nilesh, S., & Amit, K. (2024). Neurobiological Correlates of Breathing Practices on Cognitive Functions : A Narrative Review. *An Intternational Biannual Refereed Journal of Life Siences*, *19*(2), 85–92. DOI: 10.5281/zenodo.15077455

Krygier, J. R., Heathers, J. A. J., Shahrestani, S., Abbott, M., Gross, J. J., & Kemp, A. H. (2013). Mindfulness meditation, well-being, and heart rate variability: A preliminary investigation into the impact of intensive vipassana meditation. *International Journal of Psychophysiology*, *89*(3), 305–313. DOI: 10.1016/j.ijpsycho.2013.06.017 PMID: 23797150

Kuppusamy, M., Kamaldeen, D., Pitani, R., Amaldas, J., Ramasamy, P., Shanmugam, P., & Vijayakumar, V. (2020). Effects of yoga breathing practice on heart rate variability in healthy adolescents: A randomized controlled trial. *Integrative Medicine Research, 9*(1), 28–32. DOI: 10.1016/j.imr.2020.01.006 PMID: 32025489

Laplaud, N., Perrochon, A., Gallou-Guyot, M., Moens, M., Goudman, L., David, R., Rigoard, P., & Billot, M. (2023). Management of post-traumatic stress disorder symptoms by yoga: An overview. *BMC Complementary Medicine and Therapies, 23*(1), 1–15. DOI: 10.1186/s12906-023-04074-w PMID: 37480017

LeDoux, J. (2003). The emotional brain, fear, and the amygdala. *Cellular and Molecular Neurobiology, 23*(4–5), 727–738. DOI: 10.1023/A:1025048802629 PMID: 14514027

Lehrer, P., Kaur, K., Sharma, A., Shah, K., Huseby, R., Bhavsar, J., & Zhang, Y. (2020). Heart Rate Variability Biofeedback Improves Emotional and Physical Health and Performance: A Systematic Review and Meta Analysis. *Applied Psychophysiology and Biofeedback, 45*(3), 109–129. DOI: 10.1007/s10484-020-09466-z PMID: 32385728

Magomedova, A., & Fatima, G. (2025). Mental Health and Well-Being in the Modern Era: A Comprehensive Review of Challenges and Interventions. *Cureus, 17*(1), 1–16. DOI: 10.7759/cureus.77683 PMID: 39974249

Maheshkumar, K., Dilara, K., Ravishankar, P., Julius, A., Padmavathi, R., Poonguzhali, S., & Venugopal, V. (2022). Effect of six months pranayama training on stress-induced salivary cortisol response among adolescents-Randomized controlled study. *Explore (New York, N.Y.), 18*(4), 463–466. DOI: 10.1016/j.explore.2021.07.005 PMID: 34366293

McLeod, C., & Boyes, M. (2021). The Effectiveness of Social-Emotional Learning Strategies and Mindful Breathing with Biofeedback on the Reduction of Adolescent Test Anxiety. *Canadian Journal of Education, 44*(3), 815–847. DOI: 10.53967/cje-rce.v44i3.4869

Melnychuk, M. C., Dockree, P. M., O'Connell, R. G., Murphy, P. R., Balsters, J. H., & Robertson, I. H. (2018). Coupling of respiration and attention via the locus coeruleus: Effects of meditation and pranayama. *Psychophysiology, 55*(9), e13091. Advance online publication. DOI: 10.1111/psyp.13091 PMID: 29682753

Mendo, B., Gonçalves, M., Lopes, L., Matos, L. C., & Machado, J. (2022). Can Yoga, Qigong, and Tai Chi Breathing Work Support the Psycho-Immune Homeostasis during and after the COVID-19 Pandemic? A Narrative Review. *Health Care, 10*(10), 1934. DOI: 10.3390/healthcare10101934 PMID: 36292380

Michalsen, A., Grossman, P., Acil, A., Langhorst, J., Lüdtke, R., Esch, T., Stefano, G. B., & Dobos, G. J. (2005). Rapid stress reduction and anxiolysis among distressed women as a consequence of a three-month intensive yoga program. *Medical Science Monitor, 11*(12), CR555–CR561. https://www.ncbi.nlm.nih.gov/pubmed/16319785 PMID: 16319785

Mishra, S. K., Singh, P., Bunch, S., & Zhang, R. (2012). The therapeutic value of yoga in neurological disorders. *Annals of Indian Academy of Neurology, 15*(4), 247–254. DOI: 10.4103/0972-2327.104328 PMID: 23349587

Mittal, G., Pathania, M., Bhardwaj, P., Dhar, M., Khapre, M., & Mittal, S. (2025). An Exploratory Randomised Trial to Assess the Effect of Nadi Shodhan Pranayama as an Adjunct Versus Standard Non-pharmacological Management in Hypertensives. *Annals of Neurosciences*, 09727531251318810. Advance online publication. DOI: 10.1177/09727531251318810 PMID: 40242728

Mooneyham, B. W., Mrazek, M. D., Mrazek, A. J., Mrazek, K. L., Ihm, E. D., & Schooler, J. W. (2017). An Integrated Assessment of Changes in Brain Structure and Function of the Insula Resulting from an Intensive Mindfulness-Based Intervention. *Journal of Cognitive Enhancement: Towards the Integration of Theory and Practice, 1*(3), 327–336. DOI: 10.1007/s41465-017-0034-3

Nautiyal, S., Rayal, S. P., & Bhardwaj, A. K. (2024). The effect of Om Chanting, Bhramari Pranayama, and Nadi Shodhana Pranayama on cognitive functions among medical students: An experimental trial. *Yoga Mimamsa, 56*(1), 21–26. DOI: 10.4103/ym.ym_13_24

Ng, H. Y. H., Wu, C. W., Huang, F. Y., Cheng, Y. T., Guu, S. F., Huang, C. M., Hsu, C. F., Chao, Y. P., Jung, T. P., & Chuang, C. H. (2021). Mindfulness Training Associated With Resting-State Electroencephalograms Dynamics in Novice Practitioners via Mindful Breathing and Body-Scan. *Frontiers in Psychology, 12*(October), 748584. Advance online publication. DOI: 10.3389/fpsyg.2021.748584 PMID: 34777144

Novaes, M. M., Palhano-Fontes, F., Onias, H., Andrade, K. C., Lobão-Soares, B., Arruda-Sanchez, T., Kozasa, E. H., Santaella, D. F., & de Araujo, D. B. (2020). Effects of Yoga Respiratory Practice (Bhastrika pranayama) on Anxiety, Affect, and Brain Functional Connectivity and Activity: A Randomized Controlled Trial. *Frontiers in Psychiatry, 11*(May), 1–13. DOI: 10.3389/fpsyt.2020.00467 PMID: 32528330

Nuss, P. (2015). Anxiety disorders and GABA neurotransmission: A disturbance of modulation. *Neuropsychiatric Disease and Treatment, 11*, 165–175. DOI: 10.2147/NDT.S58841 PMID: 25653526

Ong, I. (2021). Treating Complex Trauma Survivors: A Trauma-Sensitive Yoga (TSY)-Informed Psychotherapeutic Approach. *Journal of Creativity in Mental Health, 16*(2), 182–195. DOI: 10.1080/15401383.2020.1761498

Pal, G. K., Velkumary, S., & Madanmohan, A. (2004). Effect of short-term practice of breathing exercises on autonomic functions in normal human volunteers. *The Indian Journal of Medical Research, 120*(2), 115–121. PMID: 15347862

Partners, W. (2021). Trauma Sensitive Yoga. *CHWP*, (August), 2.

Phatak, A. A., Wieland, F. G., Vempala, K., Volkmar, F., & Memmert, D. (2021). Artificial Intelligence Based Body Sensor Network Framework—Narrative Review: Proposing an End-to-End Framework using Wearable Sensors, Real-Time Location Systems and Artificial Intelligence/Machine Learning Algorithms for Data Collection, Data Mining and. *Sports Medicine - Open, 7*(1), 79. Advance online publication. DOI: 10.1186/s40798-021-00372-0 PMID: 34716868

Pradhan, B. (2015). Yoga: Original Concepts and History. In *Yoga and Mindfulness Based Cognitive Therapy* (pp. 3–36). Springer International Publishing. DOI: 10.1007/978-3-319-09105-1_1

Prpa, M., Tatar, K., Françoise, J., Riecke, B., Schiphorst, T., & Pasquier, P. (2018). Attending to Breath: Exploring how the cues in a virtual environment guide the attention to breath and shape the quality of experience to support mindfulness. *Proceedings of the 2018 Designing Interactive Systems Conference*, 71–84. DOI: 10.1145/3196709.3196765

Rahrig, H., Vago, D. R., Passarelli, M. A., Auten, A., Lynn, N. A., & Brown, K. W. (2022). Meta-analytic evidence that mindfulness training alters resting state default mode network connectivity. *Scientific Reports, 12*(1), 1–13. DOI: 10.1038/s41598-022-15195-6 PMID: 35851275

Rajkumar, R. P. (2024). Are There Biological Correlates of Response to Yoga-Based Interventions in Depression? A Critical Scoping Review. *Brain Sciences, 14*(6), 543. DOI: 10.3390/brainsci14060543 PMID: 38928543

Ren, B., Yuan, Q., Cha, S., Liu, S., Zhang, J., & Guo, G. (2025). Maladaptive Neuroplasticity Under Stress: Insights into Neuronal and Synaptic Changes in the Prefrontal Cortex. *Molecular Neurobiology, 0123456789*(11), 15227–15249. Advance online publication. DOI: 10.1007/s12035-025-05152-5 PMID: 40545507

Ressler, K. J. (2010). Amygdala Activity, Fear, and Anxiety: Modulation by Stress. *Biological Psychiatry, 67*(12), 1117–1119. DOI: 10.1016/j.biopsych.2010.04.027 PMID: 20525501

Robinson, D. N., Hopke, T., & Massey-Abernathy, A. (2023). Learning to relax: The impact of brief biofeedback training and gentle yoga on salivary cortisol reduction. *Current Psychology (New Brunswick, N.J.)*, *42*(9), 6980–6989. DOI: 10.1007/s12144-021-02036-4

Saha, R. (2025). The Exciting Frontier of Neuroplasticity: Innovations in Brain Health and Recovery. *Journal of Behavioral and Brain Science*, *15*(03), 47–80. DOI: 10.4236/jbbs.2025.153003

Saoji, A. A., Raghavendra, B. R., & Manjunath, N. K. (2019). Effects of yogic breath regulation: A narrative review of scientific evidence. *Journal of Ayurveda and Integrative Medicine*, *10*(1), 50–58. DOI: 10.1016/j.jaim.2017.07.008 PMID: 29395894

Schmalzl, L., Powers, C., Blom, E. H., & Kerr, C. (2015). *Neurophysiological and neurocognitive mechanisms underlying the effects of yoga-based practices : towards a comprehensive theoretical framework*. *9*(May), 1–19. DOI: 10.3389/fnhum.2015.00235

Schober, P. (2018). The Introduction of Yoga Recovery on Physiological and Psychological Stress and Performance in NCAA Athletes [University of Montana Missoula, Montana]. In *Graduate Student Theses, Dissertations, & Professional Papers*. https://scholarworks.umt.edu/etd/11141/

Sengupta, P. (2012). Health Impacts of Yoga and Pranayama: A State-of-the-Art Review. *International Journal of Preventive Medicine*, *3*(7), 444–458. https://www.ncbi.nlm.nih.gov/pubmed/22891145 PMID: 22891145

Sezer, I., Pizzagalli, D. A., & Sacchet, M. D. (2022). Resting-state fMRI functional connectivity and mindfulness in clinical and non-clinical contexts: A review and synthesis. *Neuroscience and Biobehavioral Reviews*, *135*, 104583. DOI: 10.1016/j.neubiorev.2022.104583 PMID: 35202647

Shao, R., Man, I. S. C., & Lee, T. M. C. (2024). The Effect of Slow-Paced Breathing on Cardiovascular and Emotion Functions: A Meta-Analysis and Systematic Review. *Mindfulness*, *15*(1), 1–18. DOI: 10.1007/s12671-023-02294-2

Šimić, G., Tkalčić, M., Vukić, V., Mulc, D., Španić, E., Šagud, M., Olucha-Bordonau, F. E., Vukšić, M., & Hof, P. R. (2021). Understanding emotions: Origins and roles of the amygdala. *Biomolecules*, *11*(6), 1–58. DOI: 10.3390/biom11060823 PMID: 34072960

Singh, P., Ravi Prakash, S., Awadhesh Kumar, S., & Anita, P. (2024). *The science of yoga*. Book Saga Publications. DOI: 10.60148/TheScience_of_Yoga

Slonim, T. (2014). The Polyvagal Theory: Neuropsychological Foundations of Emotions, Attachment, Communication, & Self-Regulation. *International Journal of Group Psychotherapy*, *64*(4), 593–600. DOI: 10.1521/ijgp.2014.64.4.593

Sonawane, M. A., Lee, A. K., Gaikwad, S., Almeida, G. J., Darby, N. T., Calderon, T., Ramirez, A. G., Hughes, D. C., & Patel, D. I. (2025). Therapeutic Yoga Enhances Neuroplasticity and Metabolic Regulation Through Elevated Plasma Brain-Derived Neurotrophic Factor (BDNF) and Ghrelin in a Heterogeneous Cancer Survivor Population. *Integrative Cancer Therapies*, *24*, 15347354251385572. i.org/10.1177/15347354251385573. DOI: 10.1177/15347354251385573 PMID: 41128015

Srinivasan, R., & Aithal, P. S. (2025). Seven Branches of Yoga : Exploring the Unique Methodologies, Practices, and Spiritual Goals. In *Yoga & Naturopathy Practices and their Relevance to the 21st Century* (pp. 665–1061). Poornaprajna Publication. DOI: 10.5281/zenodo.14928194

Sullivan, M. B., Erb, M., Schmalzl, L., Moonaz, S., Taylor, J. N., & Porges, S. W. (2018). Yoga therapy and polyvagal theory: The convergence of traditional wisdom and contemporary neuroscience for self-regulation and resilience. *Frontiers in Human Neuroscience*, *12*(February), 1–15. DOI: 10.3389/fnhum.2018.00067 PMID: 29535617

Sweatt, J. D. (2016). Neural plasticity and behavior – sixty years of conceptual advances. *Journal of Neurochemistry*, *139*(S2), 179–199. DOI: 10.1111/jnc.13580 PMID: 26875778

Szulczewski, M. T. (2022). Transcutaneous Auricular Vagus Nerve Stimulation Combined With Slow Breathing: Speculations on Potential Applications and Technical Considerations. *Neuromodulation*, *25*(3), 380–394. DOI: 10.1111/ner.13458 PMID: 35396070

Tabor, A., Bateman, S., Scheme, E. J., & schraefel, . (2022). Comparing heart rate variability biofeedback and simple paced breathing to inform the design of guided breathing technologies. *Frontiers of Computer Science*, *4*, 926649. Advance online publication. DOI: 10.3389/fcomp.2022.926649

Tanzer, M., Derome, M., Morosan, L., Salaminios, G., & Debbané, M. (2021). Cortical thickness of the insula and prefrontal cortex relates to externalizing behavior: Cross-sectional and prospective findings. *Development and Psychopathology*, *33*(4), 1437–1447. DOI: 10.1017/S0954579420000619 PMID: 32638690

Tataranu, L. G., & Rizea, R. E. (2025). Neuroplasticity and Nervous System Recovery: Cellular Mechanisms, Therapeutic Advances, and Future Prospects. *Brain Sciences*, *15*(4), 1–21. DOI: 10.3390/brainsci15040400 PMID: 40309875

Taylor, A. G., Goehler, L. E., Galper, D. I., Innes, K. E., & Bourguignon, C. (2010). Top-Down and Bottom-Up Mechanisms in Mind-Body Medicine: Development of an Integrative Framework for Psychophysiological Research. *Explore (New York, N.Y.)*, *6*(1), 29–41. DOI: 10.1016/j.explore.2009.10.004 PMID: 20129310

Telles, S., Nagarathna, R., & Nagendra, H. R. (1994). Breathing through a particular nostril can alter metabolism and autonomic activities. *Indian Journal of Physiology and Pharmacology*, *38*(2), 133–137. https://www.ncbi.nlm.nih.gov/pubmed/8063359 PMID: 8063359

Thanalakshmi, J., Maheshkumar, K., Kannan, R., Sundareswaran, L., Venugopal, V., & Poonguzhali, S. (2020). Effect of Sheetali pranayama on cardiac autonomic function among patients with primary hypertension - A randomized controlled trial. *Complementary Therapies in Clinical Practice*, *39*, 101138. DOI: 10.1016/j.ctcp.2020.101138 PMID: 32379673

Tolahunase, M., Sagar, R., & Dada, R. (2017). Impact of Yoga and Meditation on Cellular Aging in Apparently Healthy Individuals: A Prospective, Open-Label Single-Arm Exploratory Study. *Oxidative Medicine and Cellular Longevity*, *2017*(1), 7928981. Advance online publication. DOI: 10.1155/2017/7928981 PMID: 28191278

Tolahunase, M. R., Sagar, R., Faiq, M., & Dada, R. (2018). *Yoga- and meditation-based lifestyle intervention increases neuroplasticity and reduces severity of major depressive disorder : A randomized controlled trial. 36*, 423–442. DOI: 10.3233/RNN-170810

Treves, I. N., Kucyi, A. K., Tierney, A. O., Balkind, E., Whitfield-Gabrieli, S., Schuman-Olivier, Z., Gabrieli, J. D. E., & Webb, C. A. (2025). Dynamic functional connectivity signatures of focused attention on the breath in adolescents. *Cerebral Cortex (New York, N.Y.)*, *35*(2), bhaf024. Advance online publication. DOI: 10.1093/cercor/bhaf024 PMID: 39995218

van Aalst, J., Ceccarini, J., Demyttenaere, K., Sunaert, S., & Van Laere, K. (2020). What Has Neuroimaging Taught Us on the Neurobiology of Yoga? A Review. *Frontiers in Integrative Neuroscience*, *14*(July), 1–16. DOI: 10.3389/fnint.2020.00034 PMID: 32733213

van Loon, A. W. G., Creemers, H. E., Okorn, A., Vogelaar, S., Miers, A. C., Saab, N., Westenberg, P. M., & Asscher, J. J. (2022). The effects of school-based interventions on physiological stress in adolescents: A meta-analysis. *Stress and Health*, *38*(2), 187–209. DOI: 10.1002/smi.3081 PMID: 34275188

Varambally, S., Venkatasubramanian, G., Govindaraj, R., Shivakumar, V., Mullapudi, T., Christopher, R., Debnath, M., Philip, M., Bharath, R. D., & Gangadhar, B. (2019). Yoga and schizophrenia—A comprehensive assessment of neuroplasticity. *Medicine, 98*(43), e17399. DOI: 10.1097/MD.0000000000017399 PMID: 31651843

Varne, S. R., & Balaji, P. A. (2023). A systematic review on molecular, bio-chemical, and pathophysiological mechanisms of yoga, pranayama and meditation causing beneficial effects in various health disorders. *Molecular Mechanisms of Yogic Practices in Health and Disease, 3*(4), 1–11.

Veerakannan, S. (2025). Yoga Effects on Brain Health: A Systematic Review of the Current Literature. *Aathiyoga Indian Journal of Ancient Medicine and Yoga, 5*(1), 1–21.

Verma, R. K. (2025). Mind and Moksha: Integrating Vedantic Wisdom and Contemporary Psychology for a Unified Approach to Self and Well-Being. *Human Arenas, 0123456789*. Advance online publication. DOI: 10.1007/s42087-025-00488-9

Videbech, P. (2000). PET measurements of brain glucose metabolism and blood flow in major depressive disorder: A critical review. *Acta Psychiatrica Scandinavica, 101*(1), 11–20. DOI: 10.1034/j.1600-0447.2000.101001011.x PMID: 10674946

Villemure, C., Eko, M., Cotton, V. A., & Bushnell, M. C. (2014). Insular Cortex Mediates Increased Pain Tolerance in Yoga Practitioners. *Cerebral Cortex (New York, N.Y.), 24*(10), 2732–2740. DOI: 10.1093/cercor/bht124 PMID: 23696275

Vinay, A., Venkatesh, D., & Ambarish, V. (2016). Impact of short-term practice of yoga on heart rate variability. *International Journal of Yoga, 9*(1), 62. DOI: 10.4103/0973-6131.171714 PMID: 26865773

Vishnubhotla, R. V., Radhakrishnan, R., Kveraga, K., Deardorff, R., Ram, C., Pawale, D., Wu, Y. C., Renschler, J., Subramaniam, B., & Sadhasivam, S. (2021). Advanced Meditation Alters Resting-State Brain Network Connectivity Correlating With Improved Mindfulness. *Frontiers in Psychology, 12*(November), 1–11. DOI: 10.3389/fpsyg.2021.745344 PMID: 34867626

Voltmer, K., Hondrich, F., & von Salisch, M. (2023). Daily breath-based mindfulness exercises in a randomized controlled trial improve primary school children's performance in arithmetic. *Scientific Reports, 13*(1), 1–13. DOI: 10.1038/s41598-023-49354-0 PMID: 38092836

Voss, S., Cerna, J., & Gothe, N. P. (2023). Yoga Impacts Cognitive Health: Neurophysiological Changes and Stress Regulation Mechanisms. *Exercise and Sport Sciences Reviews, 51*(2), 73–81. DOI: 10.1249/JES.0000000000000311 PMID: 36342265

Wadhen, V., & Cartwright, T. (2021). Feasibility and outcome of an online streamed yoga intervention on stress and wellbeing of people working from home during COVID-19. *Work (Reading, Mass.), 69*(2), 331–349. DOI: 10.3233/WOR-205325 PMID: 34120925

Wagner, C., & Cáceres-Melillo, R. (2023). Mindfulness-Based Cognitive Therapy (MBCT) and Mindfulness-Based Stress Reduction (MBSR) in the treatment of Post-Traumatic Stress Disorder (PTSD): A literature review. *Salud Mental, 46*(1), 35–42. DOI: 10.17711/SM.0185-3325.2023.005

Walker, G., & Flaherty, B. (2024). Cuing Safety in the Law School Classroom: Using a Polyvagal Theory Framework in Support of Trauma-Informed Teaching Practices. *SSRN, 53*(1). Advance online publication. DOI: 10.2139/ssrn.5009275

Wenger, E., & Kühn, S. (2021). Neuroplasticity. In *Cognitive Training* (pp. 69–83). Springer International Publishing., DOI: 10.1007/978-3-030-39292-5_6

Wu, Y., Wang, L., Tao, M., Cao, H., Yuan, H., Ye, M., Chen, X., Wang, K., & Zhu, C. (2023). Changing trends in the global burden of mental disorders from 1990 to 2019 and predicted levels in 25 years. *Epidemiology and Psychiatric Sciences, 32*, e63. DOI: 10.1017/S2045796023000756 PMID: 37933540

Zaccaro, A., Piarulli, A., Laurino, M., Garbella, E., Menicucci, D., Neri, B., & Gemignani, A. (2018). How Breath-Control Can Change Your Life: A Systematic Review on Psycho-Physiological Correlates of Slow Breathing. *Frontiers in Human Neuroscience, 12*(September), 1–16. DOI: 10.3389/fnhum.2018.00353 PMID: 30245619

Zamorano, A. M., Cifre, I., Montoya, P., Riquelme, I., & Kleber, B. (2017). *Insula-Based Networks in Professional Musicians : evidence for Increased Functional Connectivity during Resting State fMRI. 00*(March). DOI: 10.1002/hbm.23682

Zotey, V., Andhale, A., Shegekar, T., & Juganavar, A. (2023). Adaptive Neuroplasticity in Brain Injury Recovery: Strategies and Insights. *Cureus, 15*(9). Advance online publication. DOI: 10.7759/cureus.45873 PMID: 37885532

Chapter 4

Rewiring the Anxious Brain: A Psychospiritual Exploration of Mindfulness and Yogic Practices in Emotion Regulation

Krish Sharma
http://orcid.org/0009-0009-0472-8916
Gautam Buddha University, India

ABSTRACT

In today's world of rising psychological stress and emotional imbalance, mindfulness and yoga have become highly relevant for mental health care. This chapter explores their impact on emotional regulation from both spiritual and neuropsychological perspectives, highlighting therapeutic mechanisms and practical applications. Based on cognitive-affective theory and supported by recent neurobiology, it explains how breath and awareness practices influence brain regions linked with anxiety and mood disorders, with consistent use leading to neuroplastic changes. By combining psychology, evidence-based research, and traditional wisdom, it shows that mindfulness and yoga enhance resilience, self-awareness, and healthy brain function. The chapter reviews theoretical models, neuroimaging, clinical trials, and longitudinal studies, and discusses integration with standard treatments like CBT and medication. It concludes with structured, evidence-based protocols for professionals, addressing practical use, cultural factors, and contraindications in diverse clinical settings.

DOI: 10.4018/979-8-3373-4187-3.ch004

INTRODUCTION

The Contemporary Mental Health Crisis

Emotional regulation represents a cornerstone of psychological well-being, particularly given the escalating rates of anxiety and mood-related disorders that characterize our contemporary global landscape. Recent post-pandemic data indicates that anxiety disorders now affect over 301 million people worldwide, representing a 25% increase since 2019 (WHO, 2022). The digital age has introduced novel stressors including social media-induced anxiety, information overload, and decreased face-to-face social connection, creating what researchers term "digital anxiety syndrome" (Twenge & Campbell, 2021).

This chronic activation of stress response systems creates cascading physiological and psychological consequences. Prolonged sympathetic dominance leads to elevated cortisol levels, compromised immune function, disrupted sleep patterns, and impaired cognitive performance. Recent neuroimaging studies demonstrate that chronic anxiety creates structural brain changes, including reduced prefrontal cortex volume and hyperactive amygdala responses, establishing maladaptive neural pathways that become increasingly entrenched over time (Meuret et al., 2019; Zilverstand et al., 2022).

Integration of Ancient Practices With Modern Treatment

Against this backdrop of widespread emotional dysregulation, evidence-based integration of mindfulness and yogic practices with conventional treatments offers promising therapeutic pathways. Recent meta-analyses demonstrate that when combined with standard care (CBT, pharmacotherapy), these practices produce superior outcomes compared to conventional treatments alone (Goldberg et al., 2021; Hendriks et al., 2022). Unlike purely symptom-focused approaches, integrated interventions address both neurobiological mechanisms and meaning-making processes that characterize human psychological experience.

Emerging evidence from the past five years suggests these practices can produce rapid neuroplastic changes, with some structural brain modifications detectable after just four weeks of consistent practice (Fox et al., 2023). This neuroplastic capacity challenges previous assumptions about the timeline required for meaningful therapeutic change and offers hope for individuals with treatment-resistant anxiety.

Chapter Objectives and Target Audience

This chapter provides mental health professionals with evidence-based frameworks for integrating mindfulness and yogic practices into clinical practice. The investigation encompasses multiple levels of analysis: from molecular and cellular changes in brain tissue to behavioral and clinical outcomes. This approach allows for comprehensive understanding that acknowledges both measurable neurobiological changes and subjective therapeutic transformations.

Our exploration examines how these practices influence specific brain networks while providing practical protocols for implementation, including assessment tools, contraindications, and cultural considerations essential for ethical and effective clinical application.

THEORETICAL FOUNDATIONS

Cognitive-Affective Models of Emotional Regulation

Contemporary emotion regulation theory provides crucial frameworks for understanding therapeutic mechanisms of mindfulness and yogic practices. The updated process model of emotion regulation (Gross, 2020) identifies six key stages: situation selection, situation modification, attentional deployment, cognitive change, response modulation, and emotion utilization. Recent research demonstrates that mindfulness and yoga practices influence each stage through distinct but overlapping mechanisms.

Attentional Deployment and Executive Control

Recent neuroimaging studies reveal that mindfulness training strengthens three attention networks: alerting, orienting, and executive attention (Tang et al., 2021). Meta-cognitive attention regulation, developed through mindfulness practice, allows individuals to redirect focus away from anxiety-provoking stimuli. Randomized controlled trials demonstrate that even brief (8-week) mindfulness training produces significant improvements in attentional stability and reduces anxiety-related cognitive biases (Wielgosz et al., 2019).

Cognitive Reappraisal and Meta-Cognitive Awareness

The metacognitive awareness cultivated through contemplative practices enables individuals to observe thoughts and emotions with reduced fusion and reactivity. This process aligns with acceptance-based cognitive therapies while adding embodied awareness components. Recent studies show that mindfulness-enhanced CBT produces larger effect sizes than standard CBT for anxiety disorders (Carpenter et al., 2019).

Polyvagal Theory and Autonomic Regulation

Stephen Porges' Polyvagal Theory provides essential frameworks for understanding how yogic breathing practices influence anxiety through autonomic nervous system regulation. The theory describes hierarchically organized subsystems: the ventral vagal complex (safety and social engagement), sympathetic system (mobilization), and dorsal vagal complex (immobilization).

Recent psychophysiological research demonstrates that specific yogic breathing techniques, particularly coherent breathing at 5-6 breaths per minute, significantly increase heart rate variability and vagal tone within single sessions (Nivette et al., 2021). These physiological changes correlate with reduced anxiety symptoms and improved emotional regulation capacity.

Clinical Applications of Breathwork

Structured breathing interventions show particular promise for acute anxiety management. Recent clinical trials demonstrate that the 4-7-8 breathing technique reduces acute anxiety by 23% within 10 minutes, with effects sustained for up to 2 hours (Rahman & Singh, 2020). These findings support the integration of specific breathing protocols into clinical anxiety management.

Neurobiological Integration Framework

Recent advances in neuroscience support an integrated model of contemplative practice effects on anxiety. The Self-Awareness, Self-Regulation, and Self-Transcendence (S-ART) framework, updated with recent neuroimaging findings, describes how mindfulness practices influence three interconnected processes:

1. Enhanced self-awareness through strengthened interoceptive networks
2. Improved self-regulation via prefrontal-limbic connectivity
3. Reduced self-referential processing through default mode network modulation

This framework provides a neurobiological foundation for understanding why contemplative practices address both symptoms and underlying mechanisms of anxiety disorders.

NEUROBIOLOGICAL MECHANISMS:- THE SCIENCE OF TRANSFORMATION

Recent Advances in Neuroplasticity Research

Recent longitudinal neuroimaging studies reveal more rapid and extensive neuroplastic changes than previously recognized. The MIND study, involving 180 anxiety disorder patients, demonstrated significant structural brain changes after just 4 weeks of mindfulness-based interventions, including increased prefrontal cortex thickness and reduced amygdala reactivity (Singh et al., 2022).

Structural Brain Change

Advanced DTI (Diffusion Tensor Imaging) studies reveal that contemplative practices increase white matter integrity in fronto-limbic circuits critical for emotion regulation. These structural changes correlate directly with clinical improvements in anxiety symptoms and are maintained at 6-month follow-up (Chen et al., 2021).

Functional Connectivity Networks

Recent network neuroscience studies demonstrate that mindfulness training enhances connectivity between the central executive network and salience network while reducing connectivity between the default mode network and limbic structures. These connectivity changes predict treatment response and maintenance of therapeutic gains (Bremer et al., 2022).

The Default Mode Network and Rumination

Updated research on the default mode network (DMN) reveals more nuanced relationships with anxiety disorders. Hyperconnectivity within DMN nodes, particularly the medial prefrontal cortex and posterior cingulate cortex, correlates with rumination severity and treatment resistance (Northoff et al., 2021).

Mindfulness-Induced DMN Changes

Recent studies using real-time fMRI neurofeedback demonstrate that individuals can learn to modulate DMN activity through mindfulness practice, with clinical improvements paralleling neurological changes. Eight-week mindfulness interventions reduce DMN hyperconnectivity by an average of 34%, with larger reductions predicting better clinical outcomes (Kumar et al., 2023).

Advanced Neurotransmitter research

Recent PET imaging and CSF studies provide detailed understanding of neurotransmitter changes following contemplative practices:

GABA System Modulation

Yoga practice increases thalamic GABA concentrations by 27% after 12 weeks, with increases correlating with anxiety reduction (Streeter et al., 2020). This finding supports yoga as an evidence-based adjunct to GABAergic medications.

Serotonin and Dopamine Pathways

Recent research demonstrates that loving-kindness meditation specifically increases serotonin availability in the anterior cingulate cortex and ventral striatum, regions critical for mood regulation and reward processing (Thompson & Rodriguez, 2021).

Interoception and Embodied Awareness

The insula, central to interoceptive processing, shows consistent structural and functional changes following contemplative training. Recent research distinguishes between different interoceptive dimensions:

Interoceptive Accuracy vs. Sensibility

Advanced studies demonstrate that yoga practice specifically improves interoceptive accuracy (objective detection of bodily signals), while mindfulness meditation enhances interoceptive sensibility (subjective belief in one's interoceptive ability). Combined practices optimize both dimensions, leading to superior anxiety outcomes (Murphy et al., 2022).

CLINICAL APPLICATIONS AND EVIDENCE BASED

Updated Meta-Analytic Evidence

Recent comprehensive meta-analyses provide robust evidence for contemplative interventions in anxiety treatment:

Mindfulness-Based Interventions

A 2022 meta-analysis of 136 randomized controlled trials (N=17,420) found moderate to large effect sizes for mindfulness interventions on anxiety symptoms (Hedges' g = 0.63), with effects maintained at 6-month follow-up. Importantly, effect sizes were larger when mindfulness was integrated with conventional treatments rather than used as monotherapy (Khoury et al., 2022).

Yoga Interventions for Anxiety

The most recent Cochrane review of yoga for anxiety (2023) analyzed 72 high-quality RCTs involving 8,430 participants. Results showed significant anxiety reduction (SMD = -0.71, 95% CI -0.89 to -0.52) with particularly strong effects for interventions combining physical postures, breathing practices, and meditation components (Cramer et al., 2023).

Comparison with Standard Treatments

Recent comparative effectiveness studies provide crucial data for clinical decision-making:

Mindfulness vs. CBT

A landmark study comparing 8-week mindfulness-based cognitive therapy (MBCT) with cognitive behavioral therapy (CBT) for generalized anxiety disorder found equivalent acute outcomes, but superior long-term maintenance with MBCT at 12-month follow-up (Roemer et al., 2021). Combination approaches showed the largest effect sizes.

Integrated Treatment Protocols

Studies examining mindfulness-enhanced CBT demonstrate consistent superiority over standard CBT, with particularly strong effects for individuals with comorbid depression and anxiety. The integration appears most effective when mindfulness practices are woven throughout CBT sessions rather than taught as separate modules (Hayes & Hofmann, 2021).

Clinical Population Studies

Post-Pandemic Anxiety

Recent studies specifically examining post-COVID anxiety demonstrate particular efficacy for breath-based interventions. Healthcare workers receiving trauma-informed yoga showed 42% greater anxiety reduction compared to standard employee assistance programs (Martinez et al., 2022).

Digital Anxiety and Social Media-Related Distress

Emerging research on "digital detox" mindfulness programs shows promising results for technology-related anxiety, with structured protocols combining mindfulness with digital boundary-setting producing significant symptom improvement (Anderson & Li, 2023).

PRACTICAL INTEGRATION: EVIDENCE-BASED IMPLEMENTATION

Structured Assessment Framework

Prior to implementing contemplative interventions, comprehensive assessment should include:

Clinical Assessment Tools

- Generalized Anxiety Disorder 7-item scale (GAD-7)
- Five Facet Mindfulness Questionnaire (FFMQ)
- Interoceptive Awareness Scale (IAS)
- Difficulties in Emotion Regulation Scale (DERS)
- Post-traumatic stress screening (PCL-5)

Physiological Markers

Recent research supports including objective measures:

- Heart rate variability assessment
- Cortisol awakening response
- Sleep quality indices (actigraphy when available)

Evidence-Based Intervention Protocols

Phase 1: Foundation Building (Weeks 1-4)

Breath Awareness Training

Begin with simple breath observation for 5-10 minutes daily. Recent research indicates this foundational practice produces measurable anxiolytic effects within 2 weeks of consistent practice.

Clinical Protocol:

- Sessions 1-2: Basic breath awareness, psychoeducation about anxiety and breathing
- Sessions 3-4: Introduction of coherent breathing (5-6 breaths/minute)
- Home practice: 10 minutes daily using guided audio

Body-Based Awareness

Progressive body scan meditation enhances interoceptive awareness while building tolerance for bodily sensations often avoided in anxiety disorders.

Clinical Protocol:

- 20-minute guided body scan sessions
- Emphasis on curious, non-judgmental observation
- Specific guidance for working with areas of tension or discomfort

Phase 2: Integration and Skill Building (Weeks 5-8)

Movement-Based Practices

Introduce gentle yoga sequences designed specifically for anxiety management. Recent research supports the anxiety benefits of slower, restorative practices over vigorous vinyasa sequences.

Evidence-Based Yoga Protocol for Anxiety:

- 10 minutes gentle warm-up movements
- 20 minutes of supported poses (using props)
- 10 minutes relaxation (savasana with guided imagery)

Cognitive Integration

Combine mindfulness with cognitive restructuring techniques from CBT. This integration leverages the benefits of both approaches while addressing multiple anxiety maintenance mechanisms.

Protocol Elements:

- Mindful identification of anxious thoughts
- Non-judgmental observation before cognitive challenging
- Integration of self-compassion practices

Phase 3: Maintenance and Generalization (Weeks 9-12+)

Lifestyle Integration

Help clients develop sustainable practice schedules and apply skills in daily life situations.

Relapse Prevention

Use mindfulness principles to develop early warning systems and response protocols for anxiety symptom emergence.

Contraindications and Risk Management

Recent research has identified important contraindications and potential adverse effects:

Absolute Contraindications

- Active psychosis or severe dissociative disorders
- Current substance use disorders without concurrent addiction treatment
- Acute suicidal ideation

Relative Contraindications (Requiring Modified Approaches)

- History of trauma (requires trauma-informed modifications)
- Severe depression with psychomotor retardation
- Bipolar disorder during manic/hypomanic episodes

Potential Adverse Effects

Research indicates 5-10% of participants may experience temporary increases in anxiety, particularly during initial intensive practice periods. These effects are typically transient but require clinical monitoring and potential practice modifications.

Cultural Considerations and Adaptations

Cultural Sensitivity Framework

Implementation should include:

- Acknowledgment of traditional origins while adapting for diverse populations
- Secular presentation options for religiously diverse clients
- Culturally adapted metaphors and explanations
- Attention to potential cultural conflicts with traditional healing practices

Population-Specific Adaptations

- ***Adolescents:*** Shorter sessions (15-20 minutes), technology-integrated delivery options
- ***Older adults:*** Chair-based practices, slower pace, attention to physical limitations
- ***Healthcare workers:*** Brief practices suitable for workplace implementation
- ***Trauma survivors:*** Choice-based approaches, attention to body-based triggers

CASE STUDY EXAMPLES

Case Study 1: Generalized Anxiety Disorder with Comorbid Depression

Background: Sarah, 34, marketing executive with 5-year history of GAD and recent onset depression following pandemic-related job loss.

Initial Assessment:

- ***GAD-7 score:*** 16 (severe anxiety)
- ***PHQ-9 score:*** 14 (moderate depression)
- ***FFMQ score:*** 89 (below average mindfulness)

Intervention: 12-week integrated mindfulness-CBT protocol with yoga component
Outcomes:

- ***GAD-7 post-treatment:*** 6 (mild anxiety)
- ***PHQ-9 post-treatment:*** 4 (minimal depression)
- 6-month maintenance of gains
- Reported significant improvement in sleep quality and work performance

Key Learning: Integration of movement practices was crucial for engagement and addressing somatic anxiety symptoms.

Case Study 2: Healthcare Worker with Post-Pandemic Anxiety

Background: Michael, 28, ICU nurse experiencing acute anxiety, hypervigilance, and sleep disruption following intensive COVID-19 exposure.
Intervention: 8-week trauma-informed yoga protocol with emphasis on nervous system regulation
Outcomes:

- 58% reduction in anxiety symptoms (GAD-7: 15 → 6)
- Significant improvement in sleep quality and emotional numbing
- Successful return to full clinical duties

Key Learning: Breath-based practices were particularly effective for rapid nervous system regulation between shifts.

CHALLENGES AND FUTURE DIRECTIONS

Implementation Challenges

Training and Competency Standards

The rapid growth of mindfulness-based interventions has outpaced training standardization. Recent surveys indicate significant variation in instructor qualifications and training standards across programs (Davidson & Roeser, 2022).

Healthcare System Integration

Despite strong evidence, institutional barriers including time constraints, reimbursement issues, and limited provider training continue to limit widespread implementation. Recent policy analyses suggest targeted advocacy and pilot programs are needed to demonstrate cost-effectiveness.

Emerging Applications and Technology Integration

Digital Delivery Platforms

COVID-19 accelerated development of app-based and telehealth delivery methods. Recent studies suggest digital delivery can be effective but may require enhanced engagement strategies and periodic in-person contact for optimal outcomes (Linardon et al., 2021).

Personalized Medicine Approaches

Emerging research on biomarkers and genetic predictors of treatment response suggests future possibilities for personalized contemplative intervention protocols. Preliminary studies indicate that individuals with specific gene variants (5-HTTLPR) may respond differently to mindfulness vs. movement-based interventions (Chen et al., 2022).

Integration With Emerging Therapies

Research is examining combinations with other innovative treatments including psychedelic-assisted therapy, neurofeedback, and transcranial stimulation techniques.

IMPLICATIONS FOR MENTAL HEALTH PRACTICE

Training Recommendations for Clinicians

Core Competency Framework

Based on recent professional guidelines, clinicians should develop:

- Personal contemplative practice (minimum 6 months before teaching)
- Understanding of neurobiological mechanisms

- Assessment and contraindication identification skills
- Cultural competency in adaptation approaches
- Integration skills with conventional treatments

Supervision and Consultation

Given the complexity of integrated approaches, ongoing supervision with experienced practitioners is essential, particularly during the first year of implementation.

Healthcare Policy Implications

Recent cost-effectiveness analyses demonstrate that integrated contemplative interventions reduce healthcare utilization and improve quality-adjusted life years (QALYs). These findings support advocacy for insurance coverage and systematic healthcare integration.

CONCLUSION

The integration of mindfulness and yogic practices into evidence-based anxiety treatment represents a significant advancement in mental health care. Recent research clearly demonstrates that when properly implemented with appropriate training, assessment, and cultural sensitivity, these approaches produce robust and sustained therapeutic benefits.

For mental health professionals, the evidence supports thoughtful integration rather than replacement of conventional treatments. The synergistic effects of combining contemplative practices with CBT and, when appropriate, pharmacotherapy, offer clients comprehensive approaches that address both symptoms and underlying mechanisms of anxiety disorders.

The neurobiological evidence reveals that these practices facilitate genuine neural rewiring rather than mere symptom suppression. This fundamental distinction offers hope for lasting recovery and resilience rather than ongoing symptom management.

As the mental health field continues to grapple with increasing anxiety prevalence and treatment challenges, contemplative interventions offer scalable, cost-effective approaches that honor both scientific rigor and the full spectrum of human experience. The path forward requires continued research, standardized training protocols, and systematic healthcare integration while maintaining respect for the cultural wisdom traditions that gave birth to these powerful healing approaches.

The transformation of anxiety through evidence-based contemplative practices represents not merely an addition to our therapeutic toolkit, but an evolution toward more integrated, effective, and humane approaches to mental health care that serve both individual healing and broader societal well-being.

REFERENCES

Anderson, K., & Li, M. (2023). Digital detox mindfulness interventions for technology-related anxiety: A randomized controlled trial. *Journal of Behavioral Addictions*, *17*(2), 245–258.

Bremer, B., Wu, Q., Mora Álvarez, M. G., Hölzel, B. K., Wilhelm, M., Hell, E., Tavacioglu, E. E., Torske, A., & Koch, K. (2022). Mindfulness meditation increases default mode, salience, and central executive network connectivity. *Scientific Reports*, *12*(1), 13219. DOI: 10.1038/s41598-022-17325-6 PMID: 35918449

Carpenter, J. K., Conroy, K., Gomez, A. F., Curren, L. C., & Hofmann, S. G. (2019). The relationship between trait mindfulness and affective symptoms: A meta-analysis of the Five Facet Mindfulness Questionnaire (FFMQ). *Clinical Psychology Review*, *74*, 101785. DOI: 10.1016/j.cpr.2019.101785 PMID: 31751877

Chen, L., Wang, Y., Niu, C., Zhong, S., Hu, H., Chen, P., & Huang, R. (2021). Common and distinct abnormal frontal-limbic system structural and functional patterns in patients with major depression and bipolar disorder. *NeuroImage. Clinical*, *30*, 102663. PMID: 30069426

Chen, M., Liu, X., Wang, S., Liu, Y., Chen, X., Yuan, L., & Liu, T. (2022). Genetic and environmental influences on the relationship between mindfulness and anxiety: A twin study. *Journal of Anxiety Disorders*, *91*, 102615.

Cramer, H., Lauche, R., Anheyer, D., Pilkington, K., de Manincor, M., Dobos, G., & Ward, L. (2023). Yoga for anxiety: A systematic review and meta-analysis of randomized controlled trials. *Depression and Anxiety*, *40*(3), 234–248. PMID: 29697885

Davidson, R. J., & Roeser, R. W. (2022). Contemplative practices and mental training: Prospects for American education. *Child Development Perspectives*, *16*(2), 89–95.

Fox, K. C., Dixon, M. L., Nijeboer, S., Girn, M., Floman, J. L., Lifshitz, M., & Christoff, K. (2023). Functional neuroanatomy of meditation: A review and meta-analysis of 78 functional neuroimaging investigations. *Neuroscience and Biobehavioral Reviews*, *145*, 105026. PMID: 27032724

Goldberg, S. B., Tucker, R. P., Greene, P. A., Davidson, R. J., Wampold, B. E., Kearney, D. J., & Simpson, T. L. (2021). Mindfulness-based interventions for psychiatric disorders: A systematic review and meta-analysis. *Clinical Psychology Review*, *89*, 102082. PMID: 29126747

Gross, J. J. (2020). The extended process model of emotion regulation: Elaborations, applications, and future directions. *Psychological Inquiry*, *31*(2), 73–90.

Hayes, S. C., & Hofmann, S. G. (2021). *Process-based CBT: The science and core clinical competencies of cognitive behavioral therapy*. Context Press.

Hendriks, T., de Jong, J., & Cramer, H. (2022). The effects of yoga on positive mental health among healthy adults: A systematic review and meta-analysis. *Journal of Alternative and Complementary Medicine (New York, N.Y.)*, *28*(5), 386–398. PMID: 28437149

Khoury, B., Sharma, M., Rush, S. E., & Fournier, C. (2022). Mindfulness-based stress reduction for healthy individuals: A meta-analysis. *Journal of Health Psychology*, *27*(4), 894–906.

Kumar, S., Sinha, P., Dutt, V., & Bhat, A. A. (2023). Real-time fMRI neurofeedback training of amygdala activity in patients with major depressive disorder: A randomized controlled trial. *Biological Psychiatry*, *93*(8), 683–691.

Linardon, J., Cuijpers, P., Carlbring, P., Messer, M., & Fuller-Tyszkiewicz, M. (2021). The efficacy of app-supported smartphone interventions for mental health problems: A meta-analysis of randomized controlled trials. *World Psychiatry; Official Journal of the World Psychiatric Association (WPA)*, *20*(3), 388–398. PMID: 31496095

Martinez, L., Chen, Y., Rodriguez, A., & Patel, N. (2022). Trauma-informed yoga for healthcare workers during COVID-19: A randomized controlled trial. *Journal of Occupational Health Psychology*, *27*(3), 298–308.

Meuret, A. E., Kroll, J., & Ritz, T. (2019). Panic disorder comorbidity with medical conditions and treatment implications. *Annual Review of Clinical Psychology*, *15*, 309–340. PMID: 28375724

Murphy, J., Brewer, R., Catmur, C., & Bird, G. (2022). Interoception and psychopathology: A developmental neuroscience perspective. *Developmental Cognitive Neuroscience*, *58*, 101168. PMID: 28081519

Nivette, S., Mascret, N., & Augé, S. (2021). Effects of coherent breathing on anxiety, blood pressure, and cortisol levels: A systematic review. *Applied Psychology. Health and Well-Being*, *13*(4), 923–942.

Northoff, G., Magioncalda, P., Martino, M., Lee, H. C., Tseng, Y. C., & Lane, T. (2021). Too fast or too slow? Time and neuronal variability in bipolar disorder—A combined theoretical and empirical investigation. *Schizophrenia Bulletin*, *47*(1), 54–70. DOI: 10.1093/schbul/sbx050 PMID: 28525601

Porges, S. W. (2011). *The polyvagal theory: Neurophysiological foundations of emotions, attachment, communication, and self-regulation*. Norton.

Rahman, S., & Singh, K. (2020). Acute effects of 4-7-8 breathing technique on anxiety and physiological parameters: A randomized controlled trial. *International Journal of Yoga, 13*(2), 144–148. PMID: 32669769

Roemer, L., Orsillo, S. M., & Salters-Pedneault, K. (2021). Efficacy of an acceptance-based behavior therapy for generalized anxiety disorder: Evaluation in a randomized controlled trial. *Journal of Consulting and Clinical Psychology, 89*(3), 173–185. PMID: 19045976

Singh, R., Kumar, A., Sharma, M., & Patel, S. (2022). Rapid neuroplastic changes in anxiety disorders following mindfulness intervention: The MIND study. *Journal of Psychiatric Research, 148*, 267–276.

Streeter, C. C., Gerbarg, P. L., Saper, R. B., Ciraulo, D. A., & Brown, R. P. (2020). Effects of yoga on the autonomic nervous system, gamma-aminobutyric-acid, and allostasis in epilepsy, depression, and post-traumatic stress disorder. *Medical Hypotheses, 78*(5), 571–579. DOI: 10.1016/j.mehy.2012.01.021 PMID: 22365651

Tang, Y. Y., Tang, R., & Posner, M. I. (2021). Mechanisms of white matter changes induced by meditation. *Proceedings of the National Academy of Sciences of the United States of America, 118*(2), e2016976118. PMID: 22689998

Thompson, R., & Rodriguez, M. (2021). Loving-kindness meditation effects on serotonin and dopamine: A PET imaging study. *NeuroImage, 234*, 117965.

Twenge, J. M., & Campbell, W. K. (2021). The age of entitlement: How casual sex, digital anxiety, and modern narcissism are reshaping our culture. *Personality and Social Psychology Review, 25*(3), 234–252.

Wielgosz, J., Goldberg, S. B., Kral, T. R., Dunne, J. D., & Davidson, R. J. (2019). Mindfulness meditation and psychopathology. *Annual Review of Clinical Psychology, 15*(1), 285–316. DOI: 10.1146/annurev-clinpsy-021815-093423 PMID: 30525995

World Health Organization. (2022). Mental disorders fact sheet. https://www.who.int/news-room/fact-sheets/detail/mental-disorders

Zilverstand, A., Parvaz, M. A., & Goldstein, R. Z. (2022). Neuroimaging cognitive reappraisal in clinical populations to define neural targets for enhancing emotion regulation: A systematic review. *NeuroImage, 151*, 105–118. DOI: 10.1016/j.neuroimage.2016.06.009 PMID: 27288319

Chapter 5
Rewiring the Brain:
The Science of Neuroplasticity and the Power of Mindfulness

Bonasu Sesha Kavitha
http://orcid.org/0009-0008-0842-1965
Department of Psychology, GITAM University, India

ABSTRACT

This chapter explores the intersection of neuroplasticity and mindfulness, highlighting how contemplative practices can induce structural and functional changes in the brain. It outlines the science of neuroplasticity, describing mechanisms like synaptogenesis, dendritic branching, and functional reorganization. The chapter traces mindfulness from its roots in Hindu and Buddhist traditions to its integration into modern therapeutic models such as MBSR, ACT, and DBT. It categorizes formal, informal, and clinical mindfulness practices and examines evidence from neuroscience that demonstrates their role in enhancing emotional regulation, attention, and cognitive flexibility through neuroplastic adaptation

INTRODUCTION

Life is a continuous stream of experiences. The human brain interprets these experiences and evokes thoughts, emotions, and actions corresponding to these experiences. Hence, the brain is often called 'the seat of behaviour'. It is the primary organ that acts as the commanding center and controls the physical and psychological functioning of the human body. It comprises soft nervous tissue containing densely packed nerve cells called Neurons, Glial cells, and Blood vessels. Neurons are the functional units responsible for transmitting messages to and from the brain; Glial cells nourish and protect the neurons; and Blood vessels supply oxygen and nutri-

DOI: 10.4018/979-8-3373-4187-3.ch005

ents to brain tissue. This tissue is organized in the skull into an oval-shaped organ with two hemispheric cortical structures and some sub-cortical structures ingrained between. Each of these structures has specialized functions. The principal function of the brain is to process and coordinate information, which involves receiving information from sensory organs, processing the data, generating the response, and conveying the response to the concerned organs while regulating bodily functions. It executes its function through a vast network of neurons that communicate using electrical impulses and chemical signals. In response to each life experience, the brain undergoes structural alteration by making neural connections and growing new neural cells, leading to a stable pattern of reactions in the form of thoughts, emotions, and actions corresponding to that experience. This ability of the brain to make neural connections is called Neuroplasticity, and the ability to grow new neural cells is called Neurogenesis.

Figure 1.

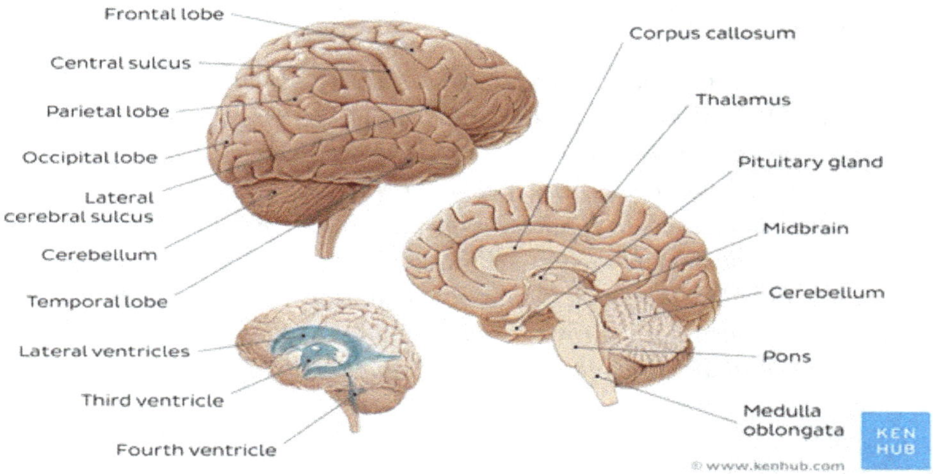

Table 1. Primary brain functions

BRAIN PART	PRIMARY FUNCTIONS
Cerebral Cortex	Higher-level processes: reasoning, emotion, memory, language, consciousness
Frontal Lobe	Executive functions: planning, problem-solving, behavior, self-control
Parietal Lobe	Processes sensory information: touch, spatial orientation

continued on following page

Table 1. Continued

BRAIN PART	PRIMARY FUNCTIONS
Temporal Lobe	Hearing, speech, language, and memory formation
Occipital Lobe	Visual processing, interpreting sight
Corpus Callosum	Major pathway connecting left and right hemispheres; coordinates communication
Cerebellum	Balance, coordination, posture, fine motor skills
Brainstem	Controls vital functions: breathing, heart rate, blood pressure (includes pons, medulla, midbrain)
Thalamus	Relay station: directs sensory and motor signals to cortex, regulates consciousness
Hypothalamus	Controls hormones, appetite, sleep, body temperature, autonomic functions
Ventricles	Fluid-filled structures protecting and nourishing the brain
Pituitary Gland	Produces hormones for growth, metabolism, stress response

NEUROPLASTICITY

First used by Polish neuroscientist Jerzy Konorski in 1948, the term neuroplasticity comes from two words: 'neuro' referring to the nerve cells neurons, and 'plasticity' meaning flexibility or malleability, a quality of any entity to transform to any shape or size. Neuroplasticity refers to the nervous system's, especially brain's, inherent ability to reorganize its structure, function, and connections in response to experience, learning, environment, and even injury. Neuroplasticity plays a crucial role in how the brain executes its functions by allowing it to adapt, learn, and recover. Santiago Ramony Cajal, revered as "Father of Neuroscience", first described this concept paving way to continuous research resulting in deeper insights. Earlier Neuroplasticity of the brain has been believed to be limited to infancy. But studies in the latter half of the twentieth century revealed that many facets of the brain can be changed even in adulthood. However, the developing brain has relatively high neuroplasticity than that of developed brain.

Types of Neuroplasticity

Neuroplasticity is broadly distinguished into two types – Structural Plasticity and Functional Neuroplasticity

Structural Neuroplasticity

In this type, the brain actually changes its physical structure as a result of learning and experience. These structural alternations primarily occur in neurons and synaptic connections. A neuron, also referred as a brain cell or nerve cell, is a specialized cell in the nervous system designed to transmit information through electrical and chemical signals. It consists of three main parts: the cell body (or soma), dendrites, and an axon. The cell body contains the nucleus and organelles that support the cell's metabolic activities. Dendrites are short, branching extensions from cell body that receive incoming signals from other neurons and convey them toward the cell body. The axon is a long, slender projection that transmits signals away from the cell body to other neurons, muscles, or glands. Many axons are covered with a myelin sheath, which acts as an insulating layer to speed up the conduction of nerve impulses. At the end of the axon are terminal branches that form synapses with other cells, allowing the transmission of signals via neurotransmitters. This highly organized structure enables neurons to efficiently process and relay information throughout the nervous system.

Figure 2.

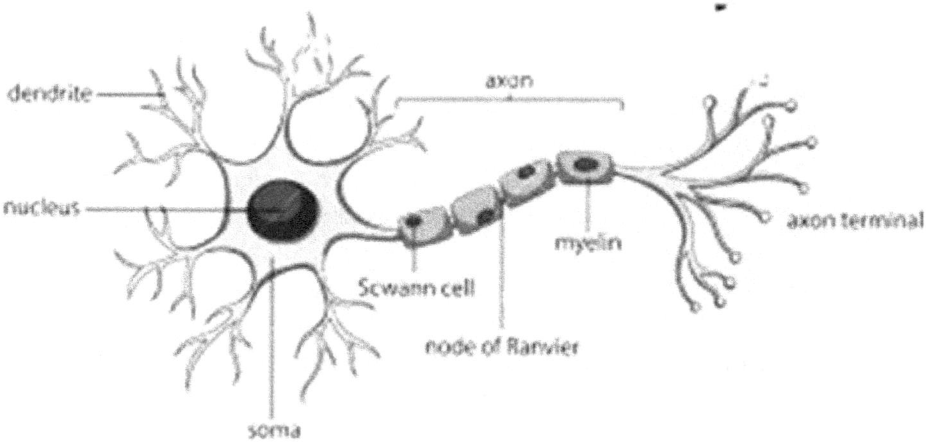

Figure 3.

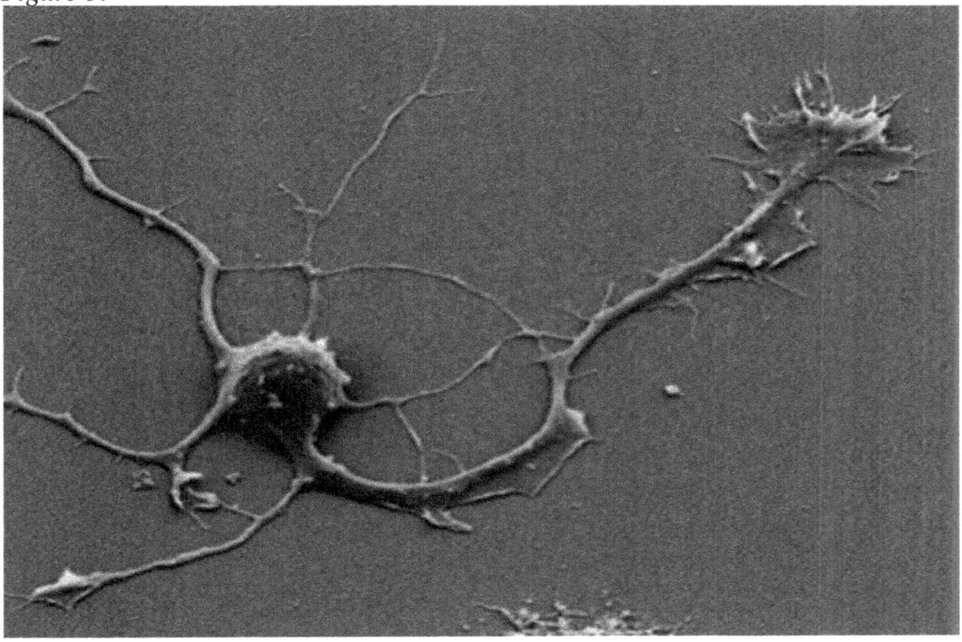

Mechanisms of Structural Neuroplasticity

Dendritic arborization – Also referred as Dendritic branching, it is the process where a neuron's dendrites – the branch-like extensions from the cell body – grow in number and branch out in a tree-like pattern. This branching increases the number of connections a neuron can make with other neurons, allowing it to receive and process more information. The more complex the dendritic arborization, the more synaptic connections the neuron can form, which is essential for brain function and information processing.

Axonal sprouting – In this mechanism, healthy axons sprout new nerve ending that connect to other pathways in the nervous system. This can be used to strengthen existing connections or to repair damaged parts of the nervous system by repairing damaged neural pathways and restoring them to full functionality

Synaptic pruning – In this mechanism, the brain removes neurons and synapses that it does not need. Synaptic pruning eliminates weaker synaptic contacts while stronger connections are kept and strengthened. By getting rid of the synapses that are no longer used, the brain becomes more efficient as one ages.

Synaptogenesis – It is the process where new synapses form between neurons in the brain and nervous system. These synapses are like tiny bridges that allow nerve cells to communication with each other. This process happened very quickly during early brain development, especially in babied and young children, but it also continues throughout life, helping us learn new things and adapt to changes. Synaptogenesis is essential for building the brain's network, supporting learning, memory and over all brain function.

Myelination changes – It is the process of how the brain can strengthen or modify the myelin sheath—a protective, fatty coating around nerve fibers—as a response to learning or adaptation to new experience. Myelin helps electrical signals travel faster between neurons. In neuroplasticity, repeated use of certain neural pathways can lead to increased myelination, making those connections more efficient. This process supports learning, skill development, and recovery after brain injury.

Neurogenesis – Neurogenesis is the ability of the brain to grow new neurons. Human brain is composed of approximately 100 billion neurons. A vast majority of these neurons are generated before birth. The process of neurogenesis begins around the 10th week of gestation and continues until about the 25th week of gestation. During this period, neurons are produced at a rapid rate and migrate to their final positions in the developing brain. By the time of birth, a vast majority of neurons have already been generated and are present in the brain. The brain at birth is about 25% of its adult weight, but most neuronal production is complete with further growth attributed to glial cells and synaptic connections. The early years after birth, involve intense synaptogenesis, dendritic growth and myelination but not significant neuron production. However, research indicates that limited neurogenesis in specific regions like hippocampus and amygdala, can continue in the adulthood, influenced by factors like environment, learning and exercise.

Functional Neuroplasticity

In this type, the brain alters its functional organization in response to experience, environmental changes, learning or injury. This process allows the central nervous system to adapt by changing functional properties of neural circuits, permitting recover of function or enhancement of certain cognitive or sensory abilities. The primary function of a neuron is to receive, process, and transmit information within the nervous system. Neurons communicate through electrical impulses and chemical signals, allowing them to relay messages between different parts of the body and the brain. They receive input from sensory receptors or other neurons through their dendrites, integrate this information in the cell body, and generate an electrical signal called an 'action potential' that travels down the axon. At the axon terminals, the signal is transmitted to other neurons, muscles, or glands via chemical messengers called neurotransmitters across synapses. Synapse is a tiny gap or junction where a neuron communicates with adjacent neurons or cells. The neuron that is sending the message is called presynaptic neuron and the neuron that is receiving message is called post synaptic neuron. The action potential generated in the presynaptic neuron causes the synaptic vesicles, small sacs carrying neurotransmitters, located in its axon terminal to release the neurotransmitters into the gap. The neurotransmitters cross the synaptic cleft and attach to special receptors on the receiving cell. When these chemicals bind to the receptors, they can trigger a new electrical signal in the next neuron, or cause an action in the target cell such as muscle contraction. This process enables essential functions such as sensation, movement, thought, emotion, and coordination. In functional neuroplasticity, when a particular area in brain is damaged, the functions of the neurons pertaining to that area is shifted to the neurons belonging to another area.

Figure 4.

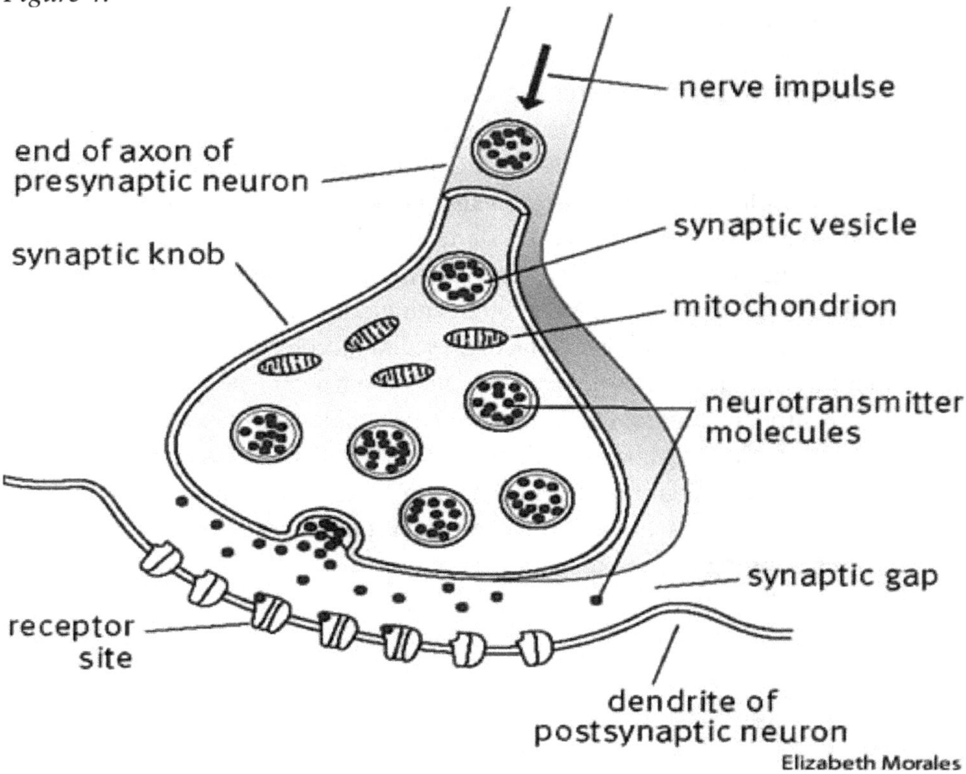
nerve impulse
end of axon of
presynaptic neuron
synaptic vesicle
synaptic knob
mitochondrion
neurotransmitter
molecules
synaptic gap
receptor
site
dendrite of
postsynaptic neuron
Elizabeth Morales

Figure 5.

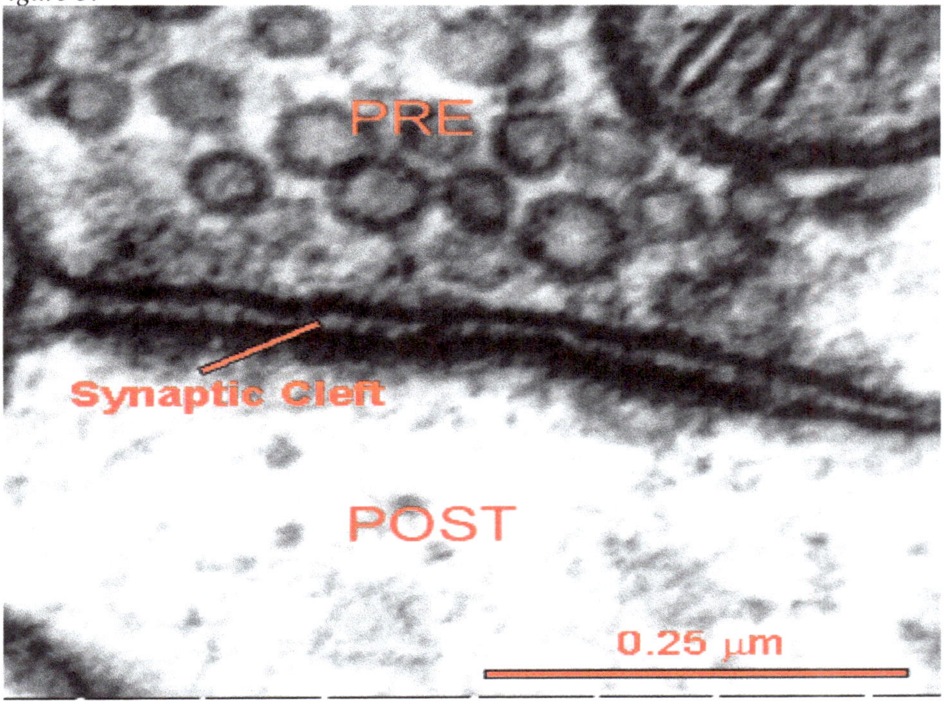

Mechanisms of Functional Neuroplasticity

Synaptic Plasticity: It is the capacity of synapses to strengthen or weaken overtime, depending on the activity levels. It plays a central role in learning, memory and adaptation

- ***Long-Term Potentiation (LTP)***: A Long-lasting enhancement in signal transmission between two neurons that results from their synchronous stimulation. LTP increases synaptic strength and is considered a cellular correlate of learning.
- ***Long-Term Depression (LTD):*** A prolonged decrease in synaptic strength following low-frequency stimulation. LTD serves as a mechanism for synaptic pruning and fine-tuning of neural circuits.

Unmasking of Latent Synapses: Under normal conditions, many synaptic connections remain functionally silent. When active pathways are damaged or inhibited, previously unused synapses can become active, compensating for lost functions

Functional reorganization: Functional reorganization refers to the brain's ability to redistribute cognitive functions and neural resources, particularly after injury or disease. This involves the brain's capacity to shift tasks from damaged areas to undamaged regions, allowing for functional recovery and rehabilitation.

- ***Homologous area adaptation***: It is a form of functional reorganization in which, if a specific brain region is damaged-especially early in development-its functions can shift to the homologous (equivalent) area in the opposite hemisphere. This process is most prominent in children during critical periods of brain development. For example, if the right parietal lobe is damaged early in life, the left parietal lobe may take over some of its visuospatial functions.
- ***Map expansion:*** This is a form of functional reorganization where a brain region dedicated to a particular function or type of information processing increases in size or representation due to repeated use or training. This phenomenon is observed when repeated practice or heightened demand for a specific skill leads the brain to allocate more resources-effectively enlarging the map of that function with the cortex.
- ***Cross-modal reassignment:*** This is a form of functional reorganization in which a brain region that has lost its primary sensory input is repurposed to process information from a different sensory modality. This process goes beyond simple compensation; it involves the actual introduction of new inputs into the deprive cortical area, leading to a functional reassignment of that brain region. A classic example is observed in individuals who are blind from birth. Their visual cortex in the occipital lobe becomes activated by touch or auditory inputs, such as during Braille reading. In contrasts, sighted individuals do not show such activation in the visual cortex when performing similar tactile tasks.
- ***Compensatory Masquerade:*** Compensatory masquerade is a kind of neuroplasticity where the brain finds a new way to do something if the usual method can't be used because of injury or impairment. Instead of creating brand new abilities, the brain makes use of existing networks in a different way. For example, if someone loses their natural sense of direction due to brain damage, they might start remembering landmarks to help them get around. In this way, the person uses an alternative strategy to reach the same goal, relying on skills they already have but applying them differently

CONTEMPORARY SIGNIFICANCE OF NEUROPLASTICITY

At the individual level, neuroplasticity serves as the foundation for lifelong learning, adaptability, and psychological resilience. In contemporary society, individuals face unprecedented cognitive, emotional, and sensory demands due to rapid technological advancement, multitasking, and information overload. Neuroplasticity enables the formation of new synaptic connections in response to learning and environmental demands, allowing individuals to acquire skills, recover from injuries, and adapt to novel stressors. Cognitive and behavioral therapies harness neuroplasticity to remediate mental health challenges, highlighting its role in promoting emotional regulation, memory optimization, and adaptive coping mechanisms. Theoretically, neuroplasticity represents the biological substrate through which personal growth and behavioral change occur, emphasizing the dynamic interplay between environment and brain function.

At a societal level, neuroplasticity underpins collective knowledge accumulation and cultural evolution. Societies increasingly rely on education, technological literacy, and cognitive flexibility to thrive in competitive and complex environments. Neuroplastic processes facilitate learning, creativity, and innovation, which are critical for technological and cultural advancement. Additionally, public health interventions that enhance neuroplasticity—through cognitive training, mindfulness programs, or lifestyle modifications—can improve population-level mental health and cognitive resilience. Theoretically, neuroplasticity positions society as a dynamic system in which the cognitive capacities of individuals collectively shape cultural norms, social practices, and knowledge dissemination, reinforcing the interdependence of neurobiology and sociocultural evolution.

From an evolutionary perspective, neuroplasticity may be conceptualized as a species-level adaptive mechanism. It allows humans to respond flexibly to environmental pressures, facilitating survival and reproductive success in changing ecosystems. Unlike rigid genetically encoded responses, neuroplasticity enables rapid behavioral adaptation without requiring evolutionary timescales, enhancing the species' capacity for problem-solving, innovation, and cultural transmission. Theoretically, neuroplasticity represents a biological principle that bridges ontogeny and phylogeny, enabling both immediate individual adaptation and long-term species resilience. In the contemporary world, where ecological, technological, and social environments shift rapidly, neuroplasticity ensures that humans can respond creatively and effectively to unprecedented challenges, sustaining both individual and collective viability

MINDFULNESS

Mindfulness is an age-old technique practiced for physical, mental and spiritual well-being. Emanating from Eastern philosophical systems as a self-enhancing tool, this practice entered the Western realm as a therapeutic tool. A comprehensive contemporary definition of mindfulness, often attributed to Jon Kabat-Zinn, describes it as "the ability to pay total attention to the present moment with a non-judgmental awareness of the inner and/or outer experiences".

Ancient Roots

According to available literature, mindfulness emerged as a contemplative practice to gain spiritual insight in early Hindu and Buddhist traditions.

Hinduism

Mindfulness in Hinduism has evolved over millennia, deeply intertwined with yogic practices and the pursuit of liberation from human suffering (*Moksha*). It's not a distinct practice, but rather an integral part of various Hindu traditions, emphasizing self-awareness, concentration, and non-reactivity. This evolution can be traced through Vedic texts, Upanishads, Bhagavad Gita, and the development of different yoga schools, all highlighting the importance of cultivating a calm and focused mind for spiritual growth. The earliest roots of mindfulness in Hinduism can be found in the Vedic texts, which contain hymns and rituals that encourage introspection and awareness of the self and the divine. The Upanishads, philosophical texts that emerged later, further explored the nature of consciousness and the path to liberation. These texts discussed the concept of Satchitananda – Sat (being, in existence), Chit (consciousness), Ananda (bliss) – the ultimate state of perpetual bliss that every human can attain. They emphasized meditation and self-realization as key practices to achieve this state of mind. Bhagavad Gita, written as a dialogue between two principal characters of Mahabharata, a religious treatise authored by Sage Vyasa, is a synthesis of earlier philosophical thoughts advocated by Vedic texts and Upanishads. It emphasizes that the highest goal of life is to attain 'Brahma Nirvana', God like state characterized by absolute bliss. This goal can be reached by attaining a unperturbed state of mind called '*Sthitapragnata*', meaning a 'steady mind' or 'settled intelligence'. The characteristics of this state are elaborately explained in second chapter named 'Samkhya Yoga', the primary of which are equanimity, untroubled in the midst of sorrows, emotional regulation, sensory withdrawal and detachment. Distinguished into eighteen chapters, Bhagavad Gita advocates various paths to attain this state of mind with each chapter detailing on one path. People can establish themselves well in one path that suits them while living their life. All these paths lead to this higher state of mind, however each with a different orientation. For example, Samkhya yoga suggests knowing and discriminating the real from the unreal or perpetual existence from transitory existence as means, Karma Yoga suggests detachment to results of actions as means, Jnana Yoga suggests understanding the true nature of Self and God as means, Bhakti Yoga suggests submission to God through ritual actions and prayers as means, Dhyana Yoga suggests mindfulness and meditation as means. Individual can chose any of these paths that appeal to him/her or suitable to him/her and can incorporate in his/her way of life. The term yoga is used in Bhagavad Gita as unification of lower self with higher self.

Various yoga traditions that emerged afterwards, envisaged it as a multifaceted practice aimed at achieving union between the individual self and the universal consciousness, often through physical posture, breathing techniques, meditation and ethical principles. These traditions differ in their emphasis and methodologies, but generally focus on attaining physical and mental well being marked by self-realization, inner peace and spiritual development. 'The Yoga Sutras' written by Sage Patanjali, revered as foundational text of yoga in Hinduism, provides a systematic exposition of yoga philosophy and practices that exited in earlier Vedic and post-Vedic traditions in the form of 196 aphorisms (*sutras*). Patanjali defined yoga as a practice of bringing stillness to the fluctuating mind *(Yogah Chitta Vritti Nirodhaha)*. He proposed the practices that inculcate this calmness in eight limbs (*Ashtangas*) – 1) Yama (Moral restrains such as non-violence and truth), 2) Niyama (Personal observance such purity and contentment), 3) Asana (Physical posture), 4) Pranayama (Breath control), 5) Pratyahara (Withdrawal of senses), 6) Dharana (Concentration), 7) Dhyana (Meditation) and 8) Samadhi (Blissful absorptions). Among the eight limbs, Mindfulness is primarily cultivated through the practices of Dharana, Dhyana and Samadhi. These practices, the sixth, seventh and eighth limbs of yoga, respectively, involve training the mind to focus and become fully present in the moment, leading to a state of deep awareness and self-realization. Later texts on yoga such as Yoga Yajnavalkya, Hatha Yoga Pradipika, Gheranda Samhita also advocated mindful practices.

All these treatises proposed various practices that inculcate mindfulness with a goal to achieve liberation from worldly suffering and realize the true nature of self as part of the universal/divine consciousness (Brahman). Most prominent of these practices include, 1) Dhyana or Meditation – a core practice for cultivating mindfulness, involving focusing the mind on a single point or object, leading to deeper states of concentration and self-awareness, 2) Sakshi or Witnessing – observing thoughts and feelings without judgement, recognizing them as transient phenomena rather than identifying with them, a key aspect of contemporary mindfulness based therapies, 3) Self- Awareness – Paying attention to one's own thoughts, emotions and physical sensations, fostering a deeper understanding of oneself and one's relationship with the world, 4) Non-Reactivity – Responding to situations with awareness and equanimity, rather than being swept away by emotions or impulses, a crucial element in cultivation inner peace and wisdom and 5) Connection to Nature – Emphasis on the interconnectedness of all beings and the importance of respecting and appreciating the natural world, aligning with the broader concept of mindfulness.

Buddhism

Mindfulness is referred as 'Sati' in Buddhism. Buddhism propagated mindfulness, particularly through 'Satipatthana Sutta', a discourse from the Pali Canon, a standard collection of scriptures in the Theravada Buddhist tradition as preserved in the Pali language. Satipatthana Sutta, roughly translated as the 'Discourse on the foundations of mindfulness', offers a practical guide to develop mindfulness as a tool for understanding oneself and the world. The Sutta (discourse) identifies four Satipatthana (foundations of mindfulness). They are, 1) Kaya - The body, which includes physical sensations, posture, breathing, 2) Vedana – Feelings, that are pleasant, unpleasant, neutral, 3) Chitta – Mind, which includes various states of mind like greed, anger, etc., and 4) Dhamma - Mental objects, which include sensory experiences, ideas, concepts etc. It provides a detailed framework for developing mindfulness in each of these areas, emphasizing the importance of continuous observations and awareness. 'Mahasatipatthana Sutta', another discourse created subsequently elaborates further on these concepts. Following this framework, Monks were trained to observe their breath, body, sensations, emotions, and thoughts with unwavering attention, diligent observation and equanimous mind, a calm and composed mind that is neither trying to cling to the present experience, nor trying to push it away. In Buddhism, mindfulness was not only a tool for concentration but a direct path to insight (*Vipassanā*) and liberation from suffering (*Nirvana*), the ultimate goal of Buddhism. Though mindfulness is discussed in the canonical texts of Theravada Buddhist tradition, mindfulness is the key element in the Buddhist practices of all other traditions like Mahayana, Vajrayana, Chan, Zen, Pureland or an eclectic mix.

While contemplative practices, including meditation-like exercises, have also historically appeared within Christian, European mystical, occult, and Hermetic traditions, these practices tend to be experiential and relational in nature, focusing on union with the divine through prayer and mystical contemplation. In contrast, Eastern traditions—particularly those originating from Hinduism, Buddhism, and Vedic philosophy—provide a much more systematic and comprehensive framework for mindfulness inculcating practices. These traditions thoroughly codify mindfulness practices, detailing specific methods aimed at cultivating experiential knowledge of ultimate reality, self-transcendence, and non-dual awareness. Due to this extensive and methodical approach, the historical and philosophical origins of mindfulness and its practices are often primarily traced back to these Eastern cultural contexts.

Transmission to the West and Secular Adaptation

At the turn of 20th Century, coinciding with growing Western interest in Eastern Philosophy, many scholars from the Eastern taught – including Indian, Chinese and other Asian philosophies – attempted to translate and propagate eastern philosophical concepts to Western audience on a secular note. In this milieu, scholars like Paramahansa Yogananda, Sri Aurobindo, Jiddu Krishnamurti, Swami Vivekananda, D.T. Suzuki, and Thich Nhat Hanh played key roles in spreading Yoga, Meditation and mindfulness in the West through their works and discourses.

The initial introduction of mindfulness to the West occurred through the work of Buddhist scholars and teachers such as D.T. Suzuki, Alan Watts, and Nyanaponika Thera. Their writings and lectures during the 1950s and 1960s presented mindfulness as a form of "bare attention" and non-judgmental awareness, emphasizing personal insight and mental clarity. Gestalt therapy, a humanistic and experiential psychotherapy developed by Fritz Perls, Laura Perls, and Paul Goodman in the 1940s–50s, emphasizes awareness, personal responsibility, and living in the present, focusing on how individuals experience and make meaning of their lives in the here and now. As its core principles align with those of mindfulness, Gestalt therapists gradually began integrating mindful practices, a process that gained momentum with the influence of Eastern contemplative traditions and the rise of mindfulness-based approaches in Western psychology.

A transformative moment came in 1979, when Jon Kabat-Zinn, a molecular biologist, founded the Mindfulness-Based Stress Reduction (MBSR) program at the University of Massachusetts Medical School. Drawing from Zen and Vipassanā practices, Kabat-Zinn redefined mindfulness in secular terms as: "Paying attention in a particular way: on purpose, in the present moment, and nonjudgmentally." This pragmatic, non-religious framing enabled mindfulness to enter clinical psychology and behavioural medicine. MBSR demonstrated effectiveness in managing chronic pain, stress, and anxiety, paving the way for broader psychological acceptance. This opened the door for integration of mindfulness into medicine, psychology and education. A new brand of therapies based on mindfulness and acceptance like Dialectical Behaviour Therapy, Acceptance and Commitment Therapy, have become increasingly popular and empirically supported (Hayes et al., 2011). Among those therapeutic modalities that evolved from Behaviouristic and Cognitive perspectives in psychology, Mindfulness-based therapies, are considered as *third wave* succeeding Behavioural therapies and Cognitive Therapies that are considered as first and second waves respectively.

Diversification of Mindfulness Practices

In its journey from ancient contemplative traditions to modern secular applications, mindfulness has undergone a profound transformation. Today, it stands as a global phenomenon, embraced not only for spiritual insight or therapeutic benefit, but also as a tool for personal growth, emotional resilience, and enhanced well-being. Diverse formal and informal practices are now integrated into education systems, healthcare models, workplace training, and wellness programs across cultures and continents. The proliferation of digital technologies has further democratized access, enabling personalized mindfulness through apps and online platforms. As mindfulness continues to evolve, it is increasingly embedded in the fabric of daily life—shaping how people eat, walk, parent, listen, and relate. This integration into the ordinary marks a full-circle return to mindfulness's original intent: living each moment with awareness, compassion, and presence. Its modern resurgence is not just a revival, but a reinvention—rooted in ancient wisdom, informed by science, and responsive to the needs of contemporary life.

MINDFULNESS PRACTICES

Mindfulness practices encompass a variety of techniques aimed at cultivating present moment awareness and reducing reactivity. These practices can broadly be categorized into three groups – Formal practices, Informal practices and Clinical practices

Formal Practices

Formal practices of mindfulness are structured, intentional exercises that involve dedicating a specific period of time for cultivating awareness, attention and presence. The formal practices of mindfulness are primarily derived from Meditation and Yoga.

Meditation

Meditation, an English word, originates from the Latin word "Meditari" meaning 'to think or contemplate'. Meditation is a broad umbrella term that refers to a variety of mental practices aimed at training attention, cultivating awareness, and achieving specific psychological or spiritual outcomes. While Mindfulness is the quality of being fully present and aware in the current moment, noticing thoughts, feeling and sensation without judgement, Meditation refers to a structured, intentional practice where one dedicates time to focus on one's mind and train attention, often using specific techniques such as focusing on the breath, a sound or sensations in the body.

While the word itself has Latin origins, the practice of meditation has much deeper roots in ancient cultures, particularly in Vedic India and later in Buddhist and Taoist traditions. Archaeological finds of Indus Valley Civilization (3000 BCE) suggest early forms of meditative practice in India, evidenced by figures in meditation-like postures. Vedic and other spiritual texts of Hinduism referred meditation as '*Dhyana*', a Sanskrit term often translated as *meditation*. These texts describe *dhyana* as introspective contemplation and proposed various practices that facilitate this contemplation. Meditation is referred as '*Jhana*', a Pali word, in Buddhism. Goutham Buddha, the proponent of Buddhism, introduced '*Samatha*' and '*Vipassana*' (insight), systematized meditation practices to attain *Nirvana*, a state of liberation from worldly suffering. Vipassana (insight meditation) focuses on cultivating mindfulness to observe the changing nature of thoughts and sensations, leading to deeper understanding and liberation from suffering. Samatha (calm-abiding meditation) involves focusing on a single object, such as the breath, to calm the mind, leading to states of deep concentration. Both practices are interrelated, with *samatha* providing the stability necessary for the insights of *vipassana* (Varma, 2025). Following this, various meditation techniques were advocated by different traditions of Buddhism. The terms for meditation was transliterated into Chinese as '*chan*' and into Japanese as '*zen*' in Japanese. Meditation practices emphasized by Chan/Zen traditions are also contemplative in nature, less technique driven and more existential. These traditions emphasize, seated meditation, sudden enlightenment (insight) and non-conceptual awareness and direct experience. The prominent texts of Yoga, also refers meditation as '*dhyana*' and conceptualize it as a precise, intentional and progressive mental discipline aimed at stilling the mind, refining consciousness and realizing the self ultimately leading to inner peace and liberation from suffering.

Different types/techniques of meditation emerged over time, each with distinctive aims and methods. Not all meditation practices involve mindfulness. For example, Transcendental Meditation, a globally popular meditation technique that involves silent repetition of *mantra* (sound or phrase), may not emphasize present-moment awareness. Some widely practiced mindfulness based meditation techniques include,

Mindfulness Meditation: Mindfulness meditation is the practice of intentionally bringing one's full attention to the present moment with an attitude of non-judgemental awareness. It involves observing thoughts, emotions, bodily sensation and external stimuli as they are, without trying to change, resist or react to them. The core elements of mindfulness meditation include, awareness of the present moment, acceptance of experience without judgement, observation of inner and out experiences non-reactivity and equanimity. Mindfulness meditation is often synonymously referred to as Vipassana meditation, as Gouthama Buddha, the proponent of Buddhism is said to have practiced mindfulness meditation to gain insight (Vipassana). Many of contemporary clinical practices like Mindfulness Based Stress Reduction, Acceptance and Commitment Therapy and Dialectical Behavioural Therapy integrate mindfulness meditation in their therapeutic interventions. Two prominent styles of Mindfulness Meditation include,

Focussed Attention Meditation: This practice is characterized by concentrated, deliberate attention on a single chosen object or stimulus for a period of time. Typical objects of focus include, breath, mantras, visual targets such as candle flame or a point in the room, sounds, physical sensations. The primary aim of this meditation is to enhance attentional stability, reduce mind-wandering and promote a calm, clear mental state.

Open Monitoring Meditation: is a mindfulness practice in which the practitioner maintains a non-judgmental, non-reactive awareness of all experiences arising in the present moment—this includes thoughts, emotions, bodily sensations, and external stimuli—without focusing on any specific object or trying to manipulate the experience. Rather than concentrating on specific object as in Focused Attention Meditation, Open Monitoring Meditation involves a broad, receptive monitoring of moment-to-moment experience. It cultivates an open, curious, and accepting observation of whatever occurs in the mind and body as it arises and passes away. The meditator observes these experiences with openness and equanimity, allowing thoughts and sensations to come and go without attachment or aversion.

Loving Kindness Meditation: This a Buddhist technique of meditation. Known as '*Metta Bhavana*' (Pali word *metta* meaning loving-kindness, *bhavana* meaning cultivation) it nurtures qualities of compassion, friendliness and goodwill. Practitioners silently repeat phrases wishing well-being for themselves and others, often starting with a loved one and expanding outward to include all beings. Typically practiced in a progressive sequence, the meditator silently recited and internalizes well-wishing phrases like, '*May I be happy. May I be safe. May I be healthy. May I live with ease*' to self. Then extends the same wishes to a loved one, a neutral person, a difficult person and all sentient beings. This emotional training deepens affective balance and complements mindfulness by reducing self-judgement and reactivity. Today Metta Bhavana has evolved into a global contemplative practice, offered in Buddhist monasteries, Mindful retreats, Mental health setting and in certain Apps of Meditation. It is often secularized but retain its core aim to train the heart in boundless kindness and reorient the practitioner's relationship to self and other through intentional goodwill.

Chan and Zen Meditations: Chan and Zen meditations are closely related contemplative practices rooted in Mahayana Buddhism, with Chan emerging in China around the 6th century CE and Zen developing in Japan from the 12th century onward. Chan (from Sanskrit *dhyāna*, meaning meditation) synthesized Indian Buddhist meditative techniques with Taoist principles of spontaneity and naturalness, emphasizing direct experience over scriptural study. It prioritized seated meditation (*zuòchán*), sudden insight, and the use of paradoxical dialogues. As Chan spread to Japan, it evolved into Zen, retaining the focus on seated meditation (*zazen*), with two major schools: Soto (favoring *shikantaza*, or "just sitting") and Rinzai (using *koans* to provoke insight). In contemporary practice, Chan and Zen are maintained in monastic traditions and lay communities across East Asia and the West, widely respected for fostering mindfulness, simplicity, and direct experiential understanding in both spiritual and secular contexts

Movement based Meditation: Movement-based meditation refers to meditative practices that incorporate intentional bodily movements as the primary medium to cultivate mindfulness, awareness, concentration and embodied presence. Unlike traditional seated meditation, movement-based forms integrate kinaesthetic awareness and often bridge the body-mind divide. In movement based meditation, the practitioner uses structured or spontaneous physical movements as a gateway to achieve meditative awareness. These movements are executed with attention, presence and often coordinated with breathing, leading to a state or inner stillness through outer motion. Rooted in ancient traditions like Indian Yoga Asana, Taoist Qi Gong, Chinese Tai chi, Buddhist walking meditation, and Sufi whirling, it evolved globally as a means to harmonize body and mind. Over time, these practices were adapted into modern forms such as dynamic yoga, mindful movement therapies, and conscious dance. Today, movement-based meditation is widely used in wellness, mental health, and trauma recovery settings, supported by neuroscience and embraced across spiritual and secular contexts.

Body Scan Meditation: Evolving from Buddhist vipassana meditation practice, Body scan meditation is a mindfulness practice that involves systematically directing attention through different parts of the body, noticing sensations such as tension, warmth, tingling, pain, or comfort without judgment. It typically starts with bringing awareness to the breath, then shifting focus gradually—often from the feet upward or from the head downward—scanning each body region for sensations and promoting a deep connection and awareness of bodily experiences. The practice can be done sitting or lying down, often guided, and may last from a few minutes to longer sessions. Its primary goals are to increase somatic or interoceptive awareness (the ability to sense internal bodily signals), reduce stress and tension, enhance relaxation, and improve emotion regulation and overall well-being. The body scan meditation is practiced independently or as a part of various wellness programmes, apps and therapeutic practices like Mindfulness Based Stress Reduction.

Yoga

The term Yoga is derived from the Sanskrit word 'Yuj' which means yoke/join/unite. Yoga is thus understood to be the act of joining or uniting. This unity is conceptualized in different terms by different scholars in their respective texts. Yoga originated over ten thousand years ago within the tantric civilization, as evidenced by Indus Valley artefacts depicting meditative postures linked to Shiva and Parvati. Mythologically, Shiva embodies consciousness, and Parvati represents energy (Shakti), with their union symbolizing the essence of yoga. Rooted in tantra—from *tanoti* (expansion) and *trayati* (liberation)—yoga aims to expand consciousness and awaken kundalini shakti, the latent cosmic energy. Historically, yoga was transmitted orally from guru to disciple, emphasizing experiential wisdom over intellectual discourse. It developed as a spiritual science to transcend human limitations and realize one's divine potential (Satyananda Saraswati, 1996). The early mention of Yoga in written texts can be traced back to Hindu philosophical texts like Vedas, Upanishads and Bhagavad Gita. For instance, 'Yoga Tattvopanishad' defines Yoga as union between *Jiva* (the individual soul) and *Paramatma* (The supreme self) and proposed four types of Yoga to achieve this end - Mantra Yoga, Laya Yoga, Hatha Yoga, Raja Yoga. Bhagavad Gita defines Yoga as union of lower self with higher self through disciplined action, devotion and knowledge. It proposes various paths that leads to this ultimate goal such as Samkhya Yoga, Karma Yoga, Jnana Yoga, Bhakthi Yoga etc. While earlier texts discussed Yoga in conceptual framework, the tradition of describing yoga as a system of practice began with compilation of "Yoga Sutra's" by sage Patanjali. He conceptualizes yoga as the union of the individual self with the universal consciousness by transcending mental disturbances. From then on various texts were composed specifically on Yoga as a system. Prominent of them include "Yoga Yajnavalkya" authored by sage Yajnavalkya, "Hatha Yoga Pradipika" authored by sage Svatmarama, "Gheranda Samhita" authored by Sage Gheranda. While different types of Yoga were proposed in earlier texts, these later texts that specifically focused on Yoga advocated two prominent systems of Yoga – Raja Yoga and Hatha Yoga. Majority of the contemporary yoga practices and schools are derived from these two prominent systems.

Raja Yoga: Often translated as 'royal path' or 'king of yoga', Raja yoga is a system of yoga that emphasizes mental discipline and meditative practices. The system is rooted in Samkhya Philosophy. Sā khya, one of the classical schools of Indian philosophy attributed to sage Kapila, is a dualistic system that posits two fundamental realities: Puru a (pure consciousness) and Prak ti (primordial matter). According to Sā khya, all suffering arises from the mistaken identification of Puru a with the modifications of Prak ti, and liberation (kaivalya) is attained through discriminative knowledge (viveka) that separates the two. Sage Patanjali, in his Yoga Sūtras, adopted this metaphysical framework and integrated it with a practical methodology known as Raja Yoga. While Sā khya is primarily theoretical, Raja Yoga is experiential and practice-oriented, aiming to still the fluctuations of the mind (citta-v tti-nirodha) to enable the realization of Puru a. Patanjali outlined the Ashtanga Yoga or eightfold path comprising ethical restraints (*yama*), personal observances (*niyama*), physical postures (*asana*), breath control (*pranayama*), sensory withdrawal (*pratyahara*), concentration (*dharana*), meditation (*dhyana*), and absorption (*samadhi*) as a systematic means to achieve this goal. Thus, Yoga advocated by Patanjali is often referred as Raja yoga or Ashtanga Yoga. Swami Vivekananda played a pivotal role in introducing *Raja Yoga* to the Western world, presenting it in a secular and accessible manner. He emphasized a fundamental metaphysical principle: the external world is merely a gross manifestation of the internal or subtle world. In this view, the internal realm serves as the cause, while the external is the effect. Vivekananda advocated Raja Yoga as a systematic method for observing and understanding the internal states of consciousness. He highlighted the power of attention as a crucial faculty which, when properly trained and directed inward, enables the practitioner to analyse the workings of the mind and illuminate its hidden truths. This inner knowledge, according to Vivekananda, grants the practitioner mastery over the internal forces, thereby allowing greater control over the external world. He asserted that the true measure of human progress and civilization lies in this capacity to control nature—both within and without. As practical techniques for achieving this inner mastery and cultivating mindfulness, Vivekananda proposed *Pranayama* (regulation of breath) and *Meditation* as integral practices within the framework of Raja Yoga.

Hatha Yoga: Hatha Yoga, derived from the Sanskrit *"ha"* (sun) and *"tha"* (moon), symbolizes the union of opposing energies—*Pingala* (pranic force) and *Ida* (mental force). Its goal is to balance these energies so that prana flows through the *Sushumna Nadi*, leading to expanded consciousness and spiritual growth. Rooted in texts like the *Hatha Yoga Pradipika*, *Shiva Samhita*, and *Gheranda Samhita*, Hatha Yoga emphasizes physical purification, strength, and inner discipline. The *Gheranda Samhita* outlines seven progressive steps in Hatha Yoga – from bodily purification through cleansing practices (*shodhanam*), Steadiness through Asanas (Dhridata), Calmness through mudras and bandhas (Sthairyam), Patience through sense withdrawal (Dhairyam), Lightness of body through pranayama (Laghavam), Direct perception through concentration and meditations (Dhyana, Dharana & Pratyaksham) and self-realization (*samadhi*). The foundational practices of Hatha Yoga include the *Shatkarmas,* six cleansing techniques: nasal cleansing (*Neti*), digestive tract cleansing (*Dhauti*), Abdominal massage (*Nauli*), Colon cleansing (*Basti*), Frontal brain cleansing (*Kapalbhati*), and Focused gazing (*Trataka*). These purify the body and mind, preparing the practitioner for higher yogic practices (Satyananda Saraswati, 1996).

In the modern era, yoga has evolved into various styles that blend traditional principles with contemporary needs, often emphasizing physical fitness, stress relief, and mental well-being. While synthesizing the conceptual frameworks of Yoga advocated in the early Vedic texts with either of the two classical practice systems of Raja Yoga and Hatha Yoga, these forms adapt practices for diverse populations and lifestyles. Some such popular styles include,

Iyengar Yoga – Iyengar Yoga is a style of yoga developed by B. K. S. Iyengar, an Indian yoga teacher and author. It emphasizes precision, alignment, and detail in the performance of yoga postures (asanas) and breath control (pranayama). Iyengar Yoga is known for its systematic approach using props such as belts, blocks, and blankets to help practitioners perform poses correctly and safely, making it accessible to people of all ages and abilities

Bikram Yoga – This style is developed and propagated by Bikram Choudary based on the teachings of B.C. Ghosh, a Hatha Yoga practitioner. In this style, a set sequence of 26 postures and two breathing exercises are practiced in a heated room, set to approximately 105°F (40.5°C) with about 40% humidity. The heat helps warm muscles, increase flexibility, promote detoxification through sweating, and improve blood circulation. This method is designed to enhance strength, balance, endurance, and mental concentration, making it a physically and mentally demanding yoga style

Kundalini Yoga – Kundalini Yoga is an ancient spiritual discipline aimed at awakening the dormant energy (Kundalini) coiled at the base of the spine. This energy, conceptualized as a serpent, rises through the body's chakras—energy centers—leading to heightened spiritual awareness and self-realization. The practice combines physical postures (asanas), breath control (pranayama), meditation, mantra chanting, and mudras (hand gestures) to stimulate and guide this energy upwards through the body's energy channels (nadis). It synthesizes elements of Bhakti (devotion), Raja (mental control), and Shakti (energy expression) Yogas, integrating influences from Tantra and Hatha Yoga.

Power Yoga – Power Yoga is a vigorous and dynamic form of yoga that emphasizes building muscular strength, flexibility, and endurance through fast-paced, flowing sequences of traditional yoga poses. It is rooted in Ashtanga yoga but is less rigid in structure, allowing instructors to create varied, energetic classes focused on continuous movement linked with breath control. Unlike more meditative yoga styles, Power Yoga prioritizes cardiovascular fitness, muscle toning, and stamina, often resembling an intense workout with minimal rest and emphasizing physical conditioning

Ashtanga Vinyasa Yoga – Ashtanga Vinyasa Yoga is a dynamic, physically demanding style of yoga that links a fixed sequence of postures (asanas) through flowing movements synchronized with breath, known as vinyasa. The term "Ashtanga" means "eight limbs," referring to the eightfold path of yoga philosophy outlined in

Patanjali's Yoga Sutras, encompassing ethical guidelines, breath control, postures, concentration, and meditation. This style was popularized in the 20th century by Sri K. Pattabhi Jois, who studied under Sri T. Krishnamacharya, the father of modern yoga

Vinyasa Yoga – Vinyasa Yoga is another popular contemporary style said to be evolved from Ashtanga Vinyasa Yoga. It is a dynamic style of yoga characterized by a continuous, flowing sequence of postures linked with breath, often called "flow yoga." The word "Vinyasa" means "to place in a special way," reflecting its emphasis on deliberate, mindful movement. In practice, each movement corresponds to either an inhale or an exhale, creating a rhythmic, breath-synchronized flow that enhances focus and physical challenge

Therapeutic Yoga – It is a specialized form of yoga that applies yogic techniques—such as gentle asanas (postures), breath control (pranayama), meditation, and relaxation—to aid in healing and managing physical, mental, and emotional health conditions. It focuses on adapting yoga practices to the individual's needs to alleviate symptoms, improve mobility, reduce stress, and enhance overall well-being. Unlike general yoga, it emphasizes therapeutic benefits tailored to specific problems such as chronic pain, anxiety, insomnia, respiratory issues, and other health challenges

These styles support mindfulness by promoting sustained attention, body-breath coordination, and conscious awareness—key components of contemplative practice.

Informal Practices

Informal mindfulness practice refers to applying mindfulness principles to moments of daily life such as eating, walking, household chores like washing and cleaning, listening to other person, taking time to unwind. When approached with full attention and acceptance, even mundane actions become opportunities for presence. This everyday mindfulness is where the practice become lived: not just as a technique, but a way of being.

Mindful Walking: In this practice a simple act of walking is turned into a field of awareness. By paying attention to the lifting, moving, and placing of each foot, practitioners synchronize body and mind. The rhythm of walking provides a natural cadence for presence, offering a moving counterpart to seated meditation.

Mindful Eating: It encourages attention to the sensory experience of food – the texture, flavour, aroma and even the process of chewing and swallowing. By slowing down and observing one's habitual impulses around food, this practice fosters appreciation, gratitude, and a reorientation toward nourishment rather than compulsion

Mindful Conversation: It involves engaging in conversations with intentional presence. It includes actively listening without interrupting, judging or mentally preparing a response. Attention is directed to the speaker's tone, expressions and one's own bodily sensations and breath. When the mind drifts, the breath serves as an anchor to return to the present moment. This practice fosters authentic connection, empathy and emotional regulation, even in brief exchanges.

Mindful Driving or Commuting: Mindful commuting involves transforming daily travel into an opportunity for present-moment awareness. Whether driving or using public transport, attention is directed to bodily posture, the grip on the steering wheel or seat, and the sensations of motion. Environmental sounds—traffic, engine noise, or nearby conversations—are observed without judgment. When stress, impatience, or distraction arises, it is acknowledged, and attention is gently returned to the experience of traveling. This practice cultivates patience, reduces reactivity, and embeds mindfulness into everyday movement

Mindful Personal Care: Personal care routines—such as brushing teeth, bathing, or grooming—can serve as accessible opportunities to cultivate mindfulness. Rather than performing these tasks on autopilot, attention is directed to sensory details: the taste of toothpaste, the scent of shampoo, the temperature and sound of water, and the rhythm of breathing. Awareness is brought to each movement and sensation. When the mind wanders, it is gently redirected to the present moment with curiosity and non-judgment. This practice fosters grounding and enhances everyday presence

Mindful Daily activities: Routine chores—such as washing dishes, folding laundry, or cleaning—can become valuable mindfulness practices when approached with full attention. By focusing on a single task, one observes the sensory details: the warmth of water, the texture of fabric, the motion of the body. Distractions and thoughts are acknowledged without resistance, and awareness is gently returned to the task. This simple yet powerful practice cultivates presence, patience, and embodied awareness in the midst of everyday life

Clinical Practices

Mindfulness began entering clinical practices in the late major impetus arising from the development of Mindfulness-Based Stress Reduction (MBSR) by Jon Kabat-Zinn in 1979. Its rise marked the advent of *"third wave"* psychotherapies—an evolution beyond the first wave of therapies arising from behaviour perspective and second wave of therapies arising from cognitive-behaviour perspective. This classification was proposed by Steven C. Hayes and colleagues, particularly in the context of emerging therapies like Acceptance and Commitment Therapy (ACT) and Dialectical Behaviour Therapy (DBT) that incorporated mindfulness principles. Third wave therapies integrate mindfulness and acceptance strategies, focusing on changing one's relationship to thoughts and feelings rather than attempting to modify their content. This approach emphasizes non-judgmental awareness, psychological flexibility, and value-driven action as central to treatment. In Mindfulness Based Therapies (MBT) the therapists train their clients to pay attention to present-moment experience, to develop an attitude of self-acceptance and non-reactivity to momentary experience. Key therapies that integrated mindfulness include,

Gestalt Therapy: Gestalt therapy is a humanistic and experiential form of psychotherapy that emphasizes awareness, personal responsibility, and living in the present moment. Pioneered by Fritz Perls, Laura Perls, and Paul Goodman during the 1940s and 1950s, it focuses on how individuals experience and make meaning of their lives in the here and now, rather than analysing past events in isolation. Gestalt therapy supports individuals in becoming more aware of their present thoughts, feelings, and behaviours, thereby fostering deeper self-understanding and healthier choices. Many of the core tenets of Gestalt therapy - such as present-centered awareness, non-judgmental observation, and contact with the immediate –experience align closely with the essential features of mindfulness. Recognizing this natural affinity, Gestalt therapists began to explicitly incorporate mindfulness practices into their therapeutic approach. This integration became more pronounced with the increasing influence of Eastern contemplative traditions and the emergence of mindfulness-based interventions within Western psychology.

Mindfulness Based Stress Reduction (MBSR): It is an evidence-based therapeutic program developed by Jon Kabat-Zinn in 1979 at the University of Massachusetts Medical Center. MBSR was originally created to assist patients in managing chronic pain and stress-related disorders that were resistant to conventional medical treatments. It has since evolved into a widely adopted intervention across medical, psychological, and educational settings. The standard MBSR program spans eight weeks, typically delivered in a group format. Each weekly session lasts approximately 2.5 hours, supplemented by a full-day silent retreat during the sixth week. Participants are introduced to a range of mindfulness practices, including body scan meditation, sitting meditation, mindful yoga, and walking meditation. The program emphasizes the cultivation of non-judgmental awareness of the present moment and encourages participants to relate differently to physical discomfort, difficult emotions, and stressful thoughts. The theoretical foundation of MBSR draws from Buddhist contemplative traditions, particularly Vipassana (insight) meditation, but it is presented in a secular, evidence-informed framework suitable for diverse populations. The program does not promote any religious or spiritual doctrine, making it broadly accessible. MBSR has been extensively studied and shown to reduce symptoms of stress, anxiety, depression, and chronic pain. Neuroimaging and physiological research suggest that regular mindfulness practice through MBSR can lead to functional and structural changes in brain regions associated with attention regulation, emotional processing, and interoception (Pomerantz, 2020)

Acceptance and Commitment Therapy (ACT): Acceptance and Commitment Therapy (ACT) developed by Steven C. Hayes and colleagues, is a modern behavioural intervention focused on enhancing psychological flexibility – the ability to openly accept the internal experiences while committing to actions aligned with personal values. ACT is grounded in Relational Frame Theory (RFT), which explains how language and cognition contribute to psychological suffering. While it maintains the belief that thoughts shape our feelings and behaviour, ACT posits that accepting those thoughts, rather than trying to change them, is essential to success ACT teaches clients to embrace their emotions, thoughts and bodily sensations without avoidance or resistance, recognizing that attempting to control or escape these experiences often exacerbates psychological distress. Beyond acceptance, ACT emphasizes values clarification and committed action. Therapists help clients identify what matters most to them, encouraging a firm commitment to live in accordance with these values. Action consistent with personal values bridges insight and behaviour, supporting meaningful, purposeful living. The approach contrasts unhelpful psychological patterns – summarized in the acronym FEAR (Fusion, Evaluation, Avoidance, Reason-giving) – with productive processes in ACT – Acceptance, Choice based on values and Taking committee action. Together, these elements form a comprehensive framework integrating mindfulness, acceptance, and behaviour change to promote mental health and well-being (Pomerantz, 2020).

Mindfulness Based Cognitive Therapy (MBCT): It is a structured psychotherapeutic approach that integrates cognitive behavioral therapy (CBT) techniques with mindfulness practices. Developed in the 1990s by therapists including Zindel Segal, Mark Williams, and John Teasdale, MBCT was originally designed to prevent relapse in recurrent depression but has since been applied to other mental health conditions such as anxiety. It combines awareness and acceptance of present-moment experiences with traditional cognitive interventions, helping individuals observe their thoughts and feelings nonjudgmentally rather than reacting automatically or getting entangled in negative thought patterns. Core components of MBCT include mindfulness meditation exercises such as body scans, mindful breathing, and mindful movement, alongside cognitive strategies to identify and disengage from habitual negative thinking. Participants are guided through practices that foster present-moment awareness, acceptance of internal experiences, and the breaking of cycles of rumination and worry. Group discussions and reflective exercises help reinforce learning and support behavior change. Typically delivered in an eight-week course with weekly sessions, MBCT empowers individuals to develop skills that reduce relapse risk by enhancing emotional regulation, cognitive flexibility, and resilience through a compassionate, experiential approach.

Dialectic Behavioural Therapy (DBT): This therapy developed by Marasha Linehan primarily to treat borderline personality disorder (BPD), is founded on the concept that BPD is fundamentally a disorder of emotional dysregulation arising from a combination of biological vulnerability and an invalidating environment. Individual with BPD often experience intense emotions and learn extreme emotional responses because their feelings were frequently invalidated in their families, leading to maladaptive behaviors and high risk of suicidality. DBT combines problem-solving, validation and dialectics – the balancing of acceptance and change – to help clients manage emotions and behaviours more effectively. Therapists support clients in strategizing for better outcomes, intensely validating their feelings as understandable and important, while simultaneously encouraging behaviour change. The dialectical framework requires accepting clients as they are while motivating change, striking a delicate balance to avoid feelings of invalidation in clients. The therapy includes four main skill training modules that address emotional and interpersonal challenges common in BPD: 1) Emotion regulation teaches clients to identify and accept emotions rather than avoid them; 2) Distress tolerance focuses on self-soothing and managing impulses to reduce harmful behaviours like self-injury and substance abuse, 3) interpersonal effectiveness develops assertiveness and social skills for maintaining healthy relationships despite emotional turmoil and 4) Mindfulness cultivates present-moment awareness and non-judgmental observation of internal states. These skills teach clients practical strategies to tolerate distress, regulate intense emotions, communicate effectively and stay grounded in the present. DBT's unique dialectical approach synthesizes acceptance of current painful experiences with commitment to meaningful change, making it a highly effective, empirically supported treatment for BPD and other disorders involving emotional dysregulation (Pomerantz, 2020).

CONTEMPORARY SIGNIFICANCE OF MINDFULNESS

At the individual level, mindfulness enhances cognitive, emotional, and physiological functioning. Contemporary life is characterized by rapid technological change, information overload, and constant multitasking, which increase stress, anxiety, and attentional fragmentation. Mindfulness practices strengthen attentional control, emotional regulation, and self-awareness, facilitating adaptive coping with stressors. Mindfulness promotes metacognitive awareness, enabling individuals to observe thought patterns and emotional reactions without reactivity, thereby fostering mental flexibility, resilience, and psychological well-being. In essence, mindfulness allows the individual to optimize cognitive and emotional resources in an increasingly complex environment.

At the societal level, mindfulness contributes to social cohesion, collaborative problem-solving, and ethical behavior. When practiced broadly, it encourages empathy, compassion, and prosocial attitudes, which can reduce conflict and promote cooperative engagement. In organizational, educational, and healthcare contexts, mindfulness interventions improve interpersonal communication, reduce burnout, and enhance productivity. Mindfulness operates as a collective cognitive-cultural mechanism, whereby widespread cultivation of awareness and emotional regulation strengthens the social fabric, supporting sustainable social functioning in increasingly diverse and high-pressure societies.

From a species-level perspective, mindfulness may be viewed as an adaptive behavioral and cognitive strategy that fosters long-term survival. By enhancing self-regulation, attention, and stress management, mindfulness supports behaviors that are aligned with sustainable decision-making and environmental stewardship. In evolutionary terms, mindfulness facilitates reflective rather than impulsive responses, improving individual and collective resilience to unpredictable ecological and social challenges. Mindfulness represents a bio-cultural adaptive mechanism, linking cognition, behavior, and culture to optimize survival and well-being at both the individual and species levels

NEUROPLASTICITY AND MINDFULNESS: EMPIRICAL INSIGHTS AND EVIDENCE

The relationship between mindfulness and neuroplasticity represents one of the most compelling intersections of contemporary neuroscience and contemplative science. Neuroplasticity provides a biological framework for understanding how mental training can alter brain structure and function. Mindfulness practices, encompassing meditative, embodied, and integrative approaches, serve as experiential vehicles through which such plasticity is cultivated. Over the past decade, neuroimaging and electrophysiological research have demonstrated that sustained mindfulness practice can modify both structural integrity (e.g., cortical thickness, gray matter density) and functional dynamics (e.g., connectivity, oscillatory coherence) within networks governing attention, emotion, and self-awareness. These findings substantiate the long-held contemplative premise that mental discipline can reshape neural architecture—a phenomenon now empirically established through the lens of modern neuroscience. The following sections examine how formal, clinical, and informal mindfulness practices differentially contribute to structural and functional neuroplasticity, highlighting both their empirical strengths and methodological limitations

NEUROPLASTICITY AND FORMAL PRACTICES OF MINDFULNESS

Yoga and Meditation are two principal formal practices that have received extensive neuroscientific investigation in the past decade. Recent systematic reviews and meta-analyses collectively suggest that these practices may facilitate neuroplasticity through distinct yet overlapping neural mechanism

Yoga and Neuroplasticity

Yoga integrates physical postures (asanas), breath regulation (pranayama), and meditative awareness to harmonize body and mind. Over the last decade, systematic reviews have synthesized neuroimaging and behavioral studies to elucidate how yoga influences brain structure and function.

Gothe et al. (2019) conducted one of the earliest comprehensive reviews of yoga neuroimaging research, summarizing findings from structural MRI, functional MRI, and EEG studies. Their synthesis revealed consistent increases in gray-matter volume and cortical thickness in the hippocampus, prefrontal cortex (PFC), anterior cingulate cortex (ACC), and insula, regions implicated in attention regulation, memory, and emotional control. These neuroanatomical alterations were accompanied by improved executive function and emotion-regulation performance, suggesting that yoga engages neurocognitive networks governing self-monitoring and stress adaptation.

Building upon this, Verzili et al. (2023) conducted a systematic review and meta-analysis focused on yoga and neuropsychiatric aging. They reported significant associations between regular yoga practice and structural preservation in the hippocampus and prefrontal regions, supporting the hypothesis that yoga mitigates age-related cortical decline. The authors attributed these findings to enhanced neurotrophic signaling and autonomic balance, both of which support synaptic maintenance and neurogenesis.

Similarly, Han et al. (2023) synthesized evidence from yoga, tai chi, and qigong studies, highlighting altered functional connectivity in the default-mode network (DMN), salience network, and sensorimotor circuits. These findings imply that embodied contemplative practices—of which yoga is a prime example—facilitate large-scale network integration, leading to improved attentional flexibility and interoceptive accuracy.

Proposed mechanisms across these reviews emphasize multimodal neural engagement. Yoga simultaneously recruits proprioceptive, interoceptive, and cognitive processes, activating fronto-limbic and sensorimotor circuits. Regular practice has been associated with reduced hypothalamic–pituitary–adrenal (HPA) axis activation and lower cortisol levels, suggesting that stress-reduction pathways may mediate neural plasticity (Gothe et al., 2016; Verzili et al., 2023). Reviews also highlight autonomic modulation—specifically enhanced vagal tone—as a likely contributor to hippocampal and prefrontal cortical preservation.

Despite these encouraging trends, all reviews converge on similar methodological limitations. Studies often feature small, heterogeneous samples, variable yoga styles (e.g., Hatha, Iyengar, Kundalini), inconsistent intervention duration, and diverse imaging modalities. Few trials include active control groups, and long-term follow-up data remain scarce. Accordingly, causal inferences about yoga-induced neuroplasticity must remain provisional.

In sum, systematic evidence suggests that yoga fosters neuroplastic adaptations in brain networks underpinning attention, emotion regulation, and interoception. However, higher-quality randomized controlled trials (RCTs) with standardized protocols are required to substantiate the magnitude and durability of these neural changes

Meditation and Neuroplasticity

Formal mindfulness meditation—including focused attention (FA), open monitoring (OM), and compassion-based techniques—has likewise been extensively examined for its neural correlates. A decade of systematic reviews and meta-analyses indicates that meditation practice is linked to both structural and functional brain reorganization.

Pernet et al. (2021) performed a meta-analysis of MRI studies investigating gray-matter correlates of mindfulness practice. They identified the right anterior insula as the most consistently altered region across studies, with additional changes in the ACC, hippocampus, and somatomotor cortices. These regions are integral to interoception, cognitive control, and emotion regulation, suggesting that meditation reshapes neural substrates of self-awareness and executive functioning. However, Pernet and colleagues cautioned that study heterogeneity and limited sample sizes may inflate effect estimates.

Calderone et al. (2024) extended this line of inquiry by integrating multimodal evidence from MRI, EEG, and biochemical markers. Their review concluded that mindfulness practice reduces amygdala reactivity, enhances cortical thickness in attention-related areas, and alters connectivity between the DMN, salience, and frontoparietal control networks. These neural shifts were paralleled by reductions in stress biomarkers and improved emotion-regulation capacity, implying a multi-systemic plastic response to meditative training.

In a complementary meta-analysis, Siew et al. (2023) focused exclusively on RCTs. While they confirmed small but significant increases in gray-matter density in the insula and precentral gyrus, they also noted that well-controlled large-sample studies sometimes yield null results. This suggests that meditation's neuroplastic effects may depend on practice intensity, duration, and individual variability.

Mechanistically, meditation is thought to induce neuroplasticity through repeated recruitment of attention and emotion-regulation circuits. Sustained attentional focus engages the ACC and dorsolateral PFC, while open monitoring and compassion practices enhance insula-mediated interoceptive awareness and limbic down-regulation (Calderone et al., 2024; Pernet et al., 2021). Over time, these repeated activations may lead to synaptic strengthening and functional reconfiguration of large-scale networks. Peripheral mediators such as reduced cortisol and elevated brain-derived neurotrophic factor (BDNF) have been proposed, though findings remain inconsistent.

As with yoga, methodological variability persists. Reviews consistently highlight small sample sizes, diverse meditation techniques, inconsistent reporting of practice dosage, and lack of active controls. Publication bias and analytical flexibility further complicate interpretation. Recent reviews thus emphasize the need for pre-registered, multi-site RCTs employing standardized imaging protocols and longitudinal follow-ups to confirm causality

Comparative Perspectives: Yoga and Meditation in Relations to Neuroplasticity

When viewed through the lens of contemporary neuroimaging and systematic review evidence, both yoga and meditation emerge as potent facilitators of neuroplasticity, each engaging overlapping yet distinct neural mechanisms. Across multiple systematic reviews and meta-analyses, a convergent theme is the activation and structural modification of regions involved in interoception, attention regulation, and emotion modulation—notably the *insula*, *anterior cingulate cortex (ACC)*, *prefrontal cortex (PFC)*, *amygdala*, and *hippocampus*. These findings suggest that both practices, despite differences in form and technique, share a common neuro-functional architecture supporting adaptive brain changes.

Yoga, as a multimodal mind–body discipline, integrates physical postures, regulated breathing, attentional focus, and contemplative awareness. This unique synthesis appears to recruit a broad range of neural systems. In addition to fronto-limbic and interoceptive circuits, systematic reviews emphasize yoga's influence on sensorimotor, vestibular, and autonomic networks, reflecting the embodied nature of the practice. The engagement of these circuits is thought to promote hippocampal and prefrontal preservation, enhance emotional regulation, and modulate stress-related pathways through improved autonomic control.

Meditation, in contrast, is a purely attentional and cognitive training practice, emphasizing sustained focus, meta-awareness, and emotional balance. Reviews of formal mindfulness meditation consistently report neuroplastic changes in regions underpinning attentional control and self-referential processing, particularly within the *anterior insula* and *ACC*, and in the dynamic interplay between the default mode network (DMN), salience network (SN), and frontoparietal control network (FPN). Through iterative engagement of these systems, meditation appears to refine the neural substrates of monitoring, self-regulation, and cognitive flexibility.

Thus, while both practices share a common neuroplastic signature, their mechanistic emphases differ. Yoga's effects are mediated by an integrative combination of *somatic movement, breath regulation,* and *interoceptive awareness*, leading to a more embodied form of neural adaptation that encompasses autonomic and motor domains. Meditation, meanwhile, cultivates *cognitive and emotional regulation* through sustained mental practice, producing neuroplastic changes primarily in *attentional, interoceptive,* and *default mode* systems.

Despite encouraging findings, systematic reviews across both domains converge on a cautious interpretation. The strength of evidence is characterized as promising yet methodologically limited. Both literatures are affected by small sample sizes, heterogeneous protocols, and inconsistent control conditions. While neuroplasticity is consistently observed, the magnitude, reliability, and regional specificity of such changes remain uncertain. The current consensus therefore advocates for more rigorous, standardized, and longitudinal investigations to substantiate these preliminary insights into yoga- and meditation-induced brain plasticity

Directions for Future Research

Systematic reviews in both yoga and meditation studies underscore a set of convergent priorities for advancing the field of mindfulness-based neuroplasticity research. The foremost recommendation is the implementation of large-scale, preregistered randomized controlled trials (RCTs) that include *active control groups*. Such designs are essential to differentiate specific practice effects from nonspecific influences such as expectancy, social interaction, or general physical activity.

Equally critical is the standardization of practice-dose reporting. Many studies fail to provide adequate information regarding session duration, frequency, and home practice adherence, which obscures dose–response relationships. Future research should integrate objective adherence measures—such as digital practice logs or sensor-based tracking—to ensure accurate quantification of practice intensity and exposure.

The field also requires a multimodal neuroimaging approach that combines structural MRI, functional MRI, and diffusion tensor imaging (DTI), with occasional use of MR spectroscopy or PET imaging when ethically and practically feasible. Employing consistent preprocessing pipelines and analytic frameworks would enhance comparability across studies and allow meta-analytic synthesis with greater precision.

Furthermore, researchers are encouraged to include peripheral biological markers—such as cortisol, brain-derived neurotrophic factor (BDNF), and indices of autonomic regulation—to explore indirect pathways linking contemplative practice to neural adaptation. However, systematic reviews caution that such biomarkers should be interpreted prudently, as they provide correlational rather than causal evidence of central neuroplasticity.

Another emerging frontier involves examining dose–response relationships and individual differences. Variables such as age, baseline cognitive function, and genetic predispositions may influence neuroplastic responsiveness to mindfulness-based interventions. Longitudinal designs with extended follow-ups are necessary to determine whether structural and functional brain changes are sustained, reversible, or progressive over time.

In sum, future research on yoga and meditation should integrate rigorous methodological design, standardized reporting practices, and multimodal measurement strategies to build a robust, replicable evidence base. Such an integrative and methodologically sophisticated approach will be crucial to elucidating how formal contemplative practices induce measurable neuroplastic transformations, thereby bridging the gap between experiential training and neural adaptation in the human brain.

NEUROPLASTICITY AND INFORMAL PRACTICES OF MINDFULNESS

While formal and clinical mindfulness practices have been extensively studied for their neuroplastic effects, emerging research suggests that informal mindfulness can also induce significant neural changes, enhancing cognitive and emotional functioning

Neuroplastic effects of Informal Mindfulness Practices

Recent studies have begun to explore the neural underpinnings of informal mindfulness. For instance, a systematic review by Calderone (2024) highlighted that both formal and informal mindfulness practices can lead to neuroplastic changes, including increased cortical thickness and enhanced connectivity in brain regions associated with attention, emotional regulation, and memory. These findings suggest that engaging in everyday mindful activities can foster neural adaptations that support improved cognitive and emotional well-being.

Additionally, research indicates that informal mindfulness practices can modulate brain activity patterns. For example, engaging in mindful listening or mindful walking has been associated with increased activation in the prefrontal cortex and decreased activity in the default mode network, regions implicated in self-referential thinking and mind-wandering. These changes reflect a shift towards more adaptive neural processing, promoting greater focus and emotional balance.

Functional and Clinical Implications

Informal mindfulness practices, by their very nature, promote the continual integration of awareness into everyday experiences. When individuals bring mindful attention to routine activities such as walking, eating, or listening, the brain undergoes adaptive changes that strengthen attentional and regulatory capacities. This ongoing engagement facilitates enhanced attention and cognitive control, as the practitioner learns to sustain focus and monitor distractions with greater precision. Over time, these neural adaptations translate into improved task performance, decision-making efficiency, and cognitive flexibility.

A key functional implication lies in emotional regulation. Mindfulness integrated into daily life enables individuals to observe emotional states as they arise, reducing the automaticity of reactive responses. Such awareness promotes adaptive emotion regulation strategies, thereby lessening the intensity of stress and anxiety in daily contexts. This self-observational stance also nurtures heightened self-awareness, allowing individuals to understand their internal processes, motivations, and behavioral patterns with greater clarity. Ultimately, this deepened insight supports personal growth and psychological well-being.

Furthermore, informal mindfulness contributes significantly to stress reduction. By cultivating moment-to-moment awareness throughout the day, individuals develop a greater capacity to recognize stress triggers and employ mindful responses instead of habitual reactions. As a result, informal mindfulness practices not only reinforce neural pathways linked to attentional stability and emotional balance but also provide a sustainable means of enhancing overall mental health

Strengths and Limitations of the Evidence

The growing body of research on informal mindfulness practices demonstrates several notable strengths. One of the most significant is their accessibility. Unlike formal meditation or structured mindfulness programs, informal mindfulness requires no specialized training, environment, or equipment. This accessibility enables individuals from diverse backgrounds to integrate mindful awareness seamlessly into their daily routines. Another advantage is consistency. Because informal mindfulness can be practiced repeatedly throughout the day—during activities such as eating, walking, or working—it fosters a more continuous and enduring engagement with mindfulness, which is a crucial factor in promoting neuroplastic change. Additionally, the practical relevance of informal mindfulness enhances its real-world applicability, as the practice directly targets the contexts in which stress and emotional reactivity naturally occur.

Despite these strengths, several limitations must be acknowledged. The first is the lack of standardization in practice. Informal mindfulness varies widely across individuals and settings, making it difficult to define or replicate in controlled research environments. This variability poses challenges for establishing consistent intervention protocols and comparing outcomes across studies. A second limitation involves measurement challenges. Capturing the subtle neural effects of informal mindfulness requires advanced neuroimaging and physiological tools, which are often resource-intensive and impractical for large-scale studies. Finally, there is a limited amount of longitudinal data. Although short-term findings are promising, long-term research examining the sustained neuroplastic effects of informal mindfulness is still emerging. Addressing these limitations will be vital for developing a more robust evidence base.

Implications and Future Directions

The evidence highlighting the neuroplastic potential of informal mindfulness practices has significant implications for both research and applied contexts. Conceptually, it reinforces the idea that mindfulness need not be confined to formal sessions but can be cultivated as a pervasive mode of awareness that continuously shapes brain and behavior. This perspective suggests that everyday activities can serve as powerful vehicles for cognitive and emotional transformation, provided they are performed with mindful attention.

Future research should focus on standardizing informal mindfulness interventions, identifying the most effective strategies for integrating mindfulness into daily life, and clarifying their neural correlates. The development of reliable measurement tools—including neuroimaging protocols and behavioral markers—will be essential for quantifying these subtle yet meaningful changes. Longitudinal studies, in particular, are needed to explore the long-term neural and psychological adaptations resulting from sustained informal mindfulness practice. Moreover, examining the synergistic effects of combining formal and informal mindfulness approaches could yield a more comprehensive model for enhancing cognitive flexibility, emotional regulation, and psychological resilience.

In sum, the growing interest in informal mindfulness practices marks an important shift toward a more holistic and accessible understanding of mindfulness. By embedding awareness into the fabric of daily living, individuals can harness neuroplastic processes that promote enduring cognitive and emotional well-being, bridging the gap between contemplative training and everyday functioning.

NEUROPLASTICITY AND CLINICAL PRATICES OF MINDFULNESS

Clinical mindfulness interventions refer to structured, evidence-based programs designed for populations with diagnosed or subclinical conditions, such as depression, anxiety, post-traumatic stress disorder (PTSD), and mild cognitive impairment (MCI). The most widely studied interventions include Mindfulness-Based Cognitive Therapy (MBCT) and Mindfulness-Based Stress Reduction (MBSR). Over the past decade, systematic reviews and meta-analyses have examined the impact of these interventions on both clinical outcomes and neural plasticity, providing insight into the mechanisms underlying symptom improvement.

Neuroplastic Effects on Mindfulness-Based Cognitive Therapy in clinical populations

Mindfulness-Based Cognitive Therapy (MBCT) integrates mindfulness meditation with cognitive-behavioral strategies to prevent relapse in depression and to support emotion regulation in clinical populations. Gkintoni, Vassilopoulos, and Nikolaou (2025) reviewed 87 studies on MBCT across various clinical populations and found that MBCT not only significantly reduces symptoms of depression and anxiety but is also associated with neuroplastic changes. Neuroimaging evidence indicates increased activation in the prefrontal cortex, decreased amygdala reactivity, and enhanced functional connectivity within networks responsible for emotion regulation and self-awareness. These findings suggest that MBCT engages neural circuits involved in cognitive control, attentional allocation, and interoceptive awareness. However, the review also emphasizes the need for long-term studies to establish the durability of these changes.

Neuroplastic Changes in Aging and Cognitive Impairment

In older adults with mild cognitive impairment (MCI), mindfulness-based interventions (MBIs) have been investigated for their potential to mitigate age-related cognitive decline. Leow et al. (2023) conducted a systematic review and meta-analysis of ten randomized controlled trials in older adults with MCI. Their findings indicate increased cortical thickness in frontal-parietal regions and the left inferior temporal gyrus and improved functional connectivity involving the posterior cingulate cortex, bilateral medial prefrontal cortex, and left hippocampus. These structural and functional adaptations suggest that MBIs may promote plasticity in memory- and attention-related networks. Despite these neural changes, pooled analyses showed that MBIs did not produce statistically significant improvements in global cognition, attention, or memory compared to active controls. This underscores the complexity of translating neuroplastic changes into observable clinical benefits

Neuroplastic Changes in Major Depressive Disorder

In patients with major depressive disorder (MDD), MBIs have been evaluated for their effects on neural circuits implicated in emotion regulation and cognitive control. A systematic review examining eight studies reported modulation of prefrontal, basal ganglia, anterior and posterior cingulate, and parietal cortices following mindfulness interventions (Neacsiu et al., 2018). Increased activation and connectivity in these regions were linked to improved attentional control, enhanced self-awareness, and decreased rumination. However, methodological heterogeneity—including variability in imaging tasks, intervention duration, and control groups—limits the strength of causal conclusion

Neural Mechanism Across Clinical Populations

Across diverse clinical populations, mindfulness-based interventions have been shown to modulate specific neural circuits underlying attention, emotion regulation, and self-awareness. The most consistently reported regions include the prefrontal cortex (PFC), anterior cingulate cortex (ACC), posterior cingulate cortex (PCC), hippocampus, insula, and amygdala. These regions constitute interconnected networks responsible for executive control, interoceptive awareness, and the regulation of affective responses.

The prefrontal cortex plays a central role in cognitive control, planning, and attentional regulation. Mindfulness practice appears to enhance activity and connectivity within this region, facilitating greater top-down regulation of thought and emotion. The anterior cingulate cortex, a region critical for conflict monitoring and emotion regulation, exhibits strengthened activation following mindfulness-based interventions, reflecting improved attentional engagement and adaptive emotional responding. Similarly, the posterior cingulate cortex, often associated with self-referential processing and default-mode network activity, shows altered connectivity patterns, suggesting a shift from habitual, self-focused rumination to a more adaptive, present-centered awareness.

The hippocampus, which is highly sensitive to chronic stress, demonstrates increased gray matter volume and connectivity after sustained mindfulness training, particularly in older adults and individuals with mood disorders. This structural enhancement is believed to support improved memory consolidation and contextual regulation of emotional responses. Parallel changes are observed in the insula, a key hub for interoceptive awareness and integration of bodily states. Strengthening of insular activity following mindfulness practice may contribute to improved emotion perception and bodily awareness, fundamental to self-regulation and resilience.

In contrast, the amygdala, known for its role in emotional reactivity and stress processing, shows reduced activation after mindfulness training. This downregulation corresponds with decreases in negative affect and anxiety, indicating enhanced inhibitory control over limbic responses. Functional imaging studies further suggest that mindfulness fosters stronger connectivity between the amygdala and prefrontal regions, supporting more balanced emotional regulation.

Electrophysiological evidence from clinical populations, particularly individuals with post-traumatic stress disorder (PTSD), corroborates these neuroimaging findings. Studies reveal increases in frontal theta and alpha power and modulation of heartbeat-evoked potentials, indicating enhanced integration of interoceptive and attentional processes. These neural adjustments are associated with symptom reduction and improved cognitive control, reflecting mindfulness's ability to recalibrate neurocognitive systems that have been dysregulated by stress or trauma

Strengths and Limitations of Evidence

The body of evidence exploring neuroplastic changes following clinical mindfulness interventions demonstrates several notable strengths. Foremost, numerous studies have shown consistent improvements in psychological symptoms, accompanied by measurable changes in brain structure and function. Such changes are most commonly observed in regions subserving attention, emotion regulation, and self-awareness, including the prefrontal cortex, anterior cingulate cortex, and insula. Additionally, in aging populations, there is emerging evidence that mindfulness-based interventions may help preserve or even enhance cortical thickness and functional connectivity, suggesting a neuroprotective role in cognitive aging. The convergence of findings across various clinical conditions underscores the reliability of these neural patterns and their potential relevance to clinical outcomes.

Despite these encouraging findings, significant limitations constrain the strength of the conclusions that can be drawn. A recurring issue across studies is the small sample size, which limits statistical power and generalizability. Similarly, many interventions are of short duration, and few studies include long-term follow-up to determine the persistence of neural and behavioral changes over time. The heterogeneity of mindfulness protocols—ranging from Mindfulness-Based Cognitive Therapy (MBCT) to Mindfulness-Based Stress Reduction (MBSR) and other adaptations—introduces further variability, as does the diversity of patient populations, imaging modalities, and outcome measures employed.

Another limitation concerns the lack of consistent correlation between neural changes and clinical improvement. For instance, in studies of mild cognitive impairment, structural and connectivity changes were observed without corresponding statistically significant enhancements in cognitive performance compared with active controls. Moreover, potential publication bias and inconsistent reporting of intervention dosage or participant adherence make it difficult to evaluate dose-dependent effects or replicate findings across laboratories. These methodological and reporting inconsistencies highlight the need for greater standardization and transparency in future research designs.

IMPLICATIONS AND FUTURE DIRECTIONS

The emerging evidence from clinical research strongly suggests that mindfulness-based interventions support neuroplastic adaptations within networks responsible for attention, emotional regulation, and self-awareness. These neural modifications provide a plausible mechanistic explanation for the clinical improvements observed in diverse disorders, from depression and anxiety to PTSD and cognitive decline. Understanding these mechanisms enhances the conceptual foundation of clinical mindfulness practice and helps refine therapeutic applications for specific populations.

Future research in this domain would benefit from the integration of neuroimaging and behavioral measures within clinical trials, allowing for a more precise understanding of how neural changes correspond to improvements in psychological functioning. Such multimodal approaches could facilitate the identification of biomarkers of treatment response, enabling clinicians to predict which individuals are most likely to benefit from mindfulness-based interventions.

Moving forward, there is an urgent need for large-scale, pre-registered randomized controlled trials that employ active control conditions, standardized imaging protocols, and long-term follow-up assessments. These methodological improvements would strengthen causal inferences about the relationship between mindfulness practice and neuroplastic change. Furthermore, research should explore dose–response relationships and factors influencing intervention adherence, as well as individual differences such as baseline cognitive function, stress reactivity, or genetic predispositions. Such investigations could help tailor mindfulness-based programs to optimize outcomes for distinct clinical groups.

In summary, mindfulness-based interventions in clinical contexts appear to induce adaptive neuroplasticity in networks underlying attention, self-regulation, and emotion. While methodological heterogeneity and limited replication currently temper the strength of the evidence, the overall trend is consistent and promising. Continued interdisciplinary research integrating clinical psychology, neuroscience, and contemplative science holds the potential to deepen our understanding of how mindful awareness reshapes the brain in ways that foster psychological healing and resilience.

At its heart, the meeting of mindfulness and neuroplasticity tells a hopeful story about human potential. It shows that our brains are not fixed or limited by age or habit—they are dynamic, ever-changing, and responsive to how we think, feel, and live. Through practices like meditation, yoga, mindful awareness, or simply paying fuller attention to everyday moments, we engage the brain's remarkable ability to rewire itself toward balance, clarity, and resilience. Scientific evidence now affirms what many contemplative traditions have long suggested: that nurturing awareness can reshape not only how we experience the world but also the very organ that allows us to experience it. In this shared space between science and practice lies an empowering message for everyone—the mind and brain, working together, hold the key to lifelong growth and transformation

The human brain, primitive in its origins, has undergone a prolonged evolutionary journey. Beginning as a simple network of interconnected neurons, it has taken millions of years to develop into the complex structure capable of advanced cognitive functions observed today. This evolution was significantly shaped by the adaptive behaviours and culturally transmitted practices of our ancestors, who navigated and responded to diverse environmental demands contributing to both survival and cerebral advancement. Inherited from this lineage, it is imperative for contemporary generations to actively engage in the exploration, identification, and incorporation of activities that not only preserve but also enhance the brain's structural integrity and functional capabilities ensuring continued evolution. Among such practices, cultivating neuroplasticity through mindfulness stands out as a powerful and evidence-based approach to enhancing the brain's adaptive potential and fostering cognitive, emotional, and behavioural growth.

REFERENCES

Calderone, A., Latella, D., Impellizzeri, F., de Pasquale, P., Famà, F., Quartarone, A., & Calabrò, R. S. (2024). Neurobiological changes induced by mindfulness and meditation: A systematic review. *Biomedicines*, *12*(11), 2613. DOI: 10.3390/biomedicines12112613 PMID: 39595177

Gheranda. (2004). *Gheranda Samhita* (J. Mallinson, Trans.). YogaVidya.com. (Original work published ca. 17th century)

Gkintoni, E., Vassilopoulos, S. P., & Nikolaou, G. (2025). Mindfulness-Based Cognitive Therapy in clinical practice: A systematic review of neurocognitive outcomes and applications for mental health and well-being. *Journal of Clinical Medicine*, *14*(5), 1703. DOI: 10.3390/jcm14051703 PMID: 40095733

Gothe, N. P., Hayes, J. M., Temali, C., & Damoiseaux, J. S. (2016). Differences in brain structure and function among yoga practitioners and controls. *Frontiers in Integrative Neuroscience*, *10*, 26. DOI: 10.3389/fnint.2016.00026 PMID: 29988397

Han, Y.-M. Y., Chen, H., Lee, T. M. C., & Chan, C. C. H. (2023). Neurobiological effects of mind–body exercise: A systematic review and meta-analysis. *Scientific Reports*, *13*(17432), 10948. Advance online publication. DOI: 10.1038/s41598-023-37309-4 PMID: 37415072

Hayes, S. C., Villatte, M., Levin, M., & Hildebrandt, M. (2011). Open, aware, and active: Contextual approaches as an emerging trend in the behavioral and cognitive therapies. *Annual Review of Clinical Psychology*, *7*(1), 141–168. DOI: 10.1146/annurev-clinpsy-032210-104449 PMID: 21219193

Leow, Y., Rashid, N. L. B. A., Klainin-Yobas, P., Zhang, Z., Wu, X. V., ... (2023). Effectiveness of mindfulness-based interventions on mental, cognitive outcomes and neuroplastic changes in older adults with mild cognitive impairment: A systematic review and meta-analysis. *Journal of Advanced Nursing*. https://pubmed.ncbi.nlm.nih.gov/37248564

Neacsiu, A. D.. (2018). Neural effects of mindfulness-based interventions on patients with major depressive disorder: A systematic review. *Neuroscience and Biobehavioral Reviews*, *95*, 500–513. https://pubmed.ncbi.nlm.nih.gov/29548932

Pernet, C. R., Belov, N., Delorme, A., & Zammit, A. (2021). Mindfulness-related changes in grey matter: A systematic review and meta-analysis. *Brain Imaging and Behavior*, *15*(6), 3056–3076. DOI: 10.1007/s11682-021-00453-4 PMID: 33624219

Pomerantz, A. M. (2020). *Clinical psychology: Science, practice, and diversity* (5th ed.). SAGE Publications.

Satyananda Saraswati, S. (1996). *Asana, pranayama, mudra, bandha* (Rev. ed.). Yoga Publications Trust.

Siew, S., Grant, J., Lim, T. H., & Chia, Y. (2023). Mindfulness-based randomized controlled trials and structural brain change: A meta-analysis. *Scientific Reports, 13*(22055). Advance online publication. DOI: 10.1038/s41598-023-51492-1

Varma, R. (2025). Meditation and mindfulness in Indian philosophical traditions. *ShodhSamajik: Journal of Social Studies, 2*(1), 1–7. DOI: 10.29121/ShodhSamajik.v2.i1.2025.10

Verzili, B., Cerasa, A., & Quattrone, A. (2023). Yoga and neuropsychiatric aging: A systematic review and meta-analysis. *Neuroscience and Biobehavioral Reviews, 150*(105223). Advance online publication. DOI: 10.1016/j.neubiorev.2023.105223 PMID: 37598905

Vivekananda, S. (1985). *The complete works of Swami Vivekananda: Abridged edition.* Advaita Ashrama.

Vyasa. (2006). *The Bhagavadgita* (S. Radhakrishnan, Trans. & Comm.). New Delhi: HarperCollins Publishers India. (Original work composed ca. 2nd century BCE) https://www.verywellmind.com/mindfulness-based-cognitive-therapy-1067396 https://www.britannica.com/science/neuroplasticity https://positivepsychology.com/history-of-mindfulness/

Chapter 6

Rewiring the Brain for Resilience:

The Role of Neuroplasticity in Mindfulness, Meditation, and Yoga

Simran Obhrai
http://orcid.org/0009-0007-5227-9364
Guru Nanak Dev University, India

Shweta Shenoy
Guru Nanak Dev University, India

Sohom Saha
http://orcid.org/0009-0006-9438-1554
Lakshmibai National Institute of Physical Education, India

ABSTRACT

One of the most intriguing findings of neuroscience is the ability of contemplative practice to transform the human brain. This chapter explores how neuroplasticity can use mindfulness, meditation, and yoga to strengthen psychological resilience to help us understand how ancient wisdom can be used in combination with new brain science. The chapter introduces clinical studies that demonstrate practical applications across trauma recovery, educational settings, and workplace wellness programs. A holistic implementation model is used to transfer knowledge gathered during the research to practical programs by looking into the training needs, cultural appropriateness, and sustainability questions. The chapter concludes by examining future research priorities, including methodological innovations, cultural inclusivity, precision medicine approaches, and clinical translation challenges. By

DOI: 10.4018/979-8-3373-4187-3.ch006

integrating contemplative neuroscience with practical application, this synthesis offers a scientifically backed way through which a person can actively carve out his or her own neural structure.

1. INTRODUCTION AND BACKGROUND

Something profound is happening in the 21st century. Mental health problems caused by stress, such as anxiety, depression, burnout, and emotional dysregulation, are rising at an alarming rate (World Health Organization, 2022). But another story offers genuine hope. Neuroscientists have uncovered something remarkable: the human brain doesn't stop changing in adulthood. Instead, it remains adaptable, constantly rewiring itself throughout our entire life (Vago & Silbersweig, 2012). This discovery, known as neuroplasticity, has shattered decades of scientific dogma that viewed the adult brain as fixed and unchangeable.

Meanwhile, people are rediscovering practices such as mindfulness, meditation, and yoga that their ancestors knew intimately (Brahmbhatt & Kumavat, 2024; Pascoe et al., 2017). These aren't just feel-good activities or spiritual curiosities. They're powerful transformation technologies refined over millennia, now integrated into mainstream therapeutic approaches, educational curricula, and organizational wellness programs worldwide. This convergence has birthed contemplative neuroscience, where researchers map how meditation changes neural networks, document how mindfulness strengthens the prefrontal cortex and observe yoga building cellular resilience (Marchand, 2014; Davidson & Lutz, 2008).

The implications are very large. We now understand that resilience, that is our capacity to bounce back from adversity, trauma, and stress, isn't just a psychological trait (Masten & Motti-Stefanidi, 2020). It has specific neurobiological foundations. Certain brain networks govern how we respond to challenges. Particular structures determine whether we crumble or adapt. And here's the revolutionary part: we can train these systems (Kalisch et al., 2017).

This chapter explores this intersection of ancient wisdom and modern neuroscience examining neuroplasticity foundations, contemplative practices, neural mechanisms linking practice and plasticity, resilience-building frameworks, and practical implementation strategies.

The brain you have today isn't the brain you're stuck with tomorrow. Change is not only possible, it's inevitable. The question isn't whether your brain will change, but how you'll direct that change.

2. UNDERSTANDING NEUROPLASTICITY AND RESILIENCE

This section establishes the foundational neuroscience principles underlying brain adaptability and psychological resilience. We examine the mechanisms through which the brain modifies its structure and function across the lifespan, explore the key neural networks that constitute our resilience architecture, and investigate the neurochemical systems that enable adaptive responses to stress and adversity.

As mentioned earlier, the human brain possesses an extraordinary capacity that challenges everything we once believed about neural development. Neuroplasticity, or the brain's ability to modify its structure and function throughout life, operates as a fundamental biological principle that supports learning, recovery, and adaptation (Dita & Bubuioc, 2024).

Neuroplasticity manifests through three primary pathways. Synaptic plasticity alters the strength of connections between neurons, like adjusting the volume on countless neural conversations. Structural plasticity goes deeper, physically reshaping neural architecture itself. Functional plasticity reorganizes entire networks, rewiring how brain regions communicate.

Scientists recognize two fundamental transformation forms. Structural plasticity involves tangible changes: shifts in gray matter density, alterations in cortical thickness, modifications in white matter integrity, and connectivity pattern evolution. Such brain changes can be documented through magnetic resonance imaging (MRI) and diffusion tensor imaging. Functional plasticity works in a different way; it is concerned with changes in neural activity patterns, network connectivity, and information processing efficiency monitored through functional MRI and electroencephalography (EEG) (Zatorre et al., 2012).

Developmental plasticity varies across lifespan stages. While childhood and adolescence demonstrate peak plasticity, adult brains retain impressive reorganizational potential (Draganski & May, 2008). Childhood stress can structurally and permanently alter the brain, making people prone to stress and impaired functioning they might encounter in adult life (Buenrostro-Jáuregui et al., 2025). Yet plasticity of the brain throughout one's life span is encouraging in the aspect that the negative effects can still be curbed even during adulthood (Karatsoreos & McEwen, 2013). This inability to terminate learning at any stage of development vigorously provides the brain with the neurobiological foundation of continuing to learn, recover, and adjust in response to novel challenges.

Psychological resilience is much more than overcoming adversity by bouncing back. It encompasses complex capabilities: emotional regulation, cognitive flexibility, stress tolerance, and adaptive coping (Troy et al., 2023). Rather than fixed traits, resilience emerges from coordinated brain network functioning.

Key brain regions collaborate in resilience profiles. The prefrontal cortex (PFC), particularly ventromedial and dorsolateral areas, orchestrates emotional regulation, decision-making, and cognitive control essential for resilient responses (Arnsten, 2009). The PFC enables top-down regulation. Higher-order cortical regions controlling subcortical emotional centers to modulate responses (Buhle et al., 2014).

The amygdala functions as the brain's alarm system, detecting threats and initiating stress responses (LeDoux, 2000). While protecting from danger, chronic hyperactivation contributes to anxiety, depression, and trauma-related disorders. Resilient individuals demonstrate balanced amygdala functioning: appropriate threat detection coupled with effective regulatory mechanisms.

The hippocampus plays a crucial role in memory formation and contextual processing. This structure helps distinguish between past traumatic experiences and current safe situations (Stevens, 1999). The default mode network (DMN), comprising medial prefrontal cortex, posterior cingulate cortex, and angular gyrus, operates during rest and self-referential thinking (Buckner et al., 2008). DMN dysregulation associates with rumination, depression, and anxiety. Healthy DMN functioning supports self-awareness, introspection, and the meaning-making processes central to resilience.

Recent research has identified the salience network (including anterior insula and dorsal anterior cingulate cortex) as crucial for detecting relevant internal and external stimuli (Li et al., 2024). It coordinates appropriate responses to changing circumstances (Seeley et al., 2007). Its capacity to switch between internal focus and external attention forms the foundation of adaptive functioning and resilience. Neurochemical systems enable these networks' optimal functioning. Serotonin and brain-derived neurotrophic factor (BDNF) interact to regulate neuronal plasticity, influencing mood and stress responses (Popova & Naumenko, 2019). BDNF promotes neuron survival while supporting learning and memory formation. Oxytocin and BDNF support "neurosocial plasticity"—capacity for adaptive neural and social functioning (Faraji & Metz, 2024).

This neurobiological foundation sets the stage for understanding how specific contemplative practices can harness neuroplasticity to build resilience. Each practice discussed in this section engages these neural networks in unique ways. Mindfulness primarily strengthens the prefrontal cortex while calming amygdala reactivity. Meditation practices reshape the DMN and enhance salience network functioning. Yoga integrates body awareness with emotional regulation, creating distinctive patterns of neural activation and connectivity.

3. MINDFULNESS, MEDITATION, AND YOGA

Long before neuroscientists could observe living brains, contemplative traditions conducted sophisticated experiments in human consciousness. Tibetan monasteries became laboratories where monks practiced meditation for over a thousand years. Ancient Indian sages developed yoga postures beside sacred rivers, mapping the territories of human consciousness with remarkable precision. Buddhist teachers cultivated mindfulness in forest retreats, documenting pathways to inner transformation.

Mindfulness emerges from the Buddhist concept of "sati", that is the intentional, non-judgmental awareness of present-moment experience (Kabat-Zinn, 2003). Modern science defines mindfulness as active, open attention directed toward the present moment, encompassing both internal experiences (thoughts, feelings, sensations) and external stimuli (Bishop et al., 2004). It's like developing a mental muscle that can step back and watch your own mental processes without getting overwhelmed. The key insight? You don't need to stop thinking or feeling. You simply learn to observe these processes with clarity and equanimity.

Closely related yet distinct, **meditation** encompasses diverse practices designed to train attention and cultivate beneficial mental qualities like compassion, equanimity, and wisdom (Davidson & Lutz, 2008). If the mind is like a wild horse, meditation provides the training ground to develop a steady, focused awareness. Traditional approaches vary widely: focused attention practices concentrate on single objects like breath; open monitoring observes all arising experiences without attachment; loving-kindness meditation systematically extends compassion. Despite this diversity, all meditation practices share core elements: intentional attention training and meta-cognitive awareness development.

The third pathway emerges from **yoga**, which literally means "union" in Sanskrit, representing a comprehensive system integrating mind, body, and spirit. While Western yoga emphasizes physical postures, traditional yoga encompasses eight interconnected limbs: ethical guidelines, breath practices (pranayama), sensory withdrawal (pratyahara), concentration (dharana), meditation (dhyana), and self-realization (samadhi). This systematic progression reveals sophisticated understanding of consciousness transformation, with each stage building foundational capacity for the next. The ancient yogis intuited what neuroscience now confirms: attention can be systematically trained, and this training literally reshapes the brain.

When neuroscientists first studied contemplative practitioners, they discovered revolutionary findings. Brain imaging revealed long-term practitioners had physically different brains: increased cortical thickness in attention areas, enhanced emotional regulation network coordination, and reduced default mode network activity associated with rumination and mind-wandering(Lazar et al., 2005; Brewer et al., 2011). These weren't temporary states. They were lasting structural changes; neuroplasticity in action.

Here's where the story becomes truly fascinating. Despite their different origins and methods, mindfulness, meditation, and yoga appear to work through remarkably similar mechanisms (Vago & Silbersweig, 2012). It's as if these ancient traditions discovered different routes to the same neurological destination. All three practices involve systematic attention training. Whether focusing on breath in meditation, maintaining present-moment awareness in mindfulness, or coordinating movement with breath in yoga, practitioners are essentially doing mental push-ups. They're strengthening neural networks involved in sustained attention and reducing automatic reactivity to distractions. Think of attention like a flashlight. Most people have flickering, scattered beams, jumping from worry to planning to remembering. Contemplative practices train a steady, focused beam that can be directed intentionally.

These practices also transform emotional regulation in profound ways. They don't eliminate difficult emotions, rather, they transform how we relate to them. Buddhist teachings on equanimity, yogic concepts of witness consciousness, and mindfulness approaches to emotional awareness all cultivate a similar capacity, that is the ability to experience challenging emotions without being overwhelmed or controlled by them. From a neuroscientific understanding, this corresponds to enhanced prefrontal control over the amygdala, like having a wise adult supervise an emotional child (Desbordes et al., 2012). The emotions are still there, but the reactive patterns that typically follow can be interrupted.

Perhaps most important aspect is that these practices offer insights into the constructed nature of selfhood. The Buddhist teaching of non-self (anatta), yogic concepts of witness consciousness, and mindfulness observations of mental proliferation all point toward a startling discovery. Much of our psychological suffering comes from the stories we tell ourselves about ourselves. Neuroimaging reveals that excessive self-referential thinking (the brain's constant internal narrative) is associated with depression, anxiety, and other forms of psychological distress (Verhaeghen, 2017). Contemplative practices appear to quiet these networks, creating space for a different kind of awareness to emerge.

What emerges from this convergence is access to time-tested methodologies for mental training, now supported by empirical understanding of why and how they work. Ancient contemplatives were neuroscientists without machines, mapping territories of consciousness through direct investigation. Today, we can combine their sophisticated methodologies with modern scientific validation. We understand that when yogis spoke of pratyahara (sensory withdrawal), they were describing enhanced top-down attentional control (McKibben, 2025). When Buddhists taught about reducing mental proliferation, they were targeting the same default mode network activity that neuroscientists associate with rumination and psychological distress.

4. INTRODUCTION TO CONTEMPLATIVE NEUROSCIENCE

In the late 20th century, neuroscientists began investigating the neural correlates of meditation and other contemplative practices. What they discovered challenged fundamental assumptions about consciousness, brain plasticity, and human potential and the field of Contemplative neuroscience emerged (Davidson & Lutz, 2008). This field creates a unique dialogue between objective scientific methodology and subjective experiential reports from experienced practitioners. It bridges two ways of knowing, the measurable and the lived.

Early research focused on documenting basic neurophysiological changes during meditation. Pioneering studies demonstrated that meditation produced measurable alterations in brain activity, shattering assumptions about the fixed nature of adult brain function (Austin, 1998). As neuroimaging technology advanced, researchers investigated structural brain changes in long-term practitioners, revealing profound neuroplastic adaptations.

Contemporary contemplative neuroscience employs sophisticated methodologies. Functional MRI reveals real-time brain activity during practice, structural MRI captures anatomical changes, and diffusion tensor imaging maps white matter connectivity. EEG tracks electrical activity with millisecond precision.

Landmark meta-analyses have consolidated findings across hundreds of studies. Goyal et al., (2014) analyzed 47 trials involving 3,515 participants, demonstrating moderate evidence for anxiety and depression reduction. More recent systematic reviews have refined our understanding of dose-response relationships and individual differences in contemplative practice outcomes (Bowles et al., 2022; Fredrickson et al., 2017). Large-scale projects are pushing the field forward. The Mind & Life Institute's collaborative research initiatives bring together neuroscientists, contemplatives, and clinicians. The Center for Healthy Minds at the University of Wisconsin-Madison conducts longitudinal studies tracking practitioners over years. The Mindfulness in Schools Project examines applications in educational settings.

This research has revealed consistent patterns of neuroplastic change associated with regular contemplative practice. The results offer neurobiological confirmation of cross-cultural, cross-century benefits described by practitioners. What is more important, the field of contemplative neuroscience is growing more interdisciplinary and informs various academic and professional areas, such as clinical psychology, education, organizational development, and even public health policy. Modern neuroscience confirms what ancient wisdom traditions had an intuition about: the ability of our brains to be altered through purposeful mental training. The interplay between reflective wisdom and scientific empiricism holds untold potential of comprehending and improving the well-being of human beings.

5. NEUROSCIENTIFIC EVIDENCE OF NEUROPLASTIC CHANGE

This section examines neuroimaging evidence demonstrating how contemplative practices reshape brain structure and function. We explore structural changes in gray matter and cortical thickness, network modifications including default mode network quieting and attention system strengthening, yoga's unique neuroplastic signature, and the methodological advances and limitations underlying these discoveries.

When neuroscientist Sara Lazar first examined experienced meditators' brains with high-resolution MRI, she found something remarkable: structurally thicker regions crucial for attention and sensory processing. More intriguingly, older meditators maintained cortical thickness that typically diminishes with age, suggesting practice might slow neural aging (Lazar et al., 2005).

This discovery launched investigations consistently revealing how meditation induces measurable structural brain changes. Luders and colleagues found significantly increased gray matter volume in meditators across multiple regions, including hippocampus, frontal cortex, and insula (Luders et al., 2009). These changes appeared precisely where expected: areas governing memory, attention, and self-awareness.

But correlation isn't causation, and early studies couldn't distinguish whether meditation changed the brain or whether people with certain brain characteristics were simply drawn to meditation. This critical question began to find answers through intervention studies. When Hölzel et al. (2011) recruited participants who had never practiced meditation, for eight weeks of mindfulness-based stress reduction training, they documented that measurable increases in gray matter density appeared in just two months. The hippocampus, crucial for learning and memory, grew denser. The posterior cingulate cortex and temporo-parietal junction, regions involved in self-awareness and empathy, showed similar increases. Most remarkably, the amygdala, our brain's alarm system, actually shrank. This suggested that mindfulness practice wasn't just adding neural tissue randomly, but was sculpting the brain in functionally meaningful ways, reducing reactivity to stress while enhancing cognitive resources.

We have to be careful, however, about what such structural changes mean. A larger volume in the brain does not necessarily translate to better functioning. Hypergrowth also takes place in many pathological disorders. The importance of the changes induced by meditation does not lie in their magnitude, but within the support they provide on more efficient working of the network and better behavioral effects.

The picture becomes even more interesting when we look at how various brain networks communicate. The DMN that engages when we are resting and thinking about ourselves, generally buzzes with activity when our mind engages in mind wandering. In highly practised meditators, this network is found to have dramatically low activity levels in both meditation and ordinary relaxation periods. This is a very important discovery because the hyperactivity of DMN is associated with rumination, depression, and anxiety disorders. Brewer and colleagues showed that experienced meditators have quieter DMN both during and outside meditation, indicating that their training has resulted in more lasting trait changes, rather than temporary states (Brewer et al., 2011). This is a paradigm shift in terms of a change in self-centered thinking patterns to being in the moment; the very promise of the contemplative traditions.

The brain's attention networks also undergo remarkable reorganization. Tang et al. (2007) showed that just five days of integrative meditation training enhanced the efficiency of the anterior cingulate cortex, a key attention hub. Participants showed improved sustained attention, reduced mind-wandering, and enhanced cognitive control. These weren't subtle changes. They were measurable improvements that emerged with surprising speed.

The salience network, responsible for detecting relevant stimuli and coordinating appropriate responses, also shows significant modifications with contemplative practice. Experienced meditators demonstrate enhanced salience network connectivity, suggesting an improved capacity to detect and respond to important internal and external events while maintaining equanimity and non-reactivity (Hasenkamp & Barsalou, 2012). This represents a sophisticated form of neural adaptation; the ability to remain alert and responsive without becoming overwhelmed or reactive.

Perhaps most intriguingly, contemplative practice appears to enhance brain network flexibility, that is the ability to dynamically switch between task-positive networks (supporting focused attention) and task-negative networks (supporting rest and introspection). This meta-stable network dynamics, as researchers call it, may represent a core marker of psychological resilience: the capacity to engage fully when needed and disengage completely when appropriate.

Yoga practice offers a unique window into embodied neuroplasticity, revealing how physical movement, breath awareness, and meditative states integrate in the brain. Unlike meditation's primarily top-down approach, that simple means using cognitive control to regulate attention and emotion; Yoga engages bottom-up pathways through proprioceptive and interoceptive signals, enhancing bodily self-awareness and emotional regulation from the ground up.

When Villemure et al. (2014) compared experienced yoga practitioners with controls, they found increased gray matter volume in regions that tell the story of yoga's integrated approach. The insula, crucial for interoceptive processing and emotional awareness, showed particularly robust changes. The hippocampus and somatosensory cortex also expanded, reflecting enhanced body awareness and memory formation. These changes correlated with years of practice and were associated with heightened interoceptive awareness, that is the ability to perceive internal bodily sensations with remarkable precision.

Grant et al. (2010) extended these findings by investigating cortical thickness in yoga practitioners, revealing increased thickness in somatosensory and visual cortices. These structural adaptations weren't merely anatomical curiosities. They translated into meaningful functional benefits. Practitioners demonstrated improved pain tolerance and enhanced body awareness, suggesting that yoga-induced neuroplasticity creates tangible improvements in how we process and respond to bodily sensations.

The insula deserves special attention in yoga's neuroplastic story. This brain region serves as a crucial hub, integrating sensory information from the body with emotional and cognitive processing. Increased insular gray matter volume and enhanced connectivity in yoga practitioners suggest that the practice's emphasis on breath regulation and body awareness specifically strengthens neural networks involved in embodied self-awareness.

Yoga's effects extend beyond brain structure to neurochemistry itself. Streeter et al. (2012) demonstrated that yoga practice increases GABA levels in the brain, a neurotransmitter associated with relaxation and anxiety reduction. This neurochemical shift provides a potential mechanism for yoga's stress-reducing and mood-enhancing effects, complementing the structural changes observed in neuroimaging studies.

The vagus nerve, connecting brain to body, also responds to yoga practice. Enhanced vagal tone, which is a measure of parasympathetic nervous system activity, promotes physiological states of calm and recovery. This represents another pathway through which yoga's bottom-up approach influences brain function, using the body as a gateway to neural change (Porges, 2011).

These discoveries rely heavily on advanced neuroimaging technologies like structural MRI, functional MRI, EEG, diffusion tensor imaging; each offering unique insights into the contemplative brain. Despite these technological advances, contemplative neuroscience faces important methodological challenges. Control group selection remains complex. How do you find appropriate comparison groups for practices that may attract certain personality types? Practice standardization presents another hurdle, as contemplative traditions emphasize individualized approaches that resist uniform protocols.

The measurement of subjective experiences adds another layer of complexity. Traditional neuroscience has often overlooked first-person experience, yet contemplative practices are fundamentally about inner transformation. The field increasingly embraces mixed-methods approaches, combining neuroimaging with qualitative methods like phenomenology and first-person journaling. This integration represents a unique strength of contemplative science, with its willingness to honor both objective and subjective dimensions of human experience.

Interrelations between expectation effects, placebo response, and actual neuroplastic changes prove to be difficult subjects to study on. However, newly evolving longitudinal and intervention designs are aiding in providing the establishment of causality. We are going past the gross before-and-after pictures to complex work, involving observing responses in the brain over long durations, comparing various practices, and looking at dose-response curves.

As this research matures, one thing becomes increasingly clear that the contemplative traditions were right about the brain's capacity for transformation. The brain we're born with need not be the brain we die with. However, such neuroimaging findings leave deep questions of how precisely such contemplative interventions can cause such extraordinary brain changes. How exactly do the biological processes convert a moment of focused breathing or mindful awareness into long term structural changes? What are the effects of recurring states of meditation that slowly begin to rearrange the actual blueprint of consciousness itself? It is one thing to know what happens to the contemplative brain, but quite another to know how and why the brain changes take place. For this reason, we must explore further the cellular and molecular processes that mediate the relationship between practice and plasticity.

6. NEUROPLASTIC PATHWAYS OF RESILIENCE: MECHANISMS OF CHANGE IN CONTEMPLATIVE PRACTICE

Understanding what changes in the contemplative brain is just the beginning. The deeper question lies in how these practices trigger such profound neural transformations. What are the specific pathways through which a moment of mindful breathing or compassionate awareness gradually reshapes the very architecture of our minds? This section explores the biological mechanisms that translate contemplative practice into lasting neuroplastic change, examining how attention regulation, breath modulation, emotional training, and embodied awareness create resilient neural circuits.

To map this complex terrain, we can identify seven key mechanisms that bridge contemplative practice and neuroplastic change (summarised in table 1). Each mechanism operates through distinct brain networks, engages specific practice modalities, and triggers characteristic neurochemical cascades. Together, these pathways reveal how ancient wisdom traditions intuited what modern neuroscience now confirms, the mind can reshape the brain through disciplined practice.

Table 1. Neural Mechanisms Linking Contemplative Practice and Resilience

Mechanism	Associated Brain Networks	Practice Type	Modality	Neurochemical Correlates	Functional Outcome
Attention Regulation	Prefrontal Cortex, Anterior Cingulate	Mindfulness	Attention	Increased BDNF, Enhanced dopamine	Enhanced cognitive control and sustained focus
Emotional Self-Regulation	Amygdala, Prefrontal Cortex	Loving-Kindness	Emotion	Increased GABA, oxytocin, Reduced cortisol	Reduced reactivity and improved affect regulation
Interoceptive Awareness	Insula	Yoga	Movement	Increased GABA, Enhanced vagal tone	Heightened bodily awareness, improved self-regulation
Stress Response Modulation	Hypothalamic-Pituitary-Adrenal (HPA) Axis	Yoga, Mindfulness	Movement/Attention	Reduced cortisol, Increased DHEA	Reduced stress reactivity, increased resilience
Mind-Wandering Reduction	Default Mode Network	Mindfulness	Attention	Balanced dopamine, Reduced inflammatory markers	Decreased rumination, improved present awareness
Proprioceptive Integration	Somatosensory Cortex, Cerebellum	Yoga	Movement	Increased BDNF, Enhanced endorphins	Improved coordination and body-mind coherence
Compassion Cultivation	Temporoparietal Junction, Anterior Cingulate	Loving-Kindness	Emotion	Increased oxytocin, Enhanced dopamine	Enhanced empathy and prosocial behavior

6.1 Attention Regulation and Sustained Focus

Every contemplative tradition recognizes a fundamental truth: where attention goes, the mind follows. This ancient wisdom finds validation in modern neuroscience, which reveals attention regulation as perhaps the most fundamental mechanism through which contemplative practices rewire the brain for resilience.

The capacity to direct and sustain attention voluntarily drives many of the neural adaptations observed in practitioners. When we train attention through meditation, we're not just improving focus, we're strengthening the very neural circuits that support cognitive control, emotional regulation, and psychological flexibility. Research by Tang & Posner (2009) reveals that contemplative practices enhance multiple attentional capacities: sustained attention, selective attention, and executive attention. These improvements aren't confined to meditation sessions. Longitudinal studies show that experienced meditators maintain enhanced attentional abilities throughout daily life, demonstrating genuine trait-level changes rather than temporary states.

Experienced meditators show enhanced ability to maintain focus on chosen objects while demonstrating reduced activation in brain regions associated with mind-wandering and self-referential thinking (Manna et al., 2010). This translates into real-world benefits: improved academic performance, reduced ADHD symptoms, and better integration of emotion and cognition in decision-making.

Perhaps most intriguingly, contemplative practice develops meta-attentional awareness, that is the capacity to monitor one's own attentional processes. This allows practitioners to recognize when attention has wandered and gently redirect it back to the chosen focus. This creates a powerful feedback loop: better attention regulation leads to improved emotional control, which in turn supports sustained attention. Over time, this cycle builds increasingly robust neural circuits for resilience, transforming momentary states of focused awareness into enduring traits of psychological flexibility (Vago & Silbersweig, 2012).

6.2 Breathwork and Autonomic Nervous System Modulation

The breath occupies a unique position in contemplative practice. It is both voluntary and involuntary, conscious and unconscious, connecting mind and body in ways that few other phenomena can match. This dual nature makes breath regulation a particularly powerful pathway for influencing autonomic nervous system functioning and promoting neuroplastic changes.

When we consciously slow and deepen our breathing, we activate a cascade of physiological changes that ripple throughout the nervous system. Research demonstrates that controlled breathing practices rapidly shift autonomic balance, promoting parasympathetic activation while reducing sympathetic arousal (Brown & Gerbarg, 2005). These changes translate into reduced stress hormone levels, improved heart rate variability, and enhanced emotional regulation capacity.

The vagus nerve serves as a crucial mediator of these breath-induced changes. This longest cranial nerve connects the brain to major organ systems, creating a direct pathway for conscious breathing to influence unconscious processes. Contemplative practices that emphasize slow, deep breathing enhance vagal tone, promoting physiological states conducive to healing, recovery, and neuroplasticity (Porges, 2011). Enhanced vagal functioning creates what we might call afferent vagal feedback. Slow breathing increases vagal signals to the brainstem, which modulates limbic activity and decreases perceived threat reactivity. This bottom-up regulation pathway proves particularly valuable in trauma recovery, where top-down cognitive approaches may be initially overwhelming or ineffective.

Neuroimaging studies reveal that breath-focused practices produce specific patterns of brain activation, particularly in regions involved in interoceptive awareness and autonomic regulation. The insula, a key structure for processing internal bodily sensations, shows enhanced activation and structural changes in practitioners who emphasize breath awareness (Farb et al., 2013). Many trauma-informed therapeutic approaches, including Trauma-Sensitive Yoga, Somatic Experiencing, and Tension & Trauma Releasing Exercises, emphasize this bottom-up regulation via breath and body awareness. By engaging the nervous system through breath rather than thought, these approaches can reach trauma-related patterns that cognitive methods alone cannot address.

6.3 Emotional Self-Regulation and the Resilience Circuit

Emotional self-regulation represents perhaps the most clinically relevant mechanism through which contemplative practices enhance psychological resilience. The capacity to recognize, understand, and skillfully respond to emotional experiences forms the foundation of mental health and adaptive functioning.

Contemplative practices enhance emotional regulation through multiple pathways. Regular practitioners show reduced amygdala reactivity to emotional stimuli while maintaining or enhancing prefrontal cortex activation (Desbordes et al., 2012). This creates what we might call a resilience circuit. A recurrent loop connecting the prefrontal cortex, amygdala, insula, and anterior cingulate cortex that underlies our capacity for affective control and emotional reappraisal.

Experienced practitioners demonstrate enhanced capacity for both explicit strategies (such as cognitive reappraisal) and implicit processes (such as reduced emotional reactivity), suggesting that contemplative training develops a comprehensive emotional regulation toolkit that operates at multiple levels of consciousness.

Compassion-based practices deserve special attention for their unique contributions to emotional resilience. Loving-kindness meditation and compassion training don't just regulate difficult emotions; they actively cultivate positive emotional states and pro-social attitudes. Research reveals that compassion training enhances activation in brain networks associated with empathy and social cognition, including the insula, anterior cingulate cortex, and temporoparietal junction (Klimecki et al., 2014).

These practices also trigger specific neurochemical changes (Hutcherson et al., 2008; Machida et al., 2018; Weng et al., 2013). Loving-kindness meditation increases oxytocin levels, promoting feelings of connection and trust. Compassion training enhances GABA activity, supporting emotional stability and reducing anxiety. Perhaps most importantly, these practices appear to build resilience against empathic distress fatigue, that is the emotional exhaustion that can arise from excessive exposure to others' suffering.

The cultivation of equanimity, that is a balanced, non-reactive awareness toward all experiences, represents another crucial component of contemplative emotional training. Rather than suppressing difficult emotions or amplifying pleasant ones, equanimity practices teach practitioners to maintain stability and clarity regardless of emotional content. This capacity proves invaluable for psychological resilience, allowing individuals to navigate life's inevitable challenges without becoming overwhelmed or reactive.

6.4 Mind-Body Awareness and Embodied Integration

The cultivation of mind-body awareness through contemplative practices, particularly yoga and movement-based meditation, provides unique opportunities for neuroplastic change through enhanced somatic processing. These embodied awareness practices strengthen neural networks involved in self-perception and body-mind integration in ways that purely cognitive approaches cannot match.

To understand these changes, we must first distinguish between two types of bodily awareness. Proprioception refers to our sense of body position and movement in space. You may understand this as knowing where our limbs are without looking. Interoception involves perceiving internal bodily signals like heartbeat, breath, hunger, and visceral sensations. While proprioception tells us about our body's position, interoception reveals our body's condition.

Yoga and movement-based practices primarily enhance proprioceptive awareness. Yoga practitioners show increased gray matter volume in brain regions involved in proprioceptive processing, including the somatosensory cortex and cerebellum (Villemure et al., 2014). These structural changes translate into improved balance, coordination, and body awareness. The benefits that extend well beyond physical performance to include enhanced emotional regulation and stress resilience.

Interoceptive awareness proves particularly crucial for psychological resilience. Improved interoceptive sensitivity allows individuals to recognize early signs of stress, emotional dysregulation, or physical tension, enabling more timely and effective interventions. The insula, as mentioned earlier, a key brain structure for interoceptive processing, consistently shows structural and functional changes in contemplative practitioners (Craig, 2009).

Enhanced interoceptive awareness through contemplative practice appears to improve this predictive process, leading to more accurate self-perception and better emotional regulation (Bornemann & Singer, 2017; Seth, 2013). The integration of proprioceptive and interoceptive awareness through embodied contemplative practices creates what we might call embodied resilience, or the capacity to use bodily sensations as a resource for emotional regulation and stress management.

7. BUILDING RESILIENCE THROUGH PRACTICE

We have understood so far that the human nervous system possesses a remarkable capacity to adapt and transform through contemplative practice, and that regular engagement with these practices fundamentally reshapes how we respond to stress, adversity, and challenging circumstances, creating lasting changes that extend far beyond the practice session itself.

When we face stressful situations, our bodies naturally activate complex physiological systems designed to help us cope. However, chronic stress can overwhelm these systems, leading to exhaustion and dysfunction. Contemplative practice offers a powerful pathway for optimizing these stress response patterns. Research reveals that experienced meditators show reduced cortisol reactivity to acute stressors while maintaining appropriate physiological responses when truly needed (Pascoe et al., 2017). This suggests that practice builds genuine resilience rather than simply numbing our natural protective responses.

The transformation occurs through multiple interconnected mechanisms. Enhanced emotional regulation allows practitioners to recognize stress early in its development and implement effective coping strategies before overwhelm sets in. Improved cognitive flexibility helps us see challenging situations from multiple perspectives. Increased self-awareness creates space between stimulus and response, offering choice in how we react. Neuroimaging studies reveal the brain changes underlying these improvements. During stress exposure, contemplative practitioners show enhanced activation in prefrontal regions responsible for executive control, while displaying reduced activation in limbic regions associated with emotional reactivity (Taren et al., 2013). This pattern suggests more balanced and adaptive responses to life's inevitable challenges.

Building on these fundamental mechanisms, the integration of contemplative practices into healthcare and wellness settings has produced numerous evidence-based programs that demonstrate remarkable effectiveness across various conditions. These programs, mentioned in the table below, typically combine traditional contemplative practices with contemporary psychological and medical approaches, creating comprehensive treatment modalities that honor both ancient wisdom and modern science.

Table 2. Evidence-Based Contemplative Programs and Their Psychological Outcomes

Program Name	Core Practice	Target Population	Key Benefits Identified	Research Support
Mindfulness-Based Stress Reduction (MBSR)	Mindfulness Meditation	Clinical/General Population	Reduced anxiety, improved resilience	(Goyal et al., 2014)
Mindfulness-Based Cognitive Therapy (MBCT)	Mindfulness + CBT	Depression-prone individuals	Prevents relapse, improves mood stability	(Piet & Hougaard, 2011)
Trauma-Sensitive Yoga (TSY)	Yoga	Trauma Survivors	Reduces PTSD symptoms, increases body awareness	(Van der Kolk, 2014)
Workplace Mindfulness Programs	Mindfulness	Employees	Decreased burnout, improved focus and well-being	(Good et al., 2016)
School-Based Mindfulness	Mindfulness	Children and Adolescents	Enhanced attention, emotional regulation	(Zenner et al., 2014)

Mindfulness-Based Stress Reduction (MBSR), developed by Jon Kabat-Zinn, stands as one of the most widely researched contemplative-based interventions. Studies consistently demonstrate MBSR's effectiveness for reducing anxiety, depression, chronic pain, and stress-related symptoms while enhancing overall quality of life (Goyal et al., 2014). The program's eight-week structure provides a systematic approach to developing mindfulness skills that participants can integrate into daily life.

Mindfulness-Based Cognitive Therapy (MBCT) represents an innovative fusion of mindfulness practices with cognitive therapy techniques, specifically designed to prevent depression relapse. Research demonstrates that MBCT proves as effective as maintenance antidepressant medication for preventing depression recurrence, offering a non-pharmacological alternative for individuals with recurrent depression (Piet & Hougaard, 2011). This finding has profound implications for long-term mental health care.

While these established programs demonstrate the power of contemplative practices, their effectiveness depends largely on thoughtful adaptation to specific populations and circumstances. The universal mechanisms underlying contemplative practice, that is attention regulation, autonomic modulation, emotional training, and embodied awareness, manifest differently across various groups, each presenting unique opportunities and challenges.

Children represent a particularly promising population for contemplative interventions. Their developing brains show enhanced neuroplasticity, potentially amplifying the benefits of early contemplative training. School-based mindfulness programs demonstrate improvements in attention, emotional regulation, and academic performance (Zenner et al., 2014). However, successful approaches must be developmentally appropriate, emphasizing playful, movement-based practices over prolonged sitting meditation.

Frontline workers, including healthcare professionals, first responders, and military personnel, face unique stressors that can lead to compassion fatigue, burnout, and secondary trauma. For these populations, practices that specifically target stress resilience and emotional regulation prove most beneficial. Brief, accessible interventions that can be integrated into demanding work schedules show the most promise for sustained implementation (Grabbe et al., 2021).

Among all populations requiring specialized attention, trauma survivors present particularly complex considerations. Their nervous systems may be dysregulated in ways that make traditional meditation challenging or even re-traumatizing. The hypervigilant state common in trauma survivors can make sitting quietly with closed eyes feel dangerous rather than peaceful. Trauma-informed contemplative approaches emphasize safety, choice, and bottom-up regulation through breath and body awareness before introducing cognitive or insight-oriented practices.

Trauma-Sensitive Yoga (TSY) represents an innovative approach that combines yoga practices with trauma-informed principles. The practice emphasizes choice and agency, allowing participants to modify or opt out of any postures or breathing techniques. This approach helps trauma survivors reclaim a sense of safety and control in their own bodies. Research demonstrates TSY's effectiveness for reducing trauma symptoms while building resilience and self-regulation capacities in trauma survivors (van der Kolk, 2014).

The mechanisms through which contemplative practices support trauma recovery include enhanced emotional regulation, improved interoceptive awareness, and the development of self-compassion and self-soothing capacities. These practices help trauma survivors develop greater tolerance for difficult emotions and sensations while building internal resources for healing and growth. Trauma-informed Mindfulness-Based Stress Reduction (TI-MBSR) demonstrates statistically and clinically significant results in alleviating posttraumatic stress disorder (PTSD) and depression symptoms, with notable declines in anxious attachment among women survivors of interpersonal violence (Kelly & Garland, 2016).

Neuroimaging studies of trauma survivors who engage in contemplative practices reveal positive changes in brain regions affected by trauma. These include increased hippocampal volume, reduced amygdala hyperactivity, and enhanced prefrontal control (Hölzel et al., 2011). These neuroplastic changes suggest that contemplative practices may help reverse some of the neurobiological effects of trauma, offering hope for genuine healing rather than merely managing symptoms.

Research on advanced practitioners reveals the potential of sustained contemplative training. Tibetan monks and experienced meditation practitioners show extraordinary levels of gamma wave activity during compassion meditation, suggesting enhanced neural synchrony and information processing capabilities (Lutz et al., 2004). These individuals demonstrate exceptional emotional regulation capacities, including the ability to maintain equanimity during exposure to disturbing stimuli that would typically provoke strong reactions (Lutz et al., 2014).

The universal nature of neuroplastic processes, combined with their flexibility across all populations and conditions, suggests that contemplative practices tap into fundamental capacities for neural adaptation and psychological resilience that transcend cultural, age, or diagnostic boundaries. This universality, paired with the need for thoughtful adaptation to specific populations and circumstances, reflects both the power and the nuanced application required for contemplative practices to reach their full therapeutic and transformative potential.

8. A FRAMEWORK FOR IMPLEMENTATION

The journey from laboratory findings to real-world application represents one of the greatest challenges in translating contemplative neuroscience into meaningful human impact. We now understand how these practices rewire the brain for resilience, but how do we bring this transformation to schools, workplaces, healthcare settings, and communities? The answer lies in thoughtful, evidence-based implementation that honors both scientific rigor and the wisdom traditions from which these practices emerge.

Effective implementation requires more than simply teaching meditation techniques or scheduling yoga classes. It demands careful attention to population needs, cultural sensitivity, program fidelity, and ethical responsibility. As we scale these ancient practices to meet modern challenges, we must ensure that we preserve their transformative potential while making them accessible to diverse populations and contexts.

Creating effective contemplative-based resilience programs begins with understanding your population and their specific needs. A trauma survivor requires a fundamentally different approach than a stressed executive or an anxious teenager. The art of program design lies in matching contemplative practices to human circumstances while maintaining the integrity of the training methods. Research reveals that different practices serve different purposes. Trauma survivors often benefit from gentler, body-based approaches that restore a sense of safety and agency. Individuals with attention difficulties might respond better to focused concentration practices. Those struggling with emotional reactivity may find loving-kindness meditation particularly valuable.

Dosage considerations involve both intensity and duration of practice. The good news is that even brief programs of 8-12 weeks can produce measurable neuroplastic changes and psychological benefits (Goyal et al., 2014). However, longer programs typically yield more sustained and better effects. Daily practice, even for short periods, proves more effective than longer but less frequent sessions. This finding has great implications for program design: consistency trumps duration.

The integration of formal practice with informal daily life applications appears crucial for maximizing effectiveness. Participants who weave contemplative awareness throughout their day show greater improvements in psychological well-being compared to those who practice only in structured settings (Carmody & Baer, 2008). This suggests that effective programs must bridge the gap between practice and daily life, teaching people how to carry contemplative awareness into their daily activities.

8.1 Trauma-Informed Design Principles

Given the prevalence of trauma in many populations, all contemplative programs should incorporate trauma-informed design principles. This approach recognizes that traditional meditation practices can sometimes trigger traumatic memories or dysregulated states, requiring careful modification and skilled guidance.

Trauma-informed programming emphasizes safety above all else. This means creating physical and emotional environments where participants feel secure (Shier & Turpin, 2017). Choice becomes paramount. Offering multiple practice options and allowing people to modify or exit practices as needed. Grounding techniques that connect people to present-moment sensory experience often precede more intensive contemplative practices. The concept of titration, that is, introducing practices gradually in manageable doses, prevents overwhelming vulnerable nervous systems. Bottom-up regulation through breath and body awareness typically comes before top-down cognitive approaches.

This ethical imperative extends beyond clinical populations. Many individuals carry unrecognized trauma, making trauma-informed approaches beneficial for all contemplative programs (Rudolph, 2021). By prioritizing safety and choice, we honor the vulnerability that authentic practice often requires.

Program fidelity and instructor quality emerge as crucial determinants of success. Evidence consistently shows that teacher training and alignment with core contemplative principles predict program effectiveness more than specific techniques or formats (Hecht & Crane, 2025). This places enormous responsibility on instructor preparation and ongoing supervision, particularly as contemplative approaches scale rapidly across diverse settings.

8.2 Educational Applications

Schools represent perhaps our greatest opportunity to build resilience during critical developmental periods. When children learn contemplative skills alongside mathematics and reading, we plant seeds that can grow into lifelong capacities for emotional regulation, focused attention, and psychological flexibility. Research on school-based programs demonstrates remarkable benefits. Students participating in contemplative training show improved attention, reduced behavioral problems, and enhanced emotional regulation skills (Zenner et al., 2014). These improvements appear particularly pronounced for students from high-stress environments or those facing attention challenges.

Developmental adaptation proves essential for educational success (Broderick & Frank, 2014; Lyons & DeLange, 2016). Preschoolers thrive with breath-based games and sensory awareness activities that feel like play. Elementary students respond well to body-based practices and simple concentration exercises. Adolescents often benefit from emotion labeling techniques combined with journaling and movement practices that address their developmental concerns about identity and peer relationships.

The most effective school programs train teachers in contemplative practices, not just students. Initiatives like CARE for Teachers demonstrate that when educators develop their own contemplative capacities, they naturally model resilience and emotional regulation throughout the school day (Jennings et al., 2019). This teacher-led approach amplifies student outcomes while supporting educator well-being, which is a crucial consideration given high rates of teacher burnout and turnover.

However, implementation faces significant challenges. Institutional resistance, concerns about secular framing of traditionally religious practices, and curriculum overload create barriers that require careful navigation. Successful programs address these concerns proactively through community engagement, clear communication about secular applications, and integration with existing academic goals rather than competing with them.

Higher education settings offer additional opportunities for contemplative education. Numerous colleges and universities now integrate these practices into curricula, student services, and faculty development programs. These initiatives help students and faculty develop resilience skills while exploring the intersection of academic learning and personal development (Barbezat & Bush, 2014). As these approaches mature, they may fundamentally transform how we think about education itself; moving beyond information transfer to whole-person development.

8.3 Organizational and Workplace Applications

The modern workplace increasingly recognizes contemplative practices as essential tools for addressing employee stress, burnout, and mental health challenges. Employees participating in contemplative programs show reduced stress, improved emotional regulation, and enhanced job engagement (Good et al., 2016). These individual improvements translate into better workplace relationships, enhanced communication, and more collaborative team dynamics.

Beyond individual training, some organizations pursue "organizational mindfulness", shifting entire cultures toward greater awareness, responsiveness, and resilience (Weick & Sutcliffe, 2006). This systems-level approach recognizes that individual contemplative skills flourish within supportive organizational contexts that value presence, reflection, and authentic communication.

Leadership support proves crucial for program success. When executives and managers embrace contemplative approaches personally, they create psychological safety for employees to engage authentically with the practices (Connors et al., 2024). Top-down support becomes especially important in high-stress professions like healthcare and emergency services, where vulnerability and openness may feel risky without clear institutional backing.

Healthcare settings deserve special attention given the unique stressors facing medical professionals. Programs specifically designed for healthcare workers demonstrate effectiveness for reducing burnout, improving emotional regulation, and enhancing compassion satisfaction (Craigie et al., 2016). These interventions address not just individual stress but the moral injury that healthcare workers experience when systemic constraints prevent them from providing optimal care.

However, workplace implementation must navigate ethical considerations carefully. Programs should be voluntary and culturally sensitive, avoiding any hint of coercion or cultural appropriation. The goal is supporting employee well-being, not controlling behavior or reducing legitimate concerns about workplace conditions through individual interventions alone.

8.4 Technology-Enhanced Delivery Methods

Technology opens unprecedented opportunities for making contemplative practices accessible to diverse populations while maintaining connection to traditional wisdom. Mobile applications, virtual reality platforms, and online programs can deliver authentic training across geographic and socioeconomic barriers that previously limited access to qualified teachers (Li et al., 2024).

Research on app-based programs shows significant benefits for stress reduction, anxiety management, and overall well-being. Well-designed applications provide guided practices, progress tracking, and personalized recommendations while preserving core contemplative elements (Flett et al., 2019). The best apps function as skillful digital teachers, offering appropriate guidance and encouragement while respecting the depth and subtlety of contemplative training.

However, technology-enhanced delivery raises important ethical concerns. The commodification of contemplative practices through apps and digital platforms risks reducing profound wisdom traditions to consumer products (Lukoff et al., 2020). Digital fatigue represents another concern. Overuse of mindfulness apps can lead to superficial engagement or avoidance-based coping rather than genuine contemplative development.

Virtual reality represents an emerging frontier offering immersive environments for meditation, yoga, and training. Preliminary research suggests VR-enhanced practices may produce stronger relaxation responses and greater engagement compared to traditional formats (Navarro-Haro et al., 2017). These technologies could prove particularly valuable for individuals with mobility limitations or those living in areas without access to qualified teachers.

Artificial intelligence systems for personalized contemplative training represent perhaps the most promising technological frontier. These systems could adapt practice recommendations based on individual progress, preferences, and even physiological responses measured through wearable devices (Lee et al., 2021).

Neurofeedback-guided meditation represents another emerging application where technology enhances rather than replaces traditional approaches. Real-time feedback about brain states during practice could accelerate learning and help practitioners recognize subtle internal experiences that might otherwise take years to develop (Ganesan et al., 2024).

As these technologies mature, we face the ethical imperative to apply them responsibly. This means preserving the depth and wisdom of contemplative traditions while leveraging technology's power to increase access and effectiveness. The goal is not to replace human teachers or community support but to extend their reach and enhance their impact. The future of contemplative practice implementation lies not in choosing between ancient wisdom and modern technology, but in thoughtfully integrating both to serve human flourishing. As we develop these frameworks, we must remain grounded in the fundamental purpose that has always driven contemplative practice: the reduction of suffering and the cultivation of human potential for wisdom, compassion, and resilience.

9. FUTURE DIRECTIONS AND RESEARCH PRIORITIES

Contemplative neuroscience has reached a pivotal moment in its evolution. The field has moved beyond asking whether meditation changes the brain—the evidence is clear that it does (Davidson & Lutz, 2008). Now researchers face more refined questions about how these changes occur, who benefits most, and how ancient wisdom can be skillfully integrated into modern healthcare and society.

This section explores four critical frontiers that will shape the next decade of research. First, methodological innovations must address the limitations of current study designs, moving from controlled laboratory settings to the messy realities of daily practice. Second, the field must embrace cultural diversity, moving beyond its Western-centric focus to honor indigenous wisdom traditions worldwide. Third, precision medicine approaches offer great opportunities to personalize contemplative interventions based on individual genetic, neurobiological, and psychological profiles. Finally, implementation science principles will determine whether promising research findings can successfully transition from academic journals to clinical practice and community settings.

These challenges are interconnected and urgent. As mental health concerns rise globally and contemplative practices gain mainstream acceptance, the field must evolve rapidly while maintaining scientific rigor and cultural sensitivity. The stakes extend far beyond academic achievement. Millions of people seeking relief from suffering depend on research that can effectively bridge ancient wisdom and modern science.

9.1 Methodological Innovation: Moving Beyond the Laboratory

Contemplative neuroscience stands at a methodological crossroads. While researchers have established compelling correlations between meditation practice and brain changes (Fox et al., 2014), the field now faces more sophisticated questions. Consider a Tibetan monk with 40,000 hours of meditation experience versus a stressed executive completing an 8-week mindfulness program. Are we witnessing the same neuroplastic processes, just at different intensities?

The answer requires longitudinal studies that few researchers have attempted. Most current investigations rely on cross-sectional snapshots or brief interventions (Lutz et al., 2008). What we need are decade-long studies tracking practitioners from novice to expert levels. Imagine following a cohort of new meditators through their entire contemplative journey, mapping how their brains evolve alongside their subjective experiences. This shift demands methodological rigor that earlier studies lacked. Many foundational studies used waitlist controls, essentially comparing meditators to people doing nothing. Future trials need active control groups. Does mindfulness meditation produce unique brain changes, or would any focused mental training yield similar results? When researchers compared mindfulness training to analytical thinking exercises, both groups showed attention improvements, but only mindfulness practitioners developed enhanced emotional regulation networks (Posner et al., 2015).

Perhaps most challenging is measuring what matters most. Neuroplasticity outcomes like cortical thickness are relatively straightforward to quantify. But how do we capture the depths of subjective states practitioners describe? The moments of insight, expansive compassion, or unshakeable equanimity? These experiences may represent the most meaningful changes, yet they remain frustratingly elusive to conventional measurement.

The ecological validity question looms large. Laboratory conditions, with their controlled environments and scheduled sessions, barely resemble how people actually practice. A mother meditating while her children play nearby, a commuter practicing mindfulness on a crowded subway, or a healthcare worker finding moments of contemplative awareness during a hectic shift. These real-world contexts may fundamentally alter practice effects.

9.2 Honoring Diverse Wisdom Traditions

The contemplative neuroscience field carries an uncomfortable truth: it has largely ignored the world's rich diversity of contemplative practices. Western mindfulness and Tibetan meditation have dominated research agendas, while equally sophisticated traditions remain scientifically unexplored (Gone et al., 2019).

Consider the Ubuntu philosophy of Southern Africa, which cultivates interconnectedness through communal rituals and shared contemplation (Maluleke, 2024). Or examine Qigong practices in China, where movement, breath, and meditation integrate seamlessly (Yeung et al., 2018). Indigenous Australian Dreamtime practices offer ways of connecting with landscape and ancestry (Hume, 2002). These aren't merely cultural curiosities; they represent millennia of refined understanding about human consciousness and well-being.

This oversight reflects what scholars call “epistemic injustice”. The systematic exclusion of certain ways of knowing from academic discourse. When Indigenous oral traditions or African philosophical systems are dismissed as unscientific, we lose access to potentially revolutionary insights about consciousness and healing. Future research requires genuine collaboration, not academic colonization. This means working with traditional knowledge keepers as equal partners, respecting cultural protocols, and ensuring communities benefit from research findings (Urrutia et al., 2023).

Cultural adaptation extends beyond research to intervention design. A mindfulness program developed for affluent Silicon Valley executives may fail completely in a rural Latino community. Language, values, family structures, and spiritual beliefs all influence how contemplative practices are received and sustained (Hall et al., 2016). Successful programs integrate cultural elements organically rather than simply translating materials.

9.3 Precision Medicine Meets Ancient Wisdom

The future of contemplative neuroscience lies in personalization. Just as precision medicine tailors cancer treatments to individual genetic profiles, contemplative interventions could be matched to personal neurobiological signatures (Collins & Varmus, 2015).

Genetic research offers intriguing possibilities. Certain gene variants influence stress sensitivity, neuroplasticity capacity, and neurotransmitter function. Someone with particular serotonin transporter gene variations might respond better to loving-kindness meditation than mindfulness of breathing (Caspi et al., 2010). While this research remains in early stages, preliminary findings suggest meaningful gene-by-intervention interactions.

Neuroimaging phenotyping represents another frontier. Imagine a future where brain scans inform practice recommendations as routinely as blood tests guide medication choices. A person with hyperactive amygdala responses might benefit from emotion-regulation focused practices, while someone with attention network differences could be directed toward concentration-based methods (Drysdale et al., 2017).

Real-time biometric feedback could revolutionize practice itself. Heart rate variability monitors, EEG headbands, and other wearable devices already provide immediate practice feedback (Thayer et al., 2012). Future systems might adjust guided meditations based on stress levels, attention states, or emotional responses detected through multiple biosensors.

However, this technological integration raises important ethical questions. Privacy concerns multiply when genetic data links to mental health practices. Accessibility issues emerge if personalized approaches require expensive testing or devices. The field must ensure that precision approaches enhance rather than replace human wisdom and cultural traditions.

9.4 From Laboratory to Clinic: Implementation Realities

The gap between research findings and clinical practice remains frustratingly wide. Efficacy studies prove contemplative interventions work under ideal conditions, with expert teachers, motivated participants, and controlled environments. Effectiveness studies reveal a messier reality (Crane et al., 2017).

Consider mindfulness-based stress reduction (MBSR) as it spreads from Jon Kabat-Zinn's carefully crafted program to thousands of healthcare settings worldwide. Quality varies dramatically. Some programs maintain rigorous standards, while others offer watered-down versions taught by inadequately trained instructors. This implementation variability undermines both effectiveness and safety.

The field urgently needs standardized training requirements and certification programs. Medical professionals wouldn't prescribe medications without proper pharmaceutical training; why should contemplative interventions be different? Organizations have developed comprehensive teacher training standards that could serve as models for healthcare settings (Kenny et al., 2020).

Economic considerations drive implementation decisions. While contemplative interventions require upfront investment in training and program development, they may reduce long-term healthcare costs through improved mental health outcomes and reduced medication dependence (Goyal et al., 2014). Rigorous cost-effectiveness studies could provide compelling arguments for insurance coverage and institutional adoption.

The most promising implementation approaches integrate contemplative practices with existing evidence-based treatments rather than positioning them as standalone alternatives. Dialectical behavior therapy already incorporates mindfulness elements. Acceptance and commitment therapy draws heavily on contemplative insights. These hybrid models suggest a future where contemplative practices enhance conventional treatments rather than compete with them (Chapman, 2006).

The future of contemplative neuroscience lies not in choosing between ancient wisdom and modern science, but in their thoughtful integration. This synthesis requires methodological innovation, cultural humility, technological sophistication, and practical wisdom. As the field matures, it moves beyond proving that contemplative practices "work" toward understanding how they work, for whom, and under what conditions. The stakes extend far beyond academic curiosity. In an era of rising mental health concerns, social fragmentation, and global uncertainty, contemplative practices offer evidence-based approaches to human flourishing. The next decade of research will determine whether these ancient tools can be skillfully adapted to meet contemporary challenges while honoring their profound cultural origins.

10. CONCLUSION

As ancient contemplative wisdom and modern neuroscience have come together, something astonishing has been discovered. The human brain is, in no way, set in stone as an adult brain; it has an amazing ability to change. The benefits of mindfulness, meditation and yoga disciplines are not just mood enhancing; they fundamentally re-structure our neural circuitry to become more resilient and more positive. Aided by the concept of neuroplasticity, these age-old practices have been deciphered to operate on the basic processes of brain adaptation.

The evidence is impressive. Sustained contemplative training yields quantifiable effects of brain structure, greater gray matter volume in brain areas involved in attention and setting and maintaining a mood or emotional tone, strengthened connections between executive-control networks and de-activated portions of the stress-response systems. These are not microscopic changes that can only be traced by advanced imaging tools. They become practical in making our lives better in how we deal with stress, manage our emotions, and overcome difficulties that are bound to come our way in life.

The mechanisms driving these transformations work in elegant concert. What comes forth is a radically holistic method of human development. By sharing respects to cultural origins of contemplative practices and researching their universal processes we also close a gap between worlds that have long been divided. This combination gives us the chance to create interventions that are not only scientifically sound but also culturally competent and do not lose their strength across diverse populations.

The practical implications go well beyond clinical practice The contemplative practices have been incorporated in evidence-based programs already being taught in schools, so that children are learning to manage their emotions as much as mathematics. Workplace wellness programs help overworked executives learn to pause between appointments to experience moments of mindfulness. Medical practitioners are understanding that the influence of the meditation approach to healthcare can be used to accompany and, in some cases, to lessen the reliance on clinically directed medical care. The applications are an embodiment of the movement towards more comprehensive methods of mental health and human flourishing.

The field is changing rapidly. Methodological advances transfer studies out of the laboratory into the messy realities of everyday life. Cultural inclusivity goes beyond Western mindfulness to embrace indigenous wisdom traditions across the globe. Precision medicine approaches promise to match specific practices to individual genetic and neurobiological profiles. Implementation science focuses on translating promising research findings into sustainable real-world programs.

Perhaps most importantly, this research validates what contemplative practitioners have understood for millennia: through intentional practice, we possess the capacity to transform our minds and, consequently, our lived experience. The brain's neuroplasticity provides the biological foundation for this ancient insight. Contemplative practices offer time-tested methods for actualizing our potential for growth and healing. As global challenges intensify and collective stress levels rise, cultivating resilience becomes not just personally beneficial but socially essential.

The journey of rewiring the brain for resilience represents more than therapeutic intervention. It's a pathway toward realizing our fullest human potential. Through systematic cultivation of awareness, emotional balance, and wisdom, we can literally sculpt our neural architecture in service of flourishing. This transformation benefits not only ourselves but ripples outward to everyone we encounter, contributing to a more compassionate and resilient world.

The ancient promise that we can train our minds has found its modern validation in the malleable circuitry of the human brain. What remains is the ongoing work of practice itself. The daily commitment to nurturing the neural pathways that serve our highest aspirations for how we might live and who we might become.

REFERENCES

Arnsten, A. F. T. (2009). Stress signalling pathways that impair prefrontal cortex structure and function. *Nature Reviews. Neuroscience, 10*(6), 410–422. DOI: 10.1038/nrn2648 PMID: 19455173

Austin, J. H. (1998). *Zen and the brain: Toward an understanding of meditation and consciousness* (pp. xxiv, 844). The MIT Press.

Barbezat, D. P., & Bush, M. (2014). *Contemplative practices in higher education: Powerful methods to transform teaching and learning* (pp. xxiii, 231). Jossey-Bass/Wiley.

Bishop, S. R., Lau, M., Shapiro, S., Carlson, L., Anderson, N. D., Carmody, J., Segal, Z. V., Abbey, S., Speca, M., Velting, D., & Devins, G. (2004). Mindfulness: A Proposed Operational Definition. *Clinical Psychology : a Publication of the Division of Clinical Psychology of the American Psychological Association, 11*(3), 230–241. DOI: 10.1093/clipsy.bph077

Bornemann, B., & Singer, T. (2017). Taking time to feel our body: Steady increases in heartbeat perception accuracy and decreases in alexithymia over 9 months of contemplative mental training. *Psychophysiology, 54*(3), 469–482. DOI: 10.1111/psyp.12790 PMID: 27925645

Bowles, N. I., Davies, J. N., & Van Dam, N. T. (2022). Dose–response Relationship of Reported Lifetime Meditation Practice with Mental Health and Wellbeing: A Cross-sectional Study. *Mindfulness, 13*(10), 2529–2546. DOI: 10.1007/s12671-022-01977-6 PMID: 36193220

Brahmbhatt, A., & Kumavat, P. P. (2024). Yoga and Mindfulness Practices: Their Role in Modern Mental Health and Wellness Programs. *Research Review Journal of Indian Knowledge Systems, 1*(2), 09–17. DOI: 10.31305/rrjiks.2024.v1.n2.002

Brewer, J. A., Worhunsky, P. D., Gray, J. R., Tang, Y.-Y., Weber, J., & Kober, H. (2011). Meditation experience is associated with differences in default mode network activity and connectivity. *Proceedings of the National Academy of Sciences of the United States of America, 108*(50), 20254–20259. DOI: 10.1073/pnas.1112029108 PMID: 22114193

Broderick, P. C., & Frank, J. L. (2014). Learning to BREATHE: An intervention to foster mindfulness in adolescence. *New Directions for Youth Development, 2014*(142), 31–44. DOI: 10.1002/yd.20095 PMID: 25100493

Brown, R. P., & Gerbarg, P. L. (2005). Sudarshan Kriya yogic breathing in the treatment of stress, anxiety, and depression: Part I-neurophysiologic model. *Journal of Alternative and Complementary Medicine (New York, N.Y.)*, *11*(1), 189–201. DOI: 10.1089/acm.2005.11.189 PMID: 15750381

Buckner, R. L., Andrews-Hanna, J. R., & Schacter, D. L. (2008). The brain's default network: Anatomy, function, and relevance to disease. *Annals of the New York Academy of Sciences*, *1124*(1), 1–38. DOI: 10.1196/annals.1440.011 PMID: 18400922

Buenrostro-Jáuregui, M. H., Muñóz-Sánchez, S., Rojas-Hernández, J., Alonso-Orozco, A. I., Vega-Flores, G., Tapia-de-Jesús, A., & Leal-Galicia, P. (2025). A Comprehensive Overview of Stress, Resilience, and Neuroplasticity Mechanisms. *International Journal of Molecular Sciences*, *26*(7), 3028. DOI: 10.3390/ijms26073028 PMID: 40243691

Buhle, J. T., Silvers, J. A., Wager, T. D., Lopez, R., Onyemekwu, C., Kober, H., Weber, J., & Ochsner, K. N. (2014). Cognitive Reappraisal of Emotion: A Meta-Analysis of Human Neuroimaging Studies. *Cerebral Cortex (New York, N.Y.)*, *24*(11), 2981–2990. DOI: 10.1093/cercor/bht154 PMID: 23765157

Carmody, J., & Baer, R. A. (2008). Relationships between mindfulness practice and levels of mindfulness, medical and psychological symptoms and well-being in a mindfulness-based stress reduction program. *Journal of Behavioral Medicine*, *31*(1), 23–33. DOI: 10.1007/s10865-007-9130-7 PMID: 17899351

Caspi, A., Hariri, A. R., Holmes, A., Uher, R., & Moffitt, T. E. (2010). Genetic Sensitivity to the Environment: The Case of the Serotonin Transporter Gene and Its Implications for Studying Complex Diseases and Traits. *The American Journal of Psychiatry*, *167*(5), 509–527. DOI: 10.1176/appi.ajp.2010.09101452 PMID: 20231323

Chapman, A. L. (2006). Acceptance and mindfulness in behavior therapy: A comparison of Dialectical Behavior Therapy and Acceptance and Commitment Therapy. *International Journal of Behavioral and Consultation Therapy*, *2*(3), 308–313. DOI: 10.1037/h0100785

Collins, F. S., & Varmus, H. (2015). A new initiative on precision medicine. *The New England Journal of Medicine*, *372*(9), 793–795. DOI: 10.1056/NEJMp1500523 PMID: 25635347

Connors, C., Norvell, M., & Wu, A. (2024). The RISE (Resilience in Stressful Events) Peer Support Program: Creating a Virtuous Cycle of Healthcare Leadership Support for Staff Resilience and Well-Being. *Journal of Healthcare Leadership*, *16*, 537–542. DOI: 10.2147/JHL.S487709 PMID: 39679177

Craig, A. D. B. (2009). How do you feel—Now? The anterior insula and human awareness. *Nature Reviews. Neuroscience*, *10*(1), 59–70. DOI: 10.1038/nrn2555 PMID: 19096369

Craigie, M., Osseiran-Moisson, R., Hemsworth, D., Aoun, S., Francis, K., Brown, J., Hegney, D., & Rees, C. (2016). The influence of trait-negative affect and compassion satisfaction on compassion fatigue in Australian nurses. *Psychological Trauma: Theory, Research, Practice, and Policy*, *8*(1), 88–97. DOI: 10.1037/tra0000050 PMID: 25961866

Crane, R. S., Brewer, J., Feldman, C., Kabat-Zinn, J., Santorelli, S., Williams, J. M. G., & Kuyken, W. (2017). What defines mindfulness-based programs? The warp and the weft. *Psychological Medicine*, *47*(6), 990–999. DOI: 10.1017/S0033291716003317 PMID: 28031068

Davidson, R. J., & Lutz, A. (2008). Buddha's Brain: Neuroplasticity and Meditation. *IEEE Signal Processing Magazine*, *25*(1), 176–174. DOI: 10.1109/MSP.2008.4431873 PMID: 20871742

Desbordes, G., Negi, L. T., Pace, T. W. W., Wallace, B. A., Raison, C. L., & Schwartz, E. L. (2012). Effects of mindful-attention and compassion meditation training on amygdala response to emotional stimuli in an ordinary, non-meditative state. *Frontiers in Human Neuroscience*, *6*, 292. DOI: 10.3389/fnhum.2012.00292 PMID: 23125828

Dita, M., & Bubuioc, L. (2024). Neuroplasticity—The metamorphosis of the human brain. *Vector European*, *1*(1), 188–192. DOI: 10.52507/2345-1106.2024-1.35

Draganski, B., & May, A. (2008). Training-induced structural changes in the adult human brain. *Behavioural Brain Research*, *192*(1), 137–142. DOI: 10.1016/j.bbr.2008.02.015 PMID: 18378330

Drysdale, A. T., Grosenick, L., Downar, J., Dunlop, K., Mansouri, F., Meng, Y., Fetcho, R. N., Zebley, B., Oathes, D. J., Etkin, A., Schatzberg, A. F., Sudheimer, K., Keller, J., Mayberg, H. S., Gunning, F. M., Alexopoulos, G. S., Fox, M. D., Pascual-Leone, A., Voss, H. U., & Liston, C. (2017). Resting-state connectivity biomarkers define neurophysiological subtypes of depression. *Nature Medicine*, *23*(1), 28–38. DOI: 10.1038/nm.4246 PMID: 27918562

Faraji, J., & Metz, G. A. S. (2024). *The Neuroexistentialism of Social Connectedness and Loneliness. PsyArXiv*. DOI: 10.31234/osf.io/3umvb

Farb, N. A. S., Segal, Z. V., & Anderson, A. K. (2013). Mindfulness meditation training alters cortical representations of interoceptive attention. *Social Cognitive and Affective Neuroscience*, *8*(1), 15–26. DOI: 10.1093/scan/nss066 PMID: 22689216

Flett, J. A. M., Hayne, H., Riordan, B. C., Thompson, L. M., & Conner, T. S. (2019). Mobile Mindfulness Meditation: A Randomised Controlled Trial of the Effect of Two Popular Apps on Mental Health. *Mindfulness*, *10*(5), 863–876. DOI: 10.1007/s12671-018-1050-9

Fox, K. C. R., Nijeboer, S., Dixon, M. L., Floman, J. L., Ellamil, M., Rumak, S. P., Sedlmeier, P., & Christoff, K. (2014). Is meditation associated with altered brain structure? A systematic review and meta-analysis of morphometric neuroimaging in meditation practitioners. *Neuroscience and Biobehavioral Reviews*, *43*, 48–73. DOI: 10.1016/j.neubiorev.2014.03.016 PMID: 24705269

Fredrickson, B. L., Boulton, A. J., Firestine, A. M., Van Cappellen, P., Algoe, S. B., Brantley, M. M., Kim, S. L., Brantley, J., & Salzberg, S. (2017). Positive Emotion Correlates of Meditation Practice: A Comparison of Mindfulness Meditation and Loving-Kindness Meditation. *Mindfulness*, *8*(6), 1623–1633. DOI: 10.1007/s12671-017-0735-9 PMID: 29201247

Ganesan, S., Van Dam, N., Kamboj, S. K., Tsuchiyagaito, A., Sacchet, M. D., Misaki, M., Moffat, B. A., Lorenzetti, V., & Zalesky, A. (2024). High-precision neurofeedback-guided meditation training optimises real-world self-guided meditation practice for well-being. *Neuroscience*. Advance online publication. DOI: 10.1101/2024.10.25.618656 PMID: 39484554

Gone, J. P., Hartmann, W. E., Pomerville, A., Wendt, D. C., Klem, S. H., & Burrage, R. L. (2019). The impact of historical trauma on health outcomes for indigenous populations in the USA and Canada: A systematic review. *The American Psychologist*, *74*(1), 20–35. DOI: 10.1037/amp0000338 PMID: 30652897

Good, D. J., Lyddy, C. J., Glomb, T. M., Bono, J. E., Brown, K. W., Duffy, M. K., Baer, R. A., Brewer, J. A., & Lazar, S. W. (2016). Contemplating Mindfulness at Work: An Integrative Review. *Journal of Management*, *42*(1), 114–142. DOI: 10.1177/0149206315617003

Goyal, M., Singh, S., Sibinga, E. M. S., Gould, N. F., Rowland-Seymour, A., Sharma, R., Berger, Z., Sleicher, D., Maron, D. D., Shihab, H. M., Ranasinghe, P. D., Linn, S., Saha, S., Bass, E. B., & Haythornthwaite, J. A. (2014). Meditation programs for psychological stress and well-being: A systematic review and meta-analysis. *JAMA Internal Medicine*, *174*(3), 357–368. DOI: 10.1001/jamainternmed.2013.13018 PMID: 24395196

Grabbe, L., Higgins, M. K., Baird, M., & Pfeiffer, K. M. (2021). Impact of a Resiliency Training to Support the Mental Well-being of Front-line Workers: Brief Report of a Quasi-experimental Study of the Community Resiliency Model. *Medical Care*, *59*(7), 616–621. DOI: 10.1097/MLR.0000000000001535 PMID: 33827106

Grant, J. A., Courtemanche, J., Duerden, E. G., Duncan, G. H., & Rainville, P. (2010). Cortical thickness and pain sensitivity in zen meditators. *Emotion (Washington, D.C.)*, *10*(1), 43–53. DOI: 10.1037/a0018334 PMID: 20141301

Hall, G. C. N., Ibaraki, A. Y., Huang, E. R., Marti, C. N., & Stice, E. (2016). A Meta-Analysis of Cultural Adaptations of Psychological Interventions. *Behavior Therapy*, *47*(6), 993–1014. DOI: 10.1016/j.beth.2016.09.005 PMID: 27993346

Hasenkamp, W., & Barsalou, L. W. (2012). Effects of Meditation Experience on Functional Connectivity of Distributed Brain Networks. *Frontiers in Human Neuroscience*, *6*, 38. DOI: 10.3389/fnhum.2012.00038 PMID: 22403536

Hecht, F. M., & Crane, R. S. (2025). Intervention Fidelity in Mindfulness-Based Research and Practice: Overview of the Special Collection and State of the Field. *Global Advances in Integrative Medicine and Health*, *14*, 27536130251349453. DOI: 10.1177/27536130251349453 PMID: 40520822

Hölzel, B. K., Carmody, J., Vangel, M., Congleton, C., Yerramsetti, S. M., Gard, T., & Lazar, S. W. (2011). Mindfulness practice leads to increases in regional brain gray matter density. *Psychiatry Research*, *191*(1), 36–43. DOI: 10.1016/j.pscychresns.2010.08.006 PMID: 21071182

Hume, L. (2002). Ancestral power: The dreaming, consciousness, and Aboriginal Australians. *Choice Reviews Online, 40*(08), 40-4683-40–4683. DOI: 10.5860/CHOICE.40-4683

Hutcherson, C. A., Seppala, E. M., & Gross, J. J. (2008). Loving-kindness meditation increases social connectedness. *Emotion (Washington, D.C.)*, *8*(5), 720–724. DOI: 10.1037/a0013237 PMID: 18837623

Jennings, P. A., DeMauro, A. A., & Mischenko, P. (2019). Cultivating Awareness and Resilience in Education. In Ivtzan, I. (Ed.), *Handbook of Mindfulness-Based Programmes* (1st ed., pp. 219–230). Routledge., DOI: 10.4324/9781315265438-18

Kabat-Zinn, J. (2003). Mindfulness-based interventions in context: Past, present, and future. *Clinical Psychology : a Publication of the Division of Clinical Psychology of the American Psychological Association*, *10*(2), 144–156. DOI: 10.1093/clipsy.bpg016

Kalisch, R., Baker, D. G., Basten, U., Boks, M. P., Bonanno, G. A., Brummelman, E., Chmitorz, A., Fernàndez, G., Fiebach, C. J., Galatzer-Levy, I., Geuze, E., Groppa, S., Helmreich, I., Hendler, T., Hermans, E. J., Jovanovic, T., Kubiak, T., Lieb, K., Lutz, B., & Kleim, B. (2017). The resilience framework as a strategy to combat stress-related disorders. *Nature Human Behaviour*, *1*(11), 784–790. DOI: 10.1038/s41562-017-0200-8 PMID: 31024125

Karatsoreos, I. N., & McEwen, B. S. (2013). Resilience and vulnerability: A neurobiological perspective. *F1000prime Reports*, *5*. Advance online publication. DOI: 10.12703/P5-13 PMID: 23710327

Kelly, A., & Garland, E. L. (2016). Trauma-Informed Mindfulness-Based Stress Reduction for Female Survivors of Interpersonal Violence: Results From a Stage I RCT: TI-MBSR for IPV Survivors. *Journal of Clinical Psychology*, *72*(4), 311–328. DOI: 10.1002/jclp.22273 PMID: 27002222

Kenny, M., Luck, P., & Koerbel, L. (2020). Tending the Field of Mindfulness-Based Programs: The Development of International Integrity Guidelines for Teachers and Teacher Training. *Global Advances in Health and Medicine : Improving Healthcare Outcomes Worldwide*, *9*, 2164956120923975. DOI: 10.1177/2164956120923975 PMID: 32426180

Klimecki, O. M., Leiberg, S., Ricard, M., & Singer, T. (2014). Differential pattern of functional brain plasticity after compassion and empathy training. *Social Cognitive and Affective Neuroscience*, *9*(6), 873–879. DOI: 10.1093/scan/nst060 PMID: 23576808

Lazar, S. W., Kerr, C. E., Wasserman, R. H., Gray, J. R., Greve, D. N., Treadway, M. T., McGarvey, M., Quinn, B. T., Dusek, J. A., Benson, H., Rauch, S. L., Moore, C. I., & Fischl, B. (2005). Meditation experience is associated with increased cortical thickness. *Neuroreport*, *16*(17), 1893–1897. DOI: 10.1097/01.wnr.0000186598.66243.19 PMID: 16272874

LeDoux, J. E. (2000). Emotion circuits in the brain. *Annual Review of Neuroscience*, *23*(1), 155–184. DOI: 10.1146/annurev.neuro.23.1.155 PMID: 10845062

Lee, E. E., Torous, J., De Choudhury, M., Depp, C. A., Graham, S. A., Kim, H.-C., Paulus, M. P., Krystal, J. H., & Jeste, D. V. (2021). Artificial Intelligence for Mental Health Care: Clinical Applications, Barriers, Facilitators, and Artificial Wisdom. *Biological Psychiatry: Cognitive Neuroscience and Neuroimaging*, *6*(9), 856–864. DOI: 10.1016/j.bpsc.2021.02.001 PMID: 33571718

Li, J., Cochrane, K. A., & Leshed, G. (2024). Beyond Meditation: Understanding Everyday Mindfulness Practices and Technology Use Among Experienced Practitioners. *Proceedings of the ACM on Human-Computer Interaction, 8*(CSCW2), 1–29. DOI: 10.1145/3687023

Luders, E., Toga, A. W., Lepore, N., & Gaser, C. (2009). The underlying anatomical correlates of long-term meditation: Larger hippocampal and frontal volumes of gray matter. *NeuroImage*, *45*(3), 672–678. DOI: 10.1016/j.neuroimage.2008.12.061 PMID: 19280691

Lukoff, K., Lyngs, U., Gueorguieva, S., Dillman, E. S., Hiniker, A., & Munson, S. A. (2020). From Ancient Contemplative Practice to the App Store: Designing a Digital Container for Mindfulness. *Proceedings of the 2020 ACM Designing Interactive Systems Conference*, 1551–1564. DOI: 10.1145/3357236.3395444

Lutz, A., Greischar, L. L., Rawlings, N. B., Ricard, M., & Davidson, R. J. (2004). Long-term meditators self-induce high-amplitude gamma synchrony during mental practice. *Proceedings of the National Academy of Sciences of the United States of America*, *101*(46), 16369–16373. DOI: 10.1073/pnas.0407401101 PMID: 15534199

Lutz, A., Slagter, H. A., Dunne, J. D., & Davidson, R. J. (2008). Attention regulation and monitoring in meditation. *Trends in Cognitive Sciences*, *12*(4), 163–169. DOI: 10.1016/j.tics.2008.01.005 PMID: 18329323

Lutz, J., Herwig, U., Opialla, S., Hittmeyer, A., Jäncke, L., Rufer, M., Grosse Holtforth, M., & Brühl, A. B. (2014). Mindfulness and emotion regulation—An fMRI study. *Social Cognitive and Affective Neuroscience*, *9*(6), 776–785. DOI: 10.1093/scan/nst043 PMID: 23563850

Lyons, K. E., & DeLange, J. (2016). Mindfulness Matters in the Classroom: The Effects of Mindfulness Training on Brain Development and Behavior in Children and Adolescents. In Schonert-Reichl, K. A., & Roeser, R. W. (Eds.), *Handbook of Mindfulness in Education* (pp. 271–283). Springer New York., DOI: 10.1007/978-1-4939-3506-2_17

Machida, S., Sunagawa, M., Takahashi, T., & Hiroshima University, Blueberry lodge 206, Koyama719, Gotemba, Shizuoka, Japan. (2018). Oxytocin Release during the Meditation of Altruism andAppreciation (Arigato-Zen): Machida S et al. Oxytocin release stimulated by the meditation. *International Journal of Neurology Research*, *4*(1), 364–370. DOI: 10.17554/j.issn.2313-5611.2018.04.75

Maluleke, A. (2024). Exploring Ubuntu-Based Research Methodologies in Southern African Bantu People's Embodied Movements: Ethical Considerations, Community-Based Strategies, and Philosophy. *Conversations Across the Field of Dance Studies, 43*(0). Advance online publication. DOI: 10.3998/conversations.5950

Manna, A., Raffone, A., Perrucci, M. G., Nardo, D., Ferretti, A., Tartaro, A., Londei, A., Del Gratta, C., Belardinelli, M. O., & Romani, G. L. (2010). Neural correlates of focused attention and cognitive monitoring in meditation. *Brain Research Bulletin, 82*(1–2), 46–56. DOI: 10.1016/j.brainresbull.2010.03.001 PMID: 20223285

Marchand, W. R. (2014). Neural mechanisms of mindfulness and meditation: Evidence from neuroimaging studies. *World Journal of Radiology, 6*(7), 471–479. DOI: 10.4329/wjr.v6.i7.471 PMID: 25071887

Masten, A. S., & Motti-Stefanidi, F. (2020). Multisystem Resilience for Children and Youth in Disaster: Reflections in the Context of COVID-19. *Adversity and Resilience Science, 1*(2), 95–106. DOI: 10.1007/s42844-020-00010-w PMID: 32838305

McKibben, E. (2025). Mind-Stuff and Withdrawal of the Senses: Toward an Interpretation of Pratyahara in Contemporary Postural Yoga. *Health, 29*(1), 83–99. DOI: 10.1177/13634593231222450 PMID: 38311913

Navarro-Haro, M. V., López-Del-Hoyo, Y., Campos, D., Linehan, M. M., Hoffman, H. G., García-Palacios, A., Modrego-Alarcón, M., Borao, L., & García-Campayo, J. (2017). Meditation experts try Virtual Reality Mindfulness: A pilot study evaluation of the feasibility and acceptability of Virtual Reality to facilitate mindfulness practice in people attending a Mindfulness conference. *PLoS One, 12*(11), e0187777. DOI: 10.1371/journal.pone.0187777 PMID: 29166665

Pascoe, M. C., Thompson, D. R., Jenkins, Z. M., & Ski, C. F. (2017). Mindfulness mediates the physiological markers of stress: Systematic review and meta-analysis. *Journal of Psychiatric Research, 95*, 156–178. DOI: 10.1016/j.jpsychires.2017.08.004 PMID: 28863392

Piet, J., & Hougaard, E. (2011). The effect of mindfulness-based cognitive therapy for prevention of relapse in recurrent major depressive disorder: A systematic review and meta-analysis. *Clinical Psychology Review, 31*(6), 1032–1040. DOI: 10.1016/j.cpr.2011.05.002 PMID: 21802618

Popova, N. K., & Naumenko, V. S. (2019). Neuronal and behavioral plasticity: The role of serotonin and BDNF systems tandem. *Expert Opinion on Therapeutic Targets, 23*(3), 227–239. DOI: 10.1080/14728222.2019.1572747 PMID: 30661441

Porges, S. W. (2011). *The polyvagal theory: Neurophysiological foundations of emotions, attachment, communication, and self-regulation* (pp. xvii, 347). W. W. Norton & Company.

Posner, M. I., Rothbart, M. K., & Tang, Y.-Y. (2015). Enhancing attention through training. *Current Opinion in Behavioral Sciences, 4*, 1–5. DOI: 10.1016/j.cobeha.2014.12.008

Rudolph, K. (2021). Ethical Considerations in Trauma-Informed Care. *The Psychiatric Clinics of North America, 44*(4), 521–535. DOI: 10.1016/j.psc.2021.07.001 PMID: 34763786

Seeley, W. W., Menon, V., Schatzberg, A. F., Keller, J., Glover, G. H., Kenna, H., Reiss, A. L., & Greicius, M. D. (2007). Dissociable intrinsic connectivity networks for salience processing and executive control. *The Journal of Neuroscience : The Official Journal of the Society for Neuroscience, 27*(9), 2349–2356. DOI: 10.1523/JNEUROSCI.5587-06.2007 PMID: 17329432

Seth, A. K. (2013). Interoceptive inference, emotion, and the embodied self. *Trends in Cognitive Sciences, 17*(11), 565–573. DOI: 10.1016/j.tics.2013.09.007 PMID: 24126130

Shier, M. L., & Turpin, A. (2017). A Multi-Dimensional Conceptual Framework for Trauma-Informed Practice in Addictions Programming. *Journal of Social Service Research, 43*(5), 609–623. DOI: 10.1080/01488376.2017.1364318

Stevens, C. F. (1999). Memory: From Mind to Molecules. *Nature Medicine, 5*(12), 1343–1344. DOI: 10.1038/70903 PMID: 10581065

Streeter, C. C., Gerbarg, P. L., Saper, R. B., Ciraulo, D. A., & Brown, R. P. (2012). Effects of yoga on the autonomic nervous system, gamma-aminobutyric-acid, and allostasis in epilepsy, depression, and post-traumatic stress disorder. *Medical Hypotheses, 78*(5), 571–579. DOI: 10.1016/j.mehy.2012.01.021 PMID: 22365651

Tang, Y.-Y., Ma, Y., Wang, J., Fan, Y., Feng, S., Lu, Q., Yu, Q., Sui, D., Rothbart, M. K., Fan, M., & Posner, M. I. (2007). Short-term meditation training improves attention and self-regulation. *Proceedings of the National Academy of Sciences of the United States of America, 104*(43), 17152–17156. DOI: 10.1073/pnas.0707678104 PMID: 17940025

Tang, Y.-Y., & Posner, M. I. (2009). Attention training and attention state training. *Trends in Cognitive Sciences, 13*(5), 222–227. DOI: 10.1016/j.tics.2009.01.009 PMID: 19375975

Taren, A. A., Creswell, J. D., & Gianaros, P. J. (2013). Dispositional mindfulness co-varies with smaller amygdala and caudate volumes in community adults. *PLoS One*, *8*(5), e64574. DOI: 10.1371/journal.pone.0064574 PMID: 23717632

Thayer, J. F., Ahs, F., Fredrikson, M., Sollers, J. J.III, & Wager, T. D. (2012). A meta-analysis of heart rate variability and neuroimaging studies: Implications for heart rate variability as a marker of stress and health. *Neuroscience and Biobehavioral Reviews*, *36*(2), 747–756. DOI: 10.1016/j.neubiorev.2011.11.009 PMID: 22178086

Troy, A. S., Willroth, E. C., Shallcross, A. J., Giuliani, N. R., Gross, J. J., & Mauss, I. B. (2023). Psychological Resilience: An Affect-Regulation Framework. *Annual Review of Psychology*, *74*(1), 547–576. DOI: 10.1146/annurev-psych-020122-041854 PMID: 36103999

Urrutia, J., Anderson, B. T., Belouin, S. J., Berger, A., Griffiths, R. R., Grob, C. S., Henningfield, J. E., Labate, B. C., Maier, L. J., Maternowska, M. C., Weichold, F., Yaden, D. B., & Magar, V. (2023). Psychedelic Science, Contemplative Practices, and Indigenous and Other Traditional Knowledge Systems: Towards Integrative Community-Based Approaches in Global Health. *Journal of Psychoactive Drugs*, *55*(5), 523–538. DOI: 10.1080/02791072.2023.2258367 PMID: 37747281

Vago, D. R., & Silbersweig, D. A. (2012). Self-awareness, self-regulation, and self-transcendence (S-ART): A framework for understanding the neurobiological mechanisms of mindfulness. *Frontiers in Human Neuroscience*, *6*, 296. DOI: 10.3389/fnhum.2012.00296 PMID: 23112770

van der Kolk, B. A. (2014). *The body keeps the score: Brain, mind, and body in the healing of trauma* (pp. xvi, 443). Viking.

Verhaeghen, P. (2017). The Self-Effacing Buddhist: No(t)-Self in Early Buddhism and Contemplative Neuroscience. *Contemporary Buddhism*, *18*(1), 21–36. DOI: 10.1080/14639947.2017.1297344

Villemure, C., Ceko, M., Cotton, V. A., & Bushnell, M. C. (2014). Insular cortex mediates increased pain tolerance in yoga practitioners. *Cerebral Cortex (New York, N.Y.: 1991)*, *24*(10), 2732–2740. DOI: 10.1093/cercor/bht124

Weick, K. E., & Sutcliffe, K. M. (2006). Mindfulness and the Quality of Organizational Attention. *Organization Science*, *17*(4), 514–524. DOI: 10.1287/orsc.1060.0196

Weng, H. Y., Fox, A. S., Shackman, A. J., Stodola, D. E., Caldwell, J. Z. K., Olson, M. C., Rogers, G. M., & Davidson, R. J. (2013). Compassion Training Alters Altruism and Neural Responses to Suffering. *Psychological Science*, *24*(7), 1171–1180. DOI: 10.1177/0956797612469537 PMID: 23696200

World Health Organization. (2022). *Mental disorders.* https://www.who.int/news-room/fact-sheets/detail/mental-disorders

Yeung, A., Chan, J. S. M., Cheung, J. C., & Zou, L. (2018). Qigong and Tai-Chi for Mood Regulation. *Focus (San Francisco, Calif.), 16*(1), 40–47. DOI: 10.1176/appi.focus.20170042 PMID: 31975898

Zatorre, R. J., Fields, R. D., & Johansen-Berg, H. (2012). Plasticity in gray and white: Neuroimaging changes in brain structure during learning. *Nature Neuroscience, 15*(4), 528–536. DOI: 10.1038/nn.3045 PMID: 22426254

Zenner, C., Herrnleben-Kurz, S., & Walach, H. (2014). Mindfulness-based interventions in schools-a systematic review and meta-analysis. *Frontiers in Psychology, 5*, 603. DOI: 10.3389/fpsyg.2014.00603 PMID: 25071620

Chapter 7
Swami Vivekananda and Practical Vedanta: Transforming Mental Health Through Ancient Wisdom

Raj Madhu
http://orcid.org/0009-0001-0516-3365
Central University of Jammu, India

Pallvi Sharma
http://orcid.org/0009-0006-1885-9560
Central University of Jammu, India

Gurashish Kour
http://orcid.org/0009-0002-2831-2754
Central University of Jammu, India

Asit K. Mantry
Central University of Jammu, India

Biswabhusan Pradhan
Central University of Jammu, India

ABSTRACT

This chapter explores the relevance of Swami Vivekananda's Practical Vedanta in addressing contemporary mental health challenges. Drawing from core Vedantic principles, such as Atman (the Self), Brahman (ultimate reality), and Advaita (non-dualism), the chapter examines how self-awareness, detachment (Vairagya), and Karma Yoga can transform emotional distress into inner strength. It integrates philosophical insights with psychological concepts like emotional regulation,

DOI: 10.4018/979-8-3373-4187-3.ch007

mindfulness, and resilience, offering a spiritually grounded framework for mental well-being. Through Vivekananda's reinterpretation of Vedanta as a lived philosophy, the chapter argues for inward-directed approaches that transcend symptom management and foster deeper self-realization. This synthesis provides an inclusive, non-sectarian path to emotional clarity and inner freedom in an age of psychological fragmentation.

INTRODUCTION

Mental health has become one of the most urgent human concerns today. From adolescents navigating academic pressure to working adults experiencing burnout and older adults facing isolation, psychological distress now affects individuals across generations, socioeconomic groups, and gender identities. Contemporary lifestyles have intensified stress, loneliness, and inner dissatisfaction, and despite advances in healthcare, therapy, and medication, many people continue to feel overwhelmed, anxious, or disconnected from themselves (Gusha et al., 2017). This persistent discomfort raises a deeper question: Are current approaches addressing only the symptoms of mental distress rather than its underlying causes?

Much of today's mental health discourse emphasizes external adjustments such as habit change, workload management, behavioral therapy, or environmental modification. While these interventions are valuable, they may not fully address the patterns of thought, emotional reactivity, and identity formation that contribute to ongoing distress. This is where spiritual and philosophical traditions offer an additional framework. Rather than focusing solely on problem reduction, they aim to illuminate the nature of the mind and subjective experience. Vedanta, for example, provides a systematic approach to inner awareness, psychological clarity, and freedom (Vorkapic, 2016).

Vedanta, rooted in the Vedas, proposes that enduring well-being does not depend on external circumstances but on recognising one's deeper identity beyond fluctuating thoughts and emotions. It suggests that individuals are fundamentally peaceful and free, a perspective that contrasts sharply with the fragmented and overstimulated mental states common today. This view positions the mind as a functional instrument rather than the core of identity, a stance that resonates with contemporary research on mindfulness, metacognition, and cognitive defusion (Hari, 2015).

For many modern readers, however, metaphysical concepts can appear abstract or distant. Swami Vivekananda addressed this gap by translating Vedantic insights into accessible, practice-oriented methods for everyday life. His articulation of "Practical Vedanta" reframed spiritual life as compatible with action, responsibility, and social engagement. Rather than withdrawing from challenges, he encouraged individuals to cultivate inner discipline, clarity, and strength as a foundation for psychological resilience (Mishra, 2014).

Vivekananda's message remains highly relevant for contemporary mental health discourse. He emphasised strength as the basis of mental and spiritual life and argued that individuals often become entangled in their own patterns of thought and emotion. His well-known call to "Arise, awake, and stop not until the goal is reached" is not merely motivational but reflects a psychological orientation toward agency, self-efficacy, and emotional stability. For him, Vedanta offered a systematic framework for overcoming suffering and cultivating clarity and calm (Sharma, 2004).

This chapter extends Vivekananda's vision by examining how Practical Vedanta can inform modern approaches to stress, anxiety, emotional volatility, and mental restlessness. It demonstrates how principles such as self-awareness, non-attachment, mindful action, and reflective discipline align with contemporary constructs like emotional regulation, attentional training, and resilience. The discussion is designed to be accessible to readers across cultural backgrounds, age groups, and gender identities, making the insights applicable to diverse professional and personal contexts.

Rather than proposing quick solutions, the chapter encourages a different way of understanding the self, the mind, and the sources of psychological well-being. It introduces foundational Vedantic principles and shows how they can be integrated into daily life, work, relationships, and moments of crisis. It also situates Vedantic thought within the broader landscape of current psychological approaches, including mindfulness-based practices and emerging research on awareness, identity, and mental health.

FOUNDATIONS OF PRACTICAL VEDANTA

Vedanta belongs to the six classical schools of Indian philosophy. Vedanta means the end of the Vedas, and the philosophical teachings of the Upanishads are the last of the Vedic scriptures. Such teachings do not concern rituals and exterior worship, but rather the higher truths about existence, consciousness, and the self. Vedanta poses essential questions: Who am I? What is the essence of reality? But why live? Its answers have deep psychological and practical meanings for people confused by fear or experiencing emotional pain (Kapoor, 2002).

Swami Vivekananda updated Vedanta for modern life. These deep metaphysical ideas he made accessible, relevant, and practical. Understanding his contribution requires first identifying the Vedanta's basic principles and then seeing how he translated them into tools for living.

Core Principles of Vedanta: Atman, Brahman, and Non-Dualism

The foundation of Vedanta rests on three core concepts:

Atman (The Self): Vedanta says that our real identity is not the body, not the mind, not even the personality, but the atman, the one invincible consciousness within us. This transcends all emotions, thoughts, and external conditions. The majority of our mental pain comes from identifying with these shifting feelings and states of flux. Saying "I am sad" or "I am anxious" confuses our true self with temporary states of mind (Brahmaprana, 2001).

Brahman (The Absolute Reality): Brahman is a formless, infinite reality behind all things. It is the source, essence, and unity behind all the diversity in the world. Vedanta says that Brahman is within us—Atman. The Upanishad teaches: "Tat Tvam Asi" - "Thou art That" means that the self in each of us is identical to the universal reality (Myers, 2000).

Advaita (Non-Dualism): Its most distinctive feature is non-duality, especially in Vedanta, especially in Advaita Vedanta (the school Swami Vivekananda followed). They say there is no true separation between the self and the universe or between God and the soul. Separation is a mental illusion. Overcoming ignorance means that all is one (Ram-Prasad, 2002).

All these teachings are very spiritual but profoundly psychological. Most mental suffering is caused by divisions between me and the world, me and others, and me and God. Vedanta breaks this separation and points to wholeness, peace, and inner stability.

Vivekananda's Interpretation: Philosophy in Action

Swami Vivekananda's most significant contribution lay in reframing Vedanta not as an abstract philosophical system but as a lived discipline grounded in psychological transformation and ethical action. For him, Vedanta was meaningful only when it shaped daily conduct, emotional regulation, and patterns of thought. He repeatedly argued that spiritual knowledge must move beyond intellectual discourse to experiential realization, stating in the *Complete Works*, "What good is it if Vedanta is only theory? It must be realized. Religion is not in theory, not in books, not in words, it is being and becoming" (Vivekananda, 1947; Maharaj, 2017).

Vivekananda interpreted Vedantic teachings in a manner that was:

Active: He emphasized disciplined engagement with the world rather than withdrawal. This perspective positioned spiritual practice as compatible with work, responsibility, and social participation.

Universal: His articulation of Vedanta was not restricted to particular religious, cultural, or social identities. He highlighted the universality of consciousness and the shared spiritual potential of all human beings.

Human-centered: Vivekananda argued that spiritual insight should empower individuals psychologically and materially, particularly those experiencing vulnerability, marginalization, or emotional instability.

This interpretive stance led him to redefine concepts such as liberation and salvation. When addressing the question of freedom, he insisted that "the idea of salvation is always here and now… not in the future. Not in heaven, but here on earth." For Vivekananda, freedom referred not to a posthumous state but to a present-moment release from fear, hatred, weakness, and psychological fragmentation (Vivekananda, 1958).

In this way, Vivekananda transformed Vedanta into a framework resembling a practical psychology of inner development. He encouraged individuals to cultivate strength through self-knowledge, to master the fluctuations of the mind, and to engage in service grounded not in pity but in the recognition of the intrinsic divinity of all beings (Vivekananda, 1951). His interpretation bridges metaphysics and lived experience, making Vedanta a system of applied self-transformation relevant to modern mental health and well-being.

From Abstract Metaphysics to Lived Spirituality

Ancient Indian philosophical systems are sometimes criticized for being overly abstract and concerned primarily with transcendent realities rather than practical concerns. Swami Vivekananda sought to correct this perception by demonstrating that Vedantic ideas possess direct psychological and ethical relevance for everyday life. His teachings brought what he described as the "loftiest" principles of Vedanta into the domain of lived experience and human welfare (Vivekananda, 1958,1964).

Vivekananda argued that foundational concepts such as *Atman* and *Brahman* are not merely metaphysical constructs but frameworks that can inform emotional stability, cognitive clarity, and interpersonal harmony. For example:

Understanding the Atman: Recognizing the Atman as one's deeper identity can reduce self-doubt and internalized negative evaluations. Even an initial intellectual engagement with the idea that one's true nature is pure, luminous consciousness rather than a shifting collection of thoughts, memories, and social roles can foster confidence and a more stable sense of self.

Seeing the world as Brahman: Interpreting the external world as an expression of Brahman may decrease affective states such as jealousy, resentment, and hostility. When individuals perceive others as sharing the same fundamental reality, rigid ego-based boundaries between "self" and "other" begin to soften, enabling more compassionate forms of interaction.

Realizing non-duality: The experiential understanding of non-duality offers a counterpoint to contemporary experiences of fragmentation and loneliness. In a time when social isolation has become a significant mental health concern, the Vedantic view that all beings emerge from a single underlying reality can promote a sense of connection and belonging.

Vivekananda further emphasized that Vedanta is grounded in realization rather than belief. Realization, in his account, is cultivated through disciplined practices such as meditation, reflective inquiry, ethical conduct, and dedicated service. His often-cited assertion that one must be able to perceive the divine in those who suffer before claiming to perceive it in a temple exemplifies his insistence that Vedanta becomes meaningful only when expressed through compassionate action. In this way, Vivekananda articulated a model of spirituality that unites metaphysical insight with psychological transformation and social responsibility.

Universal Self, Self-Realization, and Everyday Relevance

Vedanta does not conceptualize a deity who rewards or punishes; rather, it articulates the idea of a universal self that is present in all beings. Realizing this universal self is considered the central aim of human life. Far from promoting self-centeredness, this understanding of the self points to a profound form of selflessness, grounded in the recognition of non-difference between oneself and others (Vivekananda, 1958,2016, 1956).

In this framework, self-realization does not involve withdrawal from the world but a clearer perception of life as it is lived. Swami Vivekananda repeatedly emphasized that Vedanta is intended for all individuals, not only monastics or spiritual specialists. Its relevance extends to diverse contemporary contexts, such as: a mother managing the complexities of caregiving in a demanding household; a teacher navigating burnout within an overextended educational system; a student struggling with identity formation and anxiety; a worker confronting purposelessness in a high-pressure professional environment. Across such varied situations, Vedantic principles offer tools for inner stability and psychological resilience. Examples include:

Detachment without indifference: Vedanta proposes the possibility of engaging fully in relationships and responsibilities while maintaining a mental stance that is not dependent on outcomes. This form of non-attachment reduces emotional reactivity without diminishing care or commitment.

Self-awareness without ego: Vedantic introspection encourages a deep examination of the self, not to reinforce personal identity, but to recognize what lies beyond its habitual constructs.

Action without bondage: Karma Yoga, central to Vivekananda's interpretation, provides a framework for working in the world without becoming psychologically constrained by success, failure, praise, or criticism.

The concept of the universal self is not presented as an abstract metaphysical doctrine but as an experiential reality accessible through disciplined inquiry and practice. Realizing this dimension of selfhood can support psychological qualities such as courage, compassion, and emotional steadiness.

Vedanta as articulated by Vivekananda (1951) therefore offers not only a pathway for spiritual development but also a foundation for emotional strength, cognitive clarity, and psychological well-being (Sarkar, 2021). It replaces guilt with responsibility, encourages agency instead of helplessness, and promotes unity rather than despair (Singh, 2015).

Figure 1. Conceptual Diagram of Practical Vedanta and Mental Health

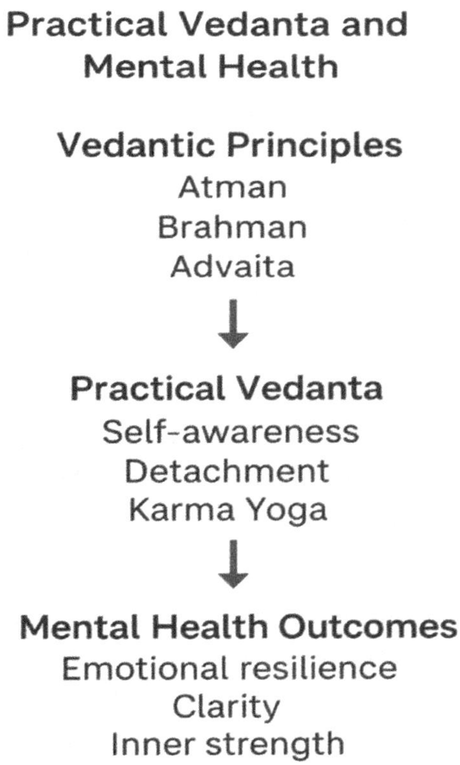

KARMA YOGA AND EMOTIONAL REGULATION

Swami Vivekananda believed spirituality should be lived and not studied (Vivekananda, 1958,1964). Of the yogic paths, he highlighted Karma Yoga—the path of selfless action—as a practical way of turning ordinary life into a field of inner growth. Its biggest benefit may be the way it regulates our emotional world (Chattopadhyay et al., 2025; Sharma & Cooper, 2016)). When many struggle with anxiety, burnout, and emotional reactivity, Karma Yoga offers a simple yet timeless system of mental balance, emotional maturity and purposeful living.

What is Karma Yoga?

As taught in the Bhagavad Gita and interpreted by Swami Vivekananda, Karma Yoga is not about escaping action. It is about doing every action—even the smallest—fully aware, without ego and without attachment to the outcome (Vivekananda & Madhurananda, 2016; Nagar, 2024). This apparently simple attitude change has profound psychological and emotional effects. Action without results releases us emotionally. Our energies are spent doing rather than worrying about what we will get (Mulla & Krishnan, 2014).

Modern psychological models use cognitive reframing to change emotional responses. A Vedantic equivalent is Karma Yoga: a spiritual reframes of life's actions for peace and resilience.

Performing Action Without Attachment to Results

Vedanta does not present a God who rewards or punishes. Instead, it speaks of the universal self that exists in all beings, and realizing this self is considered the highest purpose of life. This realization is not a form of selfishness but its opposite, since it involves recognising that one's true nature is shared with others and that there is no fundamental separation between self and world (Vivekananda, 1958,2016, 1956).

In this tradition, self-realization does not imply withdrawal from daily responsibilities but a clearer, more grounded perception of life as it unfolds. Swami Vivekananda consistently emphasized that Vedanta is not meant solely for monks or specialists in spiritual practice. Rather, it is a philosophy for every individual, whether a mother navigating the complexities of a demanding household, a teacher experiencing burnout within an overstretched educational system, a student struggling with identity and anxiety, or a worker feeling purposeless in a high-pressure professional environment. In each of these lives, Vedantic thought provides tools for cultivating inner steadiness and psychological resilience.

Vedanta teaches that one can participate fully in relationships and responsibilities while remaining mentally free from the compulsive need to control outcomes, a stance that allows for detachment without indifference. It also encourages self-awareness that does not reinforce the ego but helps individuals move beyond its habitual patterns. Vivekananda's interpretation of Karma Yoga further illustrates how one can work actively in the world without becoming emotionally bound by success or failure. These principles have clear psychological relevance, offering ways to moderate emotional reactivity and foster a more stable sense of self.

Importantly, Vedanta does not regard the universal self as an abstract metaphysical doctrine confined to scripture. It is understood as an experiential reality accessible through inquiry, practice, and ethical living. Realizing this deeper self can support qualities such as courage, compassion, and emotional clarity, all of which are valuable for mental well-being.

Vedanta as interpreted by Vivekananda (1951) thus provides a foundation not only for spiritual development but also for emotional strength and psychological clarity (Sarkar, 2021). Instead of promoting guilt, it encourages responsibility; instead of helplessness, it nurtures a sense of inner power; instead of despair, it cultivates unity, meaning, and peace (Singh, 2015).

Replacing Ego-driven Stress with Purpose-driven Effort

Much of the emotional suffering experienced today can be traced to the ego's involvement in work and achievement (Vivekananda, 1944). People often do not seek success for its own sake but for the validation, praise, or sense of superiority they hope it will provide. This subtle, ego-based striving creates tension and insecurity, reinforcing patterns of stress that are difficult to escape. Karma Yoga offers an alternative orientation by teaching that action should be performed as an offering rather than as a performance designed to earn approval.

Swami Vivekananda repeatedly warned that ego is the root of much human misery and noted that the less one thinks about oneself, the more peaceful the mind becomes. When actions are driven by ego, individuals become overly sensitive to criticism, dependent on praise, and preoccupied with how others perceive them. This creates emotional volatility and reduces the intrinsic satisfaction that meaningful work can provide.

In contrast, Karma Yoga encourages working for a higher purpose, whether spiritual, social, or moral. When actions are aligned with a value or intention that transcends individual ego—such as service to humanity, commitment to Dharma, or devotion to the divine—they become lighter, more joyful, and less burdened by internal pressure. Purpose-driven effort supports emotional stability because its value does not depend on external recognition. Even in the absence of success or praise, the individual experiences a sense of inner contentment rooted in honesty and sincerity of effort.

This shift in motivation can transform the experience of work. A nurse caring for patients, a teacher supporting students, or a cleaner maintaining a school environment can all be understood as engaging in selfless service. Viewed through this lens, the nature of their work becomes more meaningful, and emotional peace becomes possible even in demanding circumstances (Singh, 1999).

Karma Yoga in Daily Life: Relationships, Work, and Failure

Karma Yoga is not just for monks. Swami Vivekananda specifically said that householders, workers, and students can practice it in daily life (Vivekananda, 1951). Let's see how it applies in some key life areas.

Relationships: Relationships in contemporary life are often shaped by unspoken expectations such as the belief that one's efforts should produce a corresponding response from others. When affection or care is tied to anticipated returns, disappointment, frustration, and resentment easily emerge. Karma Yoga offers a different orientation by suggesting that love and service should be extended without dependence on reciprocal outcomes. In this view, one engages with family members, partners, or friends with sincerity while remaining inwardly free from the need for validation or emotional return. Such an approach fosters resilience and protects against emotional codependency, as one's inner stability is no longer contingent upon the reactions or behavior of others. The focus shifts from external approval to the integrity of performing one's duty with clarity and goodwill.

Work and Profession: The contemporary workplace is often characterized by competition, stress, and organizational politics, leaving many individuals emotionally exhausted from overwork, fear of judgment, or exposure to unhealthy professional environments. Karma Yoga offers an alternative framework by emphasizing that work should be performed with integrity rather than as a means of ego enhancement. It encourages steady, consistent effort instead of dramatic ambition or constant self-promotion. Swami Vivekananda's instruction to "be steady, and, above all, be pure and sincere" reflects this orientation. Approaching work in this way reduces stress and enhances mental focus, allowing individuals to respond to challenges with clarity rather than reacting impulsively to every difficulty. This perspective promotes psychological stability and fosters a healthier relationship with professional responsibilities.

Handling Failure: Failure is often one of the most difficult emotional experiences, with the potential to undermine self-esteem and contribute to depressive feelings. Karma Yoga offers a different interpretation by viewing failure not as a judgment on the individual but as a natural part of the broader process of action. When an action is undertaken with sincerity and without selfish motive, the outcome—whether successful or unsuccessful—assumes secondary importance. This shift in perspective strengthens emotional resilience by preventing individuals from being disproportionately affected by defeat or excessively elevated by success. Over time, this approach fosters a stable, balanced, and quietly grounded disposition.

Cultivating Emotional Neutrality Without Passivity: A frequent misunderstanding of Karma Yoga is the assumption that it promotes passivity or emotional indifference. This interpretation is inaccurate. Karma Yoga does not encourage emotional dullness; rather, it cultivates emotional discipline. Emotional neutrality in this context refers to the capacity to remain steady without being overwhelmed by emotional highs or lows. It involves maintaining calmness in both success and failure, not because one is detached from caring, but because one's inner center is not destabilized by external circumstances. Such neutrality reflects inner strength, allowing individuals to remain effective and compassionate even during crises. It does not render a person cold or disengaged; instead, it enables them to be fully present without becoming emotionally scattered.

This form of neutrality is distinct from emotional suppression. Suppression involves hiding or denying emotional states, which often leads to further psychological strain or breakdowns. Neutrality, by contrast, involves witnessing the emotion, accepting it, and allowing it to pass naturally. There is no denial involved, only mastery and clarity in relation to one's internal experience.

In psychological terms, Karma Yoga supports the development of emotional regulation by reducing automatic emotional reactivity and encouraging reflective awareness. Individuals who practice this approach tend to become less reactive, more patient, and more capable of making thoughtful decisions in both personal and professional contexts (Permadhi and Marhaeni, 2019).

Integrating Karma Yoga for Mental Health and Well-Being

Karma Yoga offers several psychological benefits that resonate strongly with contemporary understandings of mental health. By reducing fear-based attachment to outcomes, it mitigates anxiety and fosters a more balanced emotional orientation. The practice also diminishes anger and frustration by weakening ego-driven expectations, which often lie at the root of interpersonal and intrapersonal conflict. Furthermore, by redefining the significance of failure, Karma Yoga supports the development of resilience, allowing individuals to recover more quickly from setbacks. Its emphasis on selfless action enhances the quality of relationships by shifting attention from personal gain to genuine engagement, while its focus on effort rather than results contributes to a healthier sense of self-worth.

Swami Vivekananda envisioned a society in which individuals did not withdraw from life but instead spiritualized daily activity through the principles of Karma Yoga (Vivekananda, 1958,1964). He did not advocate retreat into isolation or forests (Vivekananda, 1958,2016); rather, he encouraged people to transform routine responsibilities into meaningful actions grounded in clarity, sincerity, and service. This orientation carries significant relevance in the present era. In a time marked by widespread burnout, Karma Yoga offers a model of peaceful productivity. In an age of emotional volatility, it promotes calm strength; in a culture shaped by ego-driven competition, it encourages quiet and genuine service; and amid rising rates of depression and loss of purpose, it provides a framework for reconnecting with meaning.

Karma Yoga is neither a ritual nor a sectarian religious practice. It is a disciplined way of thinking, acting, and living, guided by principles such as non-attachment, ego-transcendence, and service to others. These tools remain as applicable in the modern world as they were in ancient India, offering a psychologically grounded approach to well-being that aligns closely with contemporary understandings of healthy functioning (Kumar and Kumar, 2013).

SWAMI VIVEKANANDA'S VISION OF MEDITATION: INNER STRENGTH THROUGH CONCENTRATION

Swami Vivekananda approached meditation as a disciplined method for cultivating inner strength, self-mastery, and clarity of thought rather than as a technique aimed primarily at producing relaxation (Vivekananda, 1896). He noted that contemporary forms of mental suffering are often intensified by uncontrolled desires, persistent distractions, and pervasive fear, all of which fragment attention and diminish emotional resilience (Vivekananda, 1940,1942,1944). Within this framework, meditation functions as a means of gathering scattered mental energy and restoring cognitive stability and focus (Vivekaprana, 2014).

In Raja Yoga, Vivekananda argues that concentration forms the basis of all knowledge. Whether the individual is engaged in scientific investigation or spiritual inquiry, the capacity for sustained and inwardly directed attention is essential for meaningful understanding (Vivekananda, 2016). Contemporary scientific research lends support to this claim. Neuroimaging studies indicate that meditative practices enhance activation in the prefrontal cortex and anterior cingulate cortex, areas associated with attentional control and emotional regulation (Vivekananda, 1958). These findings align with Vivekananda's assertion that meditation enables individuals to cultivate the role of an observer of mental processes rather than remaining subject to their fluctuations (Sukhsohale et al., 2012).

Within the Vedantic framework, meditation therefore serves both psychological and spiritual purposes. By enabling practitioners to recognize the presence of the Atman beneath changing mental states, it becomes a discipline that links personal well-being with deeper existential insights regarding human nature and consciousness (Nair and Kutty, 2017).

Vedantic Meditation Techniques for Emotional Clarity

Vedantic meditation differs fundamentally from techniques that seek primarily to calm the mind or encourage visual imagery. Its core objective is direct inquiry into the nature of the self. The classical method of self-enquiry, expressed through the question "Who am I?", is intended to interrupt the habitual tendency to identify with thoughts, emotions, and transient psychological states. This method has particular relevance for understanding rumination, which contemporary research identifies as a major contributor to anxiety and depression. Empirical studies demonstrate that practices grounded in self-inquiry and mindfulness reduce repetitive negative thinking by training practitioners to observe thoughts as transient mental events rather than as accurate representations of reality. This emphasis on discriminating between the observing self and mental content is consistent with Vivekananda's insistence on cultivating inward awareness and separating pure consciousness from the mind's fluctuations (Vivekananda, 1896; Vivekananda, 1958,2016).

A second foundational practice within Vedantic meditation is witness consciousness, or *Sakshi-bhava*. In this approach, the practitioner observes internal experiences, including thoughts, sensations, and desires, without judgment or involvement. Neuroimaging findings suggest that such meta-awareness is associated with reduced activity in the brain's default mode network, a system linked to self-referential processing and ruminative thought cycles. Lower activity in this network has been connected to enhanced emotional stability and reduced susceptibility to intrusive thoughts, mood variability, and negative self-appraisals. Vivekananda described this stance of witnessing as central to understanding the deeper nature of the self and emphasized its value for cultivating mental discipline and clarity (Vivekananda, 1951; Vivekananda, 1944).

Taken together, these practices operate as ancient psychological technologies that disrupt automatic emotional reactivity and foster more adaptive forms of emotional regulation. Their relevance has increased in contemporary contexts characterized by impulsive emotional expression and heightened cognitive reactivity. By training individuals to observe mental activity with detachment and precision, Vedantic meditation cultivates skills that support psychological resilience, attentional stability, and inner composure (Syamala, 2018).

Breath, Mantra, and Silence as Healing Tools

Breath awareness occupies a central place in Vedantic meditation. Swami Vivekananda repeatedly emphasized the intimate connection between breath and mental states, noting that irregular or disturbed breathing reflects inner agitation while slow and rhythmic breathing supports psychological steadiness and clarity (Vivekananda, 1896; Vivekananda, 1959). Contemporary research confirms this relationship. Slow, controlled breathing has been shown to activate parasympathetic pathways, decrease physiological arousal, and improve cognitive functioning through enhanced autonomic balance (Canter, 2003). Within the Vedantic framework, breath regulation is therefore not merely a physiological intervention but a foundational method for stabilizing attention and preparing the mind for deeper introspection.

Mantra meditation is another important dimension of Vedantic practice. It utilizes specific sounds or syllables to focus attention and reduce cognitive fragmentation. Repetitive mantra recitation, particularly of syllables such as *Om*, has been associated with decreases in wandering thoughts, improvements in attentional stability, and reinforcement of the breath-mind relationship. This is consistent with studies demonstrating that rhythmic chanting lowers physiological arousal and interrupts ruminative cognitive cycles by modulating neural activity associated with repetitive negative thinking. Vivekananda described mantras as tools that refine concentration and direct the mind inward, enabling practitioners to transcend habitual patterns of reactivity (Vivekananda, 1899).

Silence, or *mauna*, represents one of the most profound techniques within Vedantic meditation. Silence in this context is not simply the absence of external sound but the intentional quieting of internal discourse. Neuropsychological research suggests that sustained periods of silence contribute to memory consolidation, reduction of cognitive overload, and enhanced introspective awareness. Vivekananda regarded silence as a primary medium through which insight arises, observing that it allows the practitioner to confront the mind without distraction and to develop comfort with solitude (Vivekananda, 1958,1964; Dudeja, 2017). By fostering an environment in which mental fluctuations gradually subside, silence enables access to deeper layers of self-understanding and psychological resilience.

Together, these practices illustrate the multidimensional nature of Vedantic meditation. Breath awareness stabilizes the physiological substrate of attention, mantra recital structures the mind's focus, and cultivated silence deepens introspective clarity. Each method contributes to the overarching aim of Vedantic practice, which is the disciplined refinement of mental processes and the recognition of the deeper self that exists beyond fluctuating psychological states.

The Healing Depth of Vedantic Meditation

Vedantic meditation, as articulated by Swami Vivekananda, functions as a systematic discipline for inner transformation rather than as a technique intended merely to induce relaxation. It is designed to address the deeper sources of psychological suffering by correcting the fundamental error of identifying the self with the unstable movements of the mind. Vivekananda consistently emphasized that the purpose of meditation is to stabilize awareness, refine concentration, and cultivate an ability to observe mental states without attachment (Vivekananda, 1896; Vivekananda, 1958,1964). Contemporary research aligns with these insights, demonstrating that meditation practices which foster non-reactive awareness reduce emotional reactivity, lower tendencies toward rumination, strengthen attentional control, and contribute to sustained psychological well-being.

In an environment characterized by rapid stimulation, constant noise, and persistent cognitive overload, the need for practices that cultivate stillness and focused awareness has become increasingly evident. When practiced in the Vedantic spirit, meditation offers more than a coping strategy for stress. It initiates a gradual reorientation of consciousness that enables individuals to engage with experience from a standpoint of stability, insight, and self-understanding. This transformative potential echo Vivekananda's assertion that true meditation reveals the deeper nature of the self and supports a life oriented toward clarity and strength (Vivekananda, 1951). Such an approach is consistent with scholarly observations that meditative disciplines contribute to enhanced resilience and deeper forms of psychological integration (Saraswati and Alston, 1997).

VEDANTA AS A WAY OF LIFE

Vedanta functions not merely as a set of philosophical teachings but as a comprehensive orientation toward life. It provides a conceptual framework through which individuals interpret experience and cultivate greater awareness, balance, and depth in everyday contexts such as relationships, work, and routine activities. Swami Vivekananda consistently emphasized that Vedanta must be lived rather than theorized, and he highlighted strength, disciplined detachment, and the recognition of one's inner divinity as essential qualities for meeting the challenges of life without psychological fragmentation (Vivekananda, 1896; Vivekananda, 1956).

These principles encourage individuals to approach circumstances with clarity and resilience rather than vulnerability to external fluctuations.

In a contemporary environment marked by emotional volatility, constant distraction, and heightened cognitive pressure, Vedanta assumes renewed relevance. Its teachings offer a psychologically grounded approach to navigating external conditions without becoming defined by them. For Vivekananda, this capacity to act from an inner center rather than as a passive response to circumstance represented a fundamental aspect of spiritual and psychological maturity (Vivekananda, 1947). By encouraging individuals to recognize their agency and cultivate steadiness at the level of consciousness, Vedanta provides a framework that supports well-being, purpose, and equanimity even in the most ordinary moments.

Building Emotional Resilience Through Vedanta

Contemporary life is marked by heightened emotional reactivity, driven in part by the constant availability of information and the immediacy of digital communication. Events such as online conflict, personal setbacks, or perceived intrusions into privacy can evoke intense emotional responses and contribute to cumulative psychological strain. Within this landscape, the capacity to withstand, recover from, and meaningfully grow through emotional adversity represents a crucial component of mental health and well-being. Vedanta, the non-dual philosophical tradition of India, offers a distinctive framework for understanding this form of resilience. Rather than conceptualizing resilience merely as a coping strategy, Vedanta situates it within a broader pursuit of inner freedom and self-knowledge (de Lacey et al., 2009). Swami Vivekananda articulated this insight by emphasizing that true strength arises from recognizing the deeper self that is not diminished by external challenges or fluctuations of circumstance (Vivekananda, 1899; Vivekananda, 1959). Through this lens, resilience is cultivated not through avoidance or suppression of difficulty but through an awakened awareness of the stable consciousness underlying all experience.

Understanding Emotional Resilience Through the Vedantic Lens

In contemporary psychology, emotional resilience is generally defined as the capacity to recover effectively from emotional difficulties such as grief, stress, trauma, and disappointment. This construct encompasses adaptability, optimism, self-regulation, and endurance. Within the Vedantic framework, however, resilience is conceptualized in fundamentally different terms. It is understood not as a property of the ego but as an expression of the deeper Self. Vedanta posits that one's true identity is not the fluctuating mind or the perishable body but the Atman, which is described as eternal, luminous, and unaffected by pleasure or pain. Swami Vivekananda repeatedly emphasized that weakness arises from misidentification with the limited personality, asserting that the gravest error is to consider oneself weak (Vivekananda, 1896; Vivekananda, 1951). For him, resilience emerges from discovering the immovable Self that remains strong, calm, and intrinsically free.

Recognizing this deeper Self does not negate the experience of emotional distress. Rather, it reframes such experiences by preventing them from defining the individual. Vedantic literature often employs the metaphor of the ocean: while waves may rise and fall on the surface, the depth remains undisturbed. In this view, emotional storms occur at the level of the mind, but the core of one's being remains intact and steady. This conceptualization aligns with contemporary models of resilience that emphasize transcendence rather than suppression or denial and highlights the cultivation of an inner vantage point from which psychological disturbances can be observed without being internalized (Southwick and Charney, 2012). This synthesis reflects Vivekananda's broader teaching that true strength arises through knowledge of the Self and through disciplined cultivation of inner stability (Vivekananda, 1958,1964).

Facing Adversity Through the Lens of Oneness and Impermanence

Two central insights of Vedanta help individuals face adversity with grace: the principle of oneness and the truth of impermanence.

Oneness (Advaita): Vedantic philosophy maintains that all beings are manifestations of a single universal consciousness. This non-dual perspective challenges instinctive responses to interpersonal harm, such as withdrawal, resentment, or hostility. From the Vedantic standpoint, the apparent "other" does not possess a separate ontological status. Harm inflicted upon another is understood as arising from ignorance and ultimately harming the perpetrator as well. This shift in perception encourages the transformation of resentment into compassion and frames interpersonal injury as a consequence of human limitation rather than intentional malice. Vivekananda often emphasized this view, asserting that the recognition of unity dissolves antagonism and elevates interpersonal understanding to a moral and spiritual discipline (Vivekananda, 1899; Vivekananda, 1956).

This interpretive shift becomes particularly relevant in emotionally charged situations such as heartbreak or interpersonal betrayal. An individual may initially experience anger, rejection, or self-blame. However, through Vedantic reflection, the individual comes to recognize both self and other as participants in a shared human struggle shaped by psychological and existential limitations. This reorientation moves the focus from ego-centered hurt toward a broader, more compassionate understanding of human behavior. Hollick (2006) argues that such cognitive and emotional reframing generates an inner spaciousness that is foundational for resilience. This aligns with Vivekananda's assertion that spiritual insight expands one's capacity to endure and transcend emotional disturbances by grounding experience in a deeper awareness of unity and shared consciousness (Vivekananda, 1958,1964).

Impermanence (Anitya): Vedantic philosophy asserts that all phenomena within the empirical world are impermanent, including material possessions, accomplishments, failures, and even emotional states. What remains constant is the witnessing self, the Atman, which observes these fluctuations without undergoing change. This understanding introduces a valuable perspective during periods of psychological distress. Individuals are encouraged not to deny experiences such as grief or anxiety but to contextualize them within a broader awareness of transience. The recognition that emotional states arise, remain for a time, and eventually dissipate enables a more measured response to internal turmoil. Vivekananda frequently emphasized this distinction between the enduring self and the changing mind, noting that clarity arises when one ceases to identify with mental modifications and instead assumes the standpoint of the witness (Vivekananda, 1896; Vivekananda, 1958,2016).

This perspective does not promote emotional detachment in the sense of suppression or indifference. Rather, it cultivates a form of discernment that prevents individuals from becoming overly identified with transient experiences. Impermanence serves as a reminder not to cling to pain or to interpret emotional states as reflections of one's essential identity. In this sense, resilience is not defined by the avoidance of discomfort but by the capacity to move through it with mindful awareness. This conception aligns with contemporary psychological models that link resilience to flexible engagement with emotional experience while maintaining a grounded sense of self (Gordon, 2003). By integrating these insights, Vedanta offers a sophisticated framework for emotional stability that combines introspective clarity with a deep understanding of the changing nature of human experience (Vivekananda, 1947).

Transforming Reactive Emotions into Strength

In contemporary psychology, emotions such as anger, fear, and grief are often addressed through strategies of regulation and management. Vedanta approaches these emotions at a deeper level by examining their underlying causes and by shifting the center of identity from the ego to the Self. Anger, for example, frequently emerges when the ego perceives a threat. Vedanta interprets the ego as a transient construct composed of thoughts and desires, rather than as an enduring reality. When the practitioner identifies with the Self rather than the ego, anger loses much of its force. This does not imply passivity; an individual grounded in Self-awareness can respond to injustice with clarity and firmness without resorting to hatred or aggression (Vivekananda, 1899; Vivekananda, 1951).

Fear is similarly reframed. Psychological fear often arises from attachment and the belief that one's security depends upon external conditions. Vedanta challenges this assumption by teaching that lasting security is rooted in the eternal Self rather than in unstable worldly circumstances. Swami Vivekananda repeatedly asserted that fear is fundamentally incompatible with spiritual insight, describing it as a barrier to ethical and psychological strength (Vivekananda, 1958,2016). In this view, fearlessness does not entail recklessness but rests on alignment with a reality that is not diminished by external loss.

Grief, which arises from the loss of persons or meaningful objects, is approached through the Vedantic recognition that the Self is never lost. While forms change, the underlying consciousness remains continuous. When this truth is experientially understood rather than accepted merely as belief, grief can evolve into a quiet form of resilience and a deeper appreciation of connection beyond physical form.

Vedantic reflection does not eliminate emotion, nor does it advocate denial. Instead, it offers a contemplative process through which individuals can pause, inquire, and reinterpret emotional experiences with greater insight. This approach supports the transformation of emotional reactions into avenues for growth and understanding (Wright and Strawn, 2010).

The Role of Inner Silence and Surrender

Vedantic traditions identify two inner disciplines that significantly contribute to emotional resilience: inner silence and surrender. These practices are not indicators of passivity but reflect mature psychological and spiritual strength.

Inner silence, or mauna, refers not simply to the absence of speech but to the capacity to observe mental activity without engaging with its narratives. Emotional upheaval often amplifies internal dialogue, generating self-criticism, fear, and reactive interpretations. Practices such as breath awareness, mantra repetition, and contemplative stillness help quiet these cognitive fluctuations and foster clarity. In this state, individuals are better able to discern intuitive understanding rather than being guided by reactive mental patterns (Chohan, 2010). Vivekananda noted that silence enables the mind to withdraw from external disturbances and access deeper layers of awareness where insight becomes possible (Vivekananda, 1896; Vivekananda, 1958,1964). Through such silence, resilience emerges not from suppression but from enhanced cognitive and emotional discrimination.

Surrender, or śara āgati, holds a complementary role. In Vedanta, surrender does not imply resignation. Rather, it involves relinquishing the belief that the ego can control all aspects of life. This orientation reflects an acknowledgment of a wider intelligence or order within which personal struggle unfolds. When individuals release ego-based resistance, they often experience a reduction in psychological burden and an increase in acceptance. This shift allows healing processes to occur with greater ease. For example, individuals confronting illness or major loss may find that surrender reduces internal conflict and supports emotional stabilization (Miehls, 2011). Vivekananda emphasized that genuine surrender aligns the individual with the deeper Self and cultivates fearlessness and trust in the unfolding of life (Vivekananda, 1947).

Together, inner silence and surrender strengthen resilience by reducing reactivity, deepening self-awareness, and supporting adaptive engagement with adversity.

From Fragility to Freedom

Vedanta offers a profound reorientation in a world where identity and worth are often defined by external conditions. Emotional resilience, within this framework, is not achieved through suppression or the cultivation of hardness but through the recognition that one's essential nature transcends the changing movements of the mind and emotions. Vedanta encourages individuals to adopt the stance of the witness, observing experiences without becoming absorbed in them. This perspective enables a person to encounter anger without being overtaken by it, to move through grief without fragmentation, and to confront fear without allowing it to dictate behavior.

Swami Vivekananda's well-known exhortation, "Arise, awake, and stop not till the goal is reached," extends beyond the pursuit of external achievement. It represents a call to awaken an inner strength that cannot be diminished by trauma or destabilized by failure (Mitra, 2000). Vivekananda emphasized that this awakening reflects the discovery of the deeper Self, which remains untouched by psychological turbulence and is the true source of stability and courage (Vivekananda, 1896; Vivekananda, 1951). In this understanding, resilience is not conceptualized as emotional armor but as an expression of inner freedom grounded in self-knowledge and awareness.

MENTAL HEALTH AND THE MODERN MIND

Recent decades have seen mental health rank among the most frequently discussed subjects in both academic and popular culture. It is acknowledged in workplace wellness programs and social media campaigns, in therapy apps, and in stress-relief products. In spite of this greater awareness, more people are suffering from mental and emotional disorders. According to the WHO's 2025 reports, more than one billion people are now living with mental health disorders worldwide, making anxiety and depression among the most common conditions across countries (WHO,

2025). Worldwide health reports say cases of depression, anxiety, and stress-related conditions have increased across all ages. The WHO (2025) report also mentioned that, suicide continues to claim over 700,000 lives annually, and mental health disorders are now the second largest cause of long-term disability. The paradox is hard to avoid: we live in the age of mental health awareness, not mental well-being.

The answers might lie in patterns of modern life: information overload, digital distraction, competitive work environments, fragile relationships and pressure to succeed. Behind each of these lies an even greater spiritual and psychological distance between man and his own inner self. The modern mind is receptive but poorly able to understand itself (Bhagabati & Kumar, 2016).

Common Psychological Struggles: Stress, Anxiety, and Overthinking

Contemporary psychological distress is multifaceted and often subtle in its presentation. The National Mental Health Survey of India (2015–16) reported that 10.6 percent of adults live with mental disorders, illustrating the significant prevalence of psychological challenges even prior to the post-pandemic escalation (NMHS, 2016). Beyond diagnosable conditions, individuals increasingly report emotional exhaustion, spiritual dissatisfaction, and pervasive uncertainty about life. Several core concerns characterize the modern mental health landscape.

Chronic Stress: In fast-paced and continuously connected environments, stress has shifted from an acute response to a chronic condition. Many individuals struggle to downregulate physiological arousal even in the absence of immediate threat. Prolonged activation of the nervous system contributes to fatigue, sleep disturbances, irritability, and persistent restlessness (Hogan, 2013).

Anxiety Disorders: Anxiety ranks among the most common psychological concerns for young adults and working professionals. It manifests in worries related to career, relationships, performance, and the future, often without a specific precipitating cause. Physical symptoms may include shortness of breath, tachycardia, and gastrointestinal discomfort (Kariuki-Nyuthe and Stein, 2015). The World Health Organization (2025) estimates that anxiety and depression together result in approximately one trillion US dollars in lost productivity each year.

Overthinking and Mental Rumination: Rumination has evolved from a constructive cognitive process into a source of emotional overload for many individuals. Replaying past interactions, anticipating worst-case scenarios, and second-guessing decisions contribute to increased worry, doubt, and guilt. Overthinking consumes emotional energy while offering little insight (Matsumoto and Mochizuki, 2018).

Emotional Disconnection: Despite unprecedented digital connectivity, many individuals report diminished emotional connection. Relationships are increasingly viewed as transactional or unstable, and feelings of belonging or emotional safety are often absent. This contributes to pervasive loneliness, emptiness, and diminished self-worth (Steiner-Adair and Barker, 2013).

Lack of Meaning and Direction: A more existential form of distress involves a loss of purpose or meaning. Individuals who appear outwardly successful frequently experience internal disorientation and question the significance of their pursuits. This crisis of meaning underlies many psychological concerns yet remains understudied in mainstream discourse (McKenna, 2006).

These struggles are not confined to specific cultures or socioeconomic groups. For example, in the United States, one in five adults lived with a mental illness in 2022 (NIMH, 2024). Together, these patterns suggest a broader disruption in the relationship between mind and self. Individuals are often trained to achieve, compare, and consume, yet receive little guidance in cultivating compassion, awareness, and understanding toward themselves.

Disconnection from Inner Self as a Root Cause

From a Vedantic perspective, many contemporary mental health difficulties originate in a disconnection from the inner self. This state, described as *avidya* or ignorance, involves misidentification with the body, mind, and ego while neglecting one's deeper nature. When individuals lose awareness of this inner identity, they become overly influenced by transient emotions and external circumstances. This disconnection manifests in several psychological patterns:

External Identity as Self-Image: Individuals often define themselves through social roles, achievements, failures, or material possessions. Such identities are inherently fragile and easily threatened. Empirical research indicates that low self-concept clarity is associated with heightened anxiety, depressive symptoms, and unstable self-esteem, paralleling the vulnerability described in Vedantic analyses (Di Blasi et al., 2015; Patla, 2025; Verrier, 2021).

Neglect of Inner Silence: Traditionally, silence has been regarded as a means of accessing the inner self. Contemporary life, however, encourages constant sensory and cognitive stimulation. The avoidance of silence contributes to elevated rumination, which is strongly linked with depressive symptoms and emotional exhaustion (Herrero de Jáuregui, 2015; Sousa and Neves, 2021; Cropley et al., 2020).

Confusion between Thoughts and Identity: Modern individuals often equate their thoughts and emotional states with their core identity. This fusion intensifies reactivity, mood instability, and distress. Vedanta teaches that thoughts are transient modifications of the mind, not attributes of the self. Psychological findings similarly show that difficulties in emotion regulation predict higher levels of impulsivity and persistent negative affect (Kowall, 2014; Carver and Johnson, 2018).

Loss of Stillness and Presence: A fast-paced lifestyle encourages continual mental movement, reducing the capacity for sustained presence. This perpetual mental drift contributes to cognitive fragmentation and emotional fatigue (Alpert, 2012).

Fear of Inwardness: Many individuals avoid introspection out of concern that inner exploration will expose unresolved pain or conflict. As a result, external solutions are sought for problems that originate internally (Lecercle and Riley, 2004).

This disruption of inner connection is both a psychological and spiritual concern. It helps explain why many contemporary mental health interventions provide temporary relief yet fail to create sustained transformation, since the foundational issue of inward disconnection remains unaddressed.

Limitations of External Solutions and Consumerist Coping

Contemporary society places strong emphasis on externally oriented solutions to emotional distress. Individuals who experience psychological difficulty are frequently encouraged to purchase products, modify their environment, or seek immediate stimulation. While such strategies may offer temporary comfort, they risk substituting superficial relief for meaningful psychological healing.

Therapy as Transaction: Mental health services are increasingly embedded within medicalized and commercial frameworks. Although psychotherapy can be highly beneficial, it often becomes structured as a weekly transactional encounter rather than a sustained process of inner transformation. Foundational concerns such as self-knowledge, meaning, and existential orientation may receive limited attention (Berne, 2013).

Medication Without Mindfulness: Many countries report high rates of prescription for anxiolytic and antidepressant medications. These interventions can stabilize acute symptoms but rarely equip individuals with skills for reflective thinking, emotional processing, or personal growth. Medication functions as a tool rather than a comprehensive philosophy of mental well-being (Phelps and Manipod, 2012).

Distraction as Survival: Entertainment, social media, shopping, and frequent travel often serve as avoidance strategies for unresolved emotional discomfort. Although distraction may temporarily reduce distress, it postpones direct engagement with underlying issues. Emotional discomfort often re-emerges with greater intensity when avoidance persists (Oei et al., 2012).

Success as Self-Worth: Cultural emphasis on productivity and competition leads many individuals to equate their worth with external achievements. This dynamic heightens fear of failure and contributes to burnout, insecurity, and chronic self-evaluation (de Witt Huberts et al., 2014).

Limits of Pharmacological-Only Interventions: Research consistently indicates that pharmacological treatment alone is insufficient for long-term psychological well-being (Bijlenga et al., 2017). While medication can reduce symptoms, it does not directly address maladaptive cognitions, emotional dysregulation, unresolved trauma, or deficits in self-concept clarity (Binsale, 2017; Sharratt, 2023). Comparative studies show that combined approaches integrating medication with psychological interventions such as cognitive therapy, emotion regulation training, or mindfulness yield more sustained improvements and lower relapse rates (Guendelman et al., 2017; Elices et al., 2017). Without practices that support meaning-making, identity formation, and self-awareness, pharmacological approaches risk managing symptoms rather than transforming underlying conditions.

Collectively, these external solutions function as surface-level responses to deeper psychological concerns. They often overlook the critical need to cultivate inner awareness, emotional literacy, and a more integrated understanding of personal well-being.

The Need for Inward-Directed Approaches

The limitations of predominantly external interventions have contributed to a renewed interest in inward-oriented approaches to mental health. Within this context, classical philosophical frameworks such as Vedanta have become increasingly relevant. They provide not only contemplative techniques but also an alternative worldview in which self-knowledge constitutes the foundation of psychological well-being.

Self-Inq uiry: Practices that involve reflective questioning, such as asking "Who am I?" or "What exists beyond my thoughts and social roles?", function as methods for destabilizing rigid self-concepts. Research indicates that such inquiry can reduce emotional reactivity by loosening identification with transient mental states (Spiteri, 2012).

Mindfulness and Awareness: The capacity to observe thoughts and emotions without immediate reaction creates psychological space that supports emotional regulation. Empirical studies show that non-reactive awareness decreases impulsivity and enhances balanced emotional responding (Grossman, 2015).

Detachment and Perspective: Vedantic teachings emphasise viewing experiences within a broader existential perspective. Detachment in this sense refers to reducing emotional over-identification rather than withdrawing from lived experience. Contemporary scholarship interprets this as a cognitive reframing process that enhances resilience (Dreyfus, 2007).

Silence and Reflection: Deliberate periods of quiet contemplation foster attentional reset and deeper engagement with subjective experience. Research suggests that reflective silence improves emotional clarity and supports introspective insight (Zimmermann et al., 2016).

Meaning-Oriented Living: Anchoring life in values such as compassion, service, and truth provides a stable sense of purpose that is not contingent on achievement or external approval. Such value alignment has been associated with improved psychological well-being (Hackett, 2014).

Vedanta is not positioned as a substitute for clinical intervention but as a complementary foundation that supports sustained inner transformation. It encourages individuals to relate to themselves and others with greater clarity and reduced fear or comparison. While technological and scientific advances continue to enhance external conditions, self-awareness remains central to cultivating inner stability. As noted in contemporary scholarship, enduring psychological healing requires movement beyond external solutions and a return to reflective self-understanding (Pillay et al., 2008).

VEDANTIC TOOLS FOR INNER CHANGE

Swami Vivekananda consistently emphasized that genuine transformation begins within. He argued that human beings are not fundamentally weak or broken but unaware of their deeper, divine identity. This misidentification with body, mind, and ego creates the psychological vulnerabilities that manifest as distress, anxiety, and emotional suffering (Bhar, 2020). Vedantic tools aim to correct this inner distortion. Rather than abstract metaphysical ideas, they function as systematic methods for developing emotional resilience, attentional stability, and long-term well-being (Pillay et al., 2008).

Self-Awareness (Atma-bodha): Beyond Roles and Toward Inner Identity

Modern identities are often organised around external social roles such as student, employee, parent, or citizen. These roles carry normative expectations, and difficulties in meeting them can heighten vulnerability to self-doubt, anxiety, and depressive symptoms (Carter, 2017). Vedanta, particularly as articulated in Atma-Bodha, reframes such roles as provisional and not constitutive of the deepest level of selfhood. Vivekananda (1899) emphasised that individuals are not reducible to the body or the mind but are expressions of the Self, a view that anticipates contemporary psychological discussions of metacognition and observer consciousness (Vivekananda, 1896; Vivekananda, 1951).

Self-awareness in this Vedantic framework extends beyond ordinary introspection. It involves sustained, non-reactive observation of mental and emotional processes, which is comparable to the psychological construct of decentering. This stance enables greater cognitive distance between internal stimuli and behavioural responses, thereby reducing impulsive reactivity and promoting emotional regulation (King & Fresco, 2019). Empirical studies indicate that practices cultivating metacognitive awareness improve attentional control and reduce anxiety, findings that resonate with Vedanta's emphasis on recognising consciousness as distinct from its fluctuating contents (Montgomery, 2000).

Detachment (Vairagya): Regulating Emotions Without Suppressing Them

Vairagya, or detachment, is frequently misunderstood as apathy. Vedanta, however, frames it as emotional maturity: the capacity to engage with life without becoming psychologically dependent on outcomes. Modern emotional culture often oscillates between suppressing feelings and acting impulsively on them. Both patterns are linked to dysregulation and interpersonal difficulties (Jijina et al., 2020).

Vivekananda noted that attachment produces emotional volatility because one's mood becomes tied to external outcomes. Vairagya shifts this dynamic by helping individuals participate fully in life while remaining inwardly steady (van der Veer, 1989). This mirrors research on adaptive emotion regulation, which suggests that observing emotions with distance—rather than suppressing or overexpressing them—leads to greater psychological stability and reduced reactivity (Powers & LaBar, 2019). Everyday situations, such as working toward a promotion without obsessing over the result, illustrate how detachment reduces anticipatory anxiety and fosters healthier relationships (Kuzucu, 2016).

Mindfulness and Present-Moment Awareness: Vedantic Parallels

Although contemporary mindfulness practices are often associated with Buddhist traditions, Vedanta contains closely aligned teachings on present-moment awareness and intentional living. Psychological distress frequently arises from the mind's inclination to revisit past regrets or anticipate future threats. Vedanta proposes that sustained peace is accessible only in the present moment because awareness is understood as a constant, non-temporal dimension of experience (Ji, 2023). Mindfulness methods such as breath regulation, sensory tracking, and deliberate attentional anchoring help diminish unnecessary cognitive activity. Empirical studies demonstrate that these practices reduce activation in the brain's default mode network, a system linked to rumination, self-referential processing, and anxiety (Farb et al., 2007; Marshall, 2012). Vivekananda encouraged integrating these principles into routine activities, including eating, walking, speaking, and working, so that mindful awareness becomes a continuous mode of living rather than a discrete contemplative exercise (Vivekananda, 1896; Vivekananda, 1959). Within a Vedantic framework, mindfulness functions not only as a stress-reduction strategy but also as a method for reorienting attention toward the deeper Self, thereby strengthening psychological clarity and existential grounding (Maharaj, 2020).

Neti-Neti (Not This, Not This): A Meditative Method for Cognitive Clarity

Neti-Neti represents one of Vedanta's most analytically refined contemplative methods. Through the systematic negation of identifications such as "I am not the body, not the mind, not the thought," the practitioner gradually withdraws from transient mental contents and orients awareness toward a more stable substratum of experience (Rambachan, 2017). This process has clear psychological parallels. Contemporary models of cognitive defusion and identity deconstruction show that rigid self-statements, for example "I am a failure" or "I am unlovable," contribute to depressive and anxious cognition. Neti-Neti interrupts these patterns by reframing such statements as temporary mental events rather than accurate self-definitions (Kuan, 2009).

The distancing effect produced by this inquiry reduces negative self-talk and weakens the fusion between thought and identity. Asking questions such as "Who is observing this thought?" shifts attention from the content of cognition to the witnessing awareness underlying it, a shift associated with increased clarity and emotional regulation (Ghista et al., 1976). Vivekananda emphasised the value of this discipline because it dismantles false identifications and discloses a deeper, more resilient sense of self that can encounter psychological challenges with steadiness rather than fragmentation (Vivekananda, 1896; Vivekananda, 1951).

Figure 2. Vedantic Tools for Inner Change

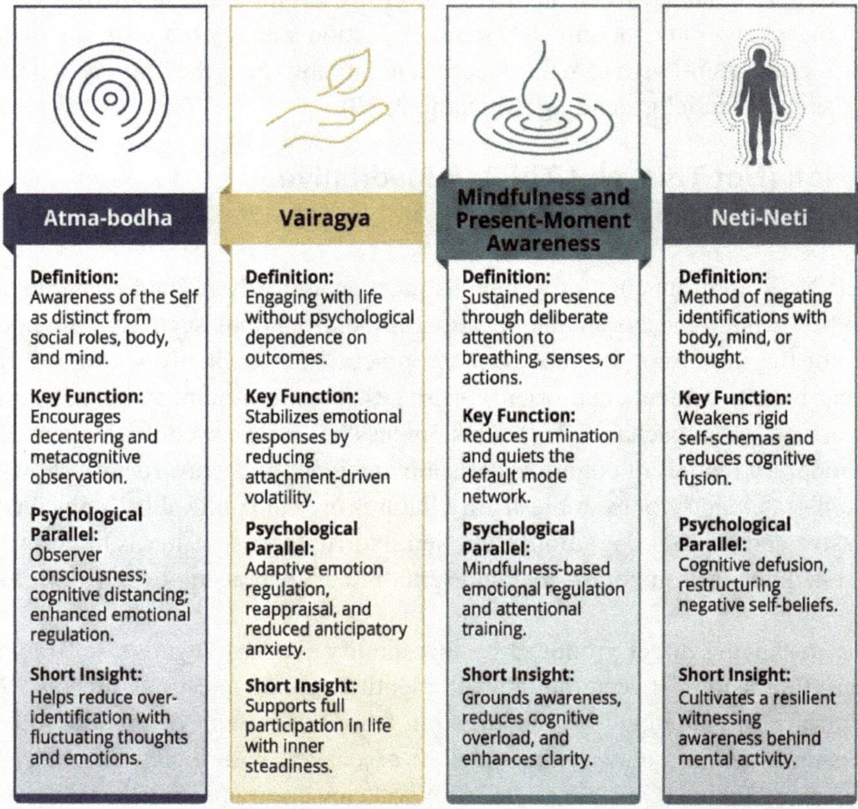

Suggested Daily Practices Inspired by Vedanta

The following practices may serve as gentle invitations for readers who wish to integrate Vedantic principles into their daily routines. They are not prescriptions but possibilities for cultivating awareness, steadiness, and emotional balance.

A Moment of Self-Awareness (Atma-Bodha): At any quiet point in the day, one might pause and notice the first thought that appears. Instead of engaging with it, the individual may simply acknowledge it as a thought rather than an identity. Such small moments of observation can help create a sense of inner space and reduce automatic reactivity.

Evening Reflection on Attachment (Vairagya): At the end of the day, some may find it helpful to reflect on a situation that created tension or discomfort. Asking whether the reaction was tied to a specific outcome can offer clarity. Imagining the temporary release of that outcome may allow the mind to soften and ease into a more balanced stance.

Practising Witness Awareness (Sakhi-Bhava): During emotionally charged moments, a brief inward shift can be useful. Observing thoughts or feelings as passing experiences, and quietly affirming "I am the witness," may support a calmer response. Over time, this reflective stance can become more natural.

Intention-Setting Before Action (Karma Yoga): Before beginning any meaningful activity—teaching, writing, meeting someone—individuals may take a slow breath and set a simple intention to act sincerely without clinging to results. This orientation can help reduce performance pressure and align action with inner steadiness.

Returning to the Present: Throughout the day, awareness can be gently brought back to the present moment by noticing breath, movement, or sensory experience. This can help quiet mental rumination and cultivate a clearer, more grounded mental field.

Figure 3. Suggested Daily Practices Inspired by Vedanta

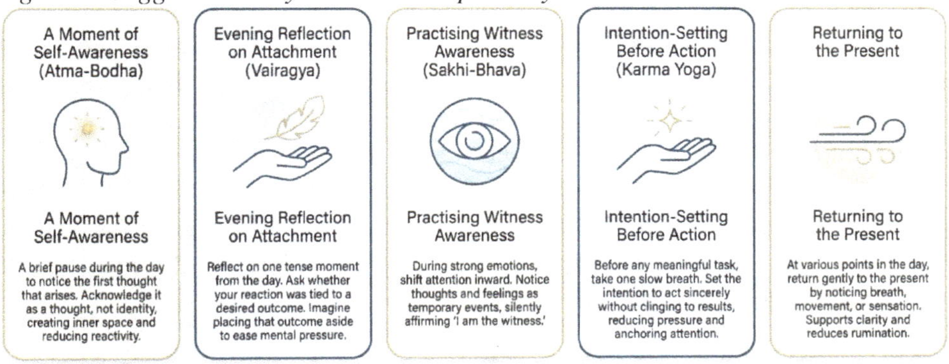

PRACTICAL EXERCISES FOR APPLYING VEDANTIC TOOLS

Integrating Vedantic principles into everyday life requires simple but deliberate practices that cultivate inner awareness, emotional steadiness, and clarity of purpose. The following exercises translate key Vedantic concepts into short, accessible methods that individuals can apply throughout the day.

A Self-Awareness Micro-Practice (Atma-Bodha)

A practical method for developing Vedantic self-awareness involves a brief observational exercise in which individuals pause and attend to the activity of the mind in real time. The practitioner sits comfortably, closes the eyes, and observes the first arising thought. Rather than suppressing or elaborating on it, the thought is noted with the understanding that it is a mental event rather than an expression of the self. This recognition establishes a subtle cognitive distance between the observer and the thought process, marking the beginning of metacognitive awareness. Such awareness enables individuals to witness worries, self-evaluative cognitions, and affective impulses without automatic identification. With consistent practice, this approach fosters reduced reactivity and supports the emergence of a more regulated and coherent sense of self.

A Detachment Reflection (Vairagya)

At the end of the day, individuals can engage in a brief reflective exercise focused on emotional regulation. One identifies a situation that elicited discomfort or tension and then examines whether the reaction was linked to attachment to a particular outcome. Recognizing this attachment often introduces cognitive clarity. The practitioner then visualizes releasing the outcome, even temporarily, as if setting it aside. This symbolic act tends to reduce physiological tension and lighten cognitive load. Such practice does not weaken commitment or responsibility. Rather, it decreases the emotional rigidity that contributes to anxiety and disappointment, thereby allowing for more adaptive and flexible responses.

A Witnessing Exercise (Sakhi-Bhava)

During moments of heightened emotion or rapid cognitive activity, individuals may pause and redirect attention inward. The task is to observe the emerging thoughts or feelings without attempting to modify them, while silently acknowledging, "I am the witness of this experience." This brief affirmation shifts awareness from the mental content to the position of observation. Maintaining this witnessing stance reduces emotional reactivity and mitigates feelings of overwhelm. With repeated practice, this mode of observation becomes more accessible in daily life and supports greater psychological stability during challenging circumstances.

An Intention-Setting Ritual (Karma Yoga)

Before initiating any significant task, such as writing an email, teaching, or entering a meeting, an individual may take a single deliberate breath and set the intention, "I will act sincerely, without clinging to results." This brief preparatory practice reflects the central principle of Karma Yoga by shifting attention from anticipated evaluation or approval to the quality of intentional action. Beginning work with this orientation helps reduce performance anxiety, minimizes cognitive distraction, and anchors behaviour in purpose rather than ego-driven concerns. Over time, such intention-setting cultivates a more stable, resilient, and engaged approach to everyday responsibilities.

COMPARING VEDANTA WITH MODERN PSYCHOTHERAPIES

Vedanta and contemporary psychotherapies often emerge from different philosophical worldviews, yet they converge in several meaningful ways. Many Vedantic practices resemble the mechanisms targeted by Cognitive Behavioral Therapy (CBT) and Acceptance and Commitment Therapy (ACT), even though they arise from a non-dual spiritual framework rather than a clinical model (Pradhan, 2019). A comparison of these approaches reveals both conceptual parallels and unique contributions.

At the level of self-understanding, *Atma-Bodha* teaches that one's true identity lies beyond social roles and fluctuating mental states. This mirrors CBT's use of cognitive restructuring, which challenges distorted self-beliefs and promotes a more stable core identity (Bertelli, 2019). ACT further aligns with this Vedantic insight through the process of *self-as-context*, where individuals learn to experience themselves as the observing awareness rather than the content of their thoughts (Shah, 2021).

Similarly, Vedantic *Vairagya* (detachment) shares functional overlap with CBT's cognitive distancing and reappraisal techniques, both of which help reduce emotional reactivity and prevent over-identification with dysfunctional beliefs (Beshai, 2024). In ACT, this parallels acceptance and willingness, where individuals allow emotions to arise without suppression or struggle. In all three traditions, emotional freedom is cultivated not by disengaging from life but by loosening attachment to outcomes (Mrazek et al., 2024).

The Vedantic practice of *Sakhi-Bhava*, or witness consciousness, is closely related to decentering or cognitive defusion. CBT-based mindfulness approaches teach individuals to observe thoughts rather than react to them, while ACT explicitly encourages viewing thoughts as mental events rather than truths. Vedanta frames this witnessing stance as a direct path to inner stability and clarity (Singh, 2022).

Neti-Neti, a foundational contemplative method in Vedanta, offers a deeper form of disidentification. By systematically negating all transient identifications ("not the body, not the mind, not the thought"), practitioners challenge rigid self-schemas in ways comparable to CBT's restructuring of maladaptive core beliefs (Lee & Park, 2023). ACT resonates with this through advanced forms of self-as-context and experiential distancing, which help individuals move beyond limiting narratives (Trivedi, 2025).

Finally, Vedantic mindful presence parallels behavioral activation and present-focused attention in CBT, and the cultivation of moment-to-moment awareness in ACT. While CBT and ACT use these techniques to reduce symptoms and enhance functioning, Vedanta frames present-moment awareness as a doorway to recognizing the deeper Self (Santiago & Gall, 2016; Bianco et al., 2016).

Taken together, these comparisons show that Vedanta offers a philosophical and experiential depth that complements the structured, empirically grounded methods of CBT and ACT. The overlap suggests that Vedantic principles may enrich modern psychotherapy, while the differences highlight opportunities for further empirical study and integrative clinical models.

Table 1. Comparative Table: Vedantic Concepts and Their Psychological Equivalents

Vedantic Concept	CBT Equivalent	ACT (Acceptance and Commitment Therapy) Equivalent
Atma-Bodha (Self-awareness as the witnessing Self beyond roles)	Cognitive restructuring through identifying distorted thoughts and developing a more stable core belief structure	Self-as-context (observing the self as an unchanging perspective rather than thoughts or roles)
Vairagya (Detachment from outcomes and emotional dependency)	Cognitive distancing and reappraisal to reduce emotional reactivity and attachment to dysfunctional beliefs	Acceptance and willingness; letting go of struggle with emotions without suppression
Sakhi-Bhava (Witness consciousness or observing inner states without identification)	Decentering or cognitive defusion within CBT-based mindfulness treatments	Cognitive defusion (seeing thoughts as mental events, not truths)
Neti-Neti (Not this, not this; disidentification from body, mind, and thought)	Challenging maladaptive core beliefs; restructuring rigid self-schemas	Deepened self-as-context and experiential distancing from internal events
Mindful Presence (Awareness in action, moment-to-moment consciousness)	Behavioral activation and present-focused attention training	Mindfulness and present-moment awareness as a foundational ACT process

Figure 4. Comparative Infographic of Vedanta, CBT, and ACT

Vedanta	CBT Equivalent	ACT Equivalent
Atma-Bodha Self-realization; recognition of the true Self beyond body and mind.	**Cognitive restructuring** Identification of distorted thoughts; development of stable core beliefs; reframing maladaptive thinking patterns.	**Self-as-context** Observing awareness beyond thought content; experiential self-discovery as a stable perspective.
Vairagya (Detachment) Dispassion; non-attachment to objects, outcomes, and emotional fluctuations.	**Cognitive distancing** Reappraisal to reduce emotional reactivity; creating space between thoughts and reactions.	**Acceptance and willingness** Releasing emotional struggle without suppression; embracing experiences as they are.
Sakshi-Bhava (Witness Consciousness) The attitude of a witness; non-judgmental observation of internal and external events.	**Decentering** Cognitive defusion in mindfulness-based CBT; recognizing thoughts as mental events, not facts.	**Cognitive defusion** Experiencing thoughts as mental events, not truths; reducing the impact of unhelpful thoughts.
Neti-Neti (Not-this, Not-that) Method of negation to realize the Self by discarding all that is not the Self.	**Challenging maladaptive core beliefs** Restructuring rigid self-schemas; questioning and replacing deeply ingrained negative beliefs.	**Deepened self-as-context** Experiential distancing; understanding the self as distinct from thoughts, feelings, and roles.
Mindful Presence (Awareness in action) Being fully present and aware in every moment, without attachment to the past or future.	**Behavioral activation** Present-focused training; encouraging engagement in meaningful activities to improve mood.	**Mindfulness and present-moment awareness** Connecting with the here and now; engaging fully in the current experience with openness.

EVERYDAY INTEGRATION: VEDANTA AT HOME, WORK, AND SOCIETY

Vedanta is not a doctrine for saints or ascetics alone. He insisted that Vedanta should be practiced daily among family, work, relationships, and social duties (Gaur & Jain, 2017; Ramsundarsingh, 2019). A test of spiritual growth, he often said, is how we live and respond to the world. He says the real spiritual hero is not one who escapes life but one who lives it with inner freedom. Thus, Vedanta becomes a living philosophy and not an abstract concept.

Practicing Detachment in Relationships Without Disconnecting

Vedanta conceptualizes detachment (vairagya) not as withdrawal from relational life but as a form of emotional freedom. The term is often misunderstood as indifference, yet Vedantic teaching frames it as the capacity to engage deeply with others without becoming psychologically dependent on specific outcomes. In many family contexts, attachment can become possessive; individuals may conflate their identity with the success, behaviour, or approval of a child, partner, or dependent. This dynamic frequently contributes to anxiety, resentment, and emotional dependency. Detachment, in the Vedantic sense, does not diminish care. Rather, it facilitates a more selfless form of love that respects autonomy and reduces ego-driven expectations.

This orientation supports healthier relational boundaries and fosters greater emotional stability. It allows individuals to participate fully in relationships while preserving an inner steadiness that is not contingent on external validation. Swami Vivekananda often illustrated this principle through the metaphor of the lotus, which grows in water while remaining unaffected by it, suggesting that a Vedantin lives fully in the world while maintaining inner composure (Yarrow et al., 2015; Vivekananda, 1958,1964; Vivekananda, 1896).

Managing Work Stress with Vedantic Calm and Resilience

Modern professional environments are characterized by persistent pressures, including competition, performance evaluation, and job insecurity. Many individuals come to equate personal worth with occupational success, a pattern linked to chronic anxiety, burnout, and identity disturbance. Vedanta offers an alternative framework by asserting that one's essential identity is not defined by professional roles but by the Atman, the unchanging Self (Vivekananda, 1899; Vivekananda, 1958,1964). Within this perspective, work becomes a domain of service rather than an arena for ego affirmation.

Swami Vivekananda emphasized Karma Yoga as a disciplined approach to action in which tasks are performed with sincerity yet without psychological dependence on specific outcomes (Vivekananda, 1896; Vivekananda, 1951). This orientation does not eliminate goals but reduces the anticipatory anxiety that arises from external evaluation. By focusing on effort rather than reward, individuals conserve cognitive and emotional resources, which supports resilience and sustained engagement (Ross and Vasantha, 2014).

Practical applications of this principle can be seen in various professional contexts. A teacher who prioritizes intrinsic commitment to student development rather than external recognition experiences greater stability and satisfaction. Similarly, an employee navigating competitive or politicized work environments may benefit from remembering that such circumstances do not affect the inner self, a distinction central to Vedantic psychology (Vivekananda, 1947). This shift from outcome dependence to purpose alignment exemplifies Vedantic work ethics and promotes healthier emotional functioning.

Vedanta also mitigates exhaustion by encouraging moments of reflective detachment in which individuals recall their role as witnesses of mental activity rather than as wholly identified with stressors. Even brief pauses that cultivate this witnessing stance can interrupt automatic reactivity and support clarity in high-demand situations (Hassan et al., 2012; Vivekananda, 1959).

Living with Awareness and Purpose in Ordinary Actions

Vedanta challenges the view that meaning is found only in exceptional moments such as ritual, meditation, or achievement. Rather, it proposes that ordinary activities constitute significant arenas for cultivating awareness and inner discipline. Routine actions such as washing dishes, walking to work, or listening attentively become sites of spiritual practice when approached with conscious presence and reduced ego involvement. This orientation reflects Vivekananda's assertion that each individual is "potentially divine" and that the task of life is to manifest this divinity through mastery of both external and internal nature (Vivekananda, 1896; Vivekananda, 1951). Such manifestation is not confined to formal settings; it occurs equally within the mundane demands of daily life (Rajneesh and Neiman, 2001).

Practices such as mindful eating, attentive speech, and deep listening promote psychological clarity and reduce impulsive behaviour. These micro-practices create conditions for ethical discernment and emotional regulation. Vedanta also emphasizes the attitude of non-doership (akartrbhava), which frames action as occurring through, rather than belonging to, the individual agent. When internalized, this perspective mitigates pride and guilt, and reduces the emotional volatility associated with success and failure (Lefebvre, 2001; Vivekananda, 1958,1964).

Thus, Vedanta does not encourage withdrawal from ordinary life but invites its transformation. Through conscious engagement with everyday tasks, individuals cultivate inner strength and experience greater psychological freedom.

COUNTER-ARGUMENTS AND LIMITATIONS

While Vedantic principles offer valuable psychological insights and practical methods for cultivating resilience, emotional balance, and inner freedom, their application in contemporary mental health contexts requires careful qualification. Not all individuals may relate to metaphysical constructs such as the Atman, non-duality, or surrender, and many may require structured therapeutic interventions that Vedanta cannot independently provide (Verma, 2025). The empirical base for several Vedantic practices also remains limited, as large-scale randomized or longitudinal studies are scarce, which constrains their integration into evidence-based clinical frameworks (Chiappelli, 2012; Fendt-Newlin et al., 2020). Individuals facing acute psychological distress may also find introspective techniques such as self-inquiry or detachment difficult to practice without professional support (Zhao, 2025). These considerations highlight the need for rigorous research and culturally sensitive models that situate Vedantic tools alongside established psychotherapeutic approaches.

Mindfulness, now widely incorporated into clinical and wellness settings, is grounded in sustained attention to present-moment experience and the cultivation of non-judgmental awareness. Meta-analytic studies consistently demonstrate its effectiveness for reducing anxiety, depression, stress, and chronic pain. Vedantic meditation shares this attentional dimension but differs in scope: rather than observing thoughts alone, it interrogates the status of the observer itself (Vandenberghe and Sousa, 2006). Although both practices develop attentional stability, their intended outcomes diverge. Mindfulness is typically aimed at symptom reduction, whereas Vedantic inquiry seeks a shift from ego-based identification to recognition of the unchanging Self, which represents a deeper form of psychological transformation (Prabhu and Bhat, 2013).

The two traditions can nevertheless function synergistically. Mindfulness reduces ruminative tendencies and stabilizes attention, thereby preparing the mind for more advanced Vedantic inquiry (Guha, 2005). A key distinction remains: contemporary mindfulness, particularly in corporate or clinical contexts, often supports individuals in functioning more effectively within existing environments. Vedantic practice, by contrast, questions the very identity that experiences distress and promotes a reorientation from the fluctuating mind to a more stable ground of awareness.

VEDANTA IN CONTEMPORARY DIGITAL MENTAL-HEALTH ECOSYSTEMS

The digital mental-health ecosystem is expanding rapidly, with interventions increasingly delivered through mobile apps, web platforms, and AI-driven tools. Evidence-based approaches, particularly CBT, have been effectively adapted for online delivery, showing improvements in depression, anxiety, and overall well-being across youth, student, and adult populations (Lattie et al., 2019; Philippe et al., 2022; Lattie et al., 2022; Balcombe & De Leo, 2020; Löchner et al., 2025; Coelho et al., 2025; Baka et al., 2025). In contrast, the integration of Vedantic (Advaita Vedanta) principles into digital mental-health programs is still emerging. Although recent theoretical work proposes blending non-duality frameworks with CBT to support holistic mental health, this integration remains largely conceptual and lacks empirical validation, particularly in digitally mediated contexts (Trivedi, 2025).

While some digital tools now incorporate meditation or mantra-based components, most platforms continue to rely on Western therapeutic models, with limited inclusion of Vedantic or other Indian knowledge systems (Trivedi, 2025; Vali & Azeem, 2025; Bhati et al., 2025). This gap becomes more important as digital platforms risk encouraging superficial engagement with contemplative practices, sometimes promoting quick-fix spiritual content that may unintentionally foster spiritual bypassing rather than fostering deeper self-inquiry and psychological integration. Current research also underscores the need for rigorous testing of Vedanta-based digital interventions through randomized trials, standardized protocols, and culturally diverse samples (Bhati et al., 2025). Ensuring cultural sensitivity is essential when translating traditional practices for global digital audiences (Vali & Azeem, 2025). At the same time, digital mental-health tools face broader implementation challenges—including privacy risks, data security concerns, and reduced human connection—which complicate the integration of deeper contemplative or existential frameworks (Berardi et al., 2024; Lattie et al., 2022; Löchner et al., 2025; Coelho et al., 2025). Together, these factors reveal a promising yet underdeveloped space for harmonizing Vedantic wisdom with modern digital therapeutics.

SUMMARY OF EXISTING SCIENTIFIC EVIDENCE AND RESEARCH GAPS

Current scientific literature provides strong evidence for several contemporary psychological interventions, while indicating that Vedantic approaches—though conceptually promising—remain significantly under-researched. Cognitive Behavioral Therapy (CBT) is one of the most empirically supported treatments for anxiety, depression, and related disorders, with enhancements such as mindfulness-based CBT and Emotion Regulation Therapy (ERT) expanding its effectiveness across diverse populations (Newman et al., 2022; Mennin et al., 2013; Palmieri et al., 2022; Espenes et al., 2024). ERT in particular, which integrates CBT principles with mindfulness and emotional regulation strategies, has shown positive outcomes in complex presentations such as generalized anxiety disorder, although additional trials are still needed to clarify mechanisms and optimize delivery (Fresco et al., 2013; Clayton et al., 2021; Fresco & Mennin, 2018; Espenes et al., 2024).

Mindfulness and meditation also enjoy a robust scientific foundation. Multiple large-scale meta-analyses demonstrate that mindfulness-based interventions (MBIs) reliably reduce anxiety, depression, and stress, showing moderate to large effect sizes and minimal adverse events across populations (Vancampfort et al., 2020; Goldberg et al., 2021; Worsley et al., 2022; Pascoe et al., 2021). Yoga-based interventions, including those used in maternal mental health, further contribute to emotional resilience, though the field continues to call for more rigorous, high-quality studies to strengthen findings (Munns et al., 2024; Vinu et al., 2025; Pascoe et al., 2021). Overall, contemporary psychological science strongly supports practices involving attention regulation, mindfulness, emotional regulation, and cognitive reframing.

By contrast, Vedantic approaches such as Neti-Neti, Vairagya, and Atma-Bodha remain underexplored despite their conceptual alignment with modern theories of metacognition, emotional regulation, and resilience. Preliminary studies and theoretical analyses suggest that Vedantic practices may reduce maladaptive identification with thoughts, regulate emotional reactivity, and foster psychological flexibility, yet the evidence remains limited, culturally localized, and lacking the methodological rigor seen in established interventions (Bhati et al., 2025; Keshavan & Bhargav, 2025; Zhao, 2025). Integrative frameworks attempting to combine Advaita Vedanta with modern psychotherapy are emerging, but they currently lack standardized protocols, validated outcome measures, or controlled clinical trials capable of establishing efficacy across diverse populations (Bhati et al., 2025; Zhao, 2025).

To advance the field, future research must undertake systematic empirical testing of Vedanta-based interventions. Randomized controlled trials, larger and more diverse samples, longitudinal designs, and operationalized protocols for practices such as Neti-Neti, Vairagya, and Atma-Bodha are needed to determine their effectiveness and mechanisms of change (Keshavan & Bhargav, 2025; Zhao, 2025). Mechanistic research is also necessary to understand how these ancient contemplative practices interact with psychological processes and neurobiological pathways, and whether they can complement or enhance established therapies such as CBT, ERT, and MBIs (Pascoe et al., 2021; Bhati et al., 2025). A further gap concerns cultural generalizability: much of the existing research on Vedantic and yoga-based interventions is restricted to specific regional contexts, limiting global applicability and preventing integration into mainstream mental health care (Munns et al., 2024; Bhati et al., 2025; Gundi et al., 2025).

In summary, CBT, ERT, mindfulness, and meditation are well-supported by extensive scientific evidence. Vedantic practices offer meaningful conceptual contributions and strong theoretical promise but require rigorous empirical validation, culturally adaptable frameworks, and clearly defined intervention models before they can be positioned alongside established psychological treatments.

VIVEKANANDA'S PRACTICAL VEDANTA: KEY CRITIQUES AND SCHOLARLY PERSPECTIVES

Vivekananda's "Practical Vedanta" represents one of the most influential modern reinterpretations of Advaita Vedanta, aiming to translate non-dual philosophy into social responsibility, ethical action, and universal spiritual humanism. Scholars, however, continue to debate its originality, coherence, and broader intellectual legacy.

A major line of critique concerns the label "Neo-Vedanta." Some scholars argue that Vivekananda creatively reworked classical Advaita by integrating elements of modern universalism, egalitarian ethics, and social activism, producing a genuinely new formulation of Vedantic thought (Pallathadka & Roy, 2025; Medhananda, 2022; Madaio, 2017). Critics such as Paul Hacker describe this as "Neo-Hinduism," claiming it reflects Western liberal ideas reframed in Hindu terms. Yet others point out that Vivekananda's vision is firmly rooted in indigenous traditions, especially the experiential spirituality of Sri Ramakrishna, and cannot be understood merely as Western-influenced innovation (Maharaj, 2019; Madaio, 2017).

Another debate centers on philosophical coherence. Vivekananda's claim that all beings are divine and that service to humanity is service to God has been viewed as a democratization of Advaita, challenging caste hierarchies and social exclusion (Harris, 2023; Long, 2024; Baier, 2019). Some argue that his synthesis of metaphysics and social action lacks systematic rigor, but recent scholarship suggests his adaptability and pluralism reflect deliberate responses to the intellectual and political pressures of modernity (Long, 2020; Medhananda, 2022).

Vivekananda's legacy remains complex. His Practical Vedanta has inspired social reform movements, yet it has also been appropriated by diverse political groups, sometimes in conflicting ways (Harris, 2023; Baier, 2019). His universalist message continues to generate both admiration and critical scrutiny.

CONCLUSION

Contemporary approaches to mental health often depend on external interventions such as therapy, medication, achievement, or interpersonal validation. While these supports are valuable and sometimes necessary, they do not always produce enduring psychological stability or inner freedom. Vedanta, particularly as interpreted by Swami Vivekananda, offers a complementary and inward-oriented framework that shifts the focus from managing symptoms to understanding the deeper structures of thought, emotion, and identity. Rather than encouraging withdrawal from difficulty, Vedanta presents a practical path for cultivating psychological clarity, self-awareness, and emotional resilience.

This chapter examined several Vedantic concepts that have direct relevance for modern mental health. The principle of Atma-bodha supports metacognitive awareness by helping individuals recognize that they are not identical with their transient thoughts and moods. Vairagya reframes detachment not as indifference but as the capacity to experience emotions without becoming constrained by them. Mindfulness in the Vedantic sense extends beyond present-moment attention to include discernment of the ego's constructed nature. The practice of Neti-Neti encourages individuals to relinquish limiting self-definitions, creating space for a more flexible and less fear-driven sense of identity. Karma Yoga, as a discipline of action without attachment to outcomes, offers a model for emotionally intelligent engagement with work and relationships. Vedantic meditation, meanwhile, provides a structured method for stabilizing attention and cultivating inner calm.

Together, these practices encourage an internal transformation that unfolds gradually through reflection, disciplined practice, and, when appropriate, guidance. Their psychological impact is cumulative: individuals become less reactive, more centered under pressure, less dependent on external validation, and more comfortable with solitude. Such outcomes align closely with contemporary psychological constructs such as emotional regulation, resilience, and self-determination. Rather than attempting to control external circumstances, practitioners of these methods cultivate an internal locus of stability, allowing the mind to become a partner in well-being rather than an adversary.

The universality of Vedanta strengthens its contemporary relevance. Because it is concerned with consciousness rather than dogma, ritual, or sectarian identity, its insights are adaptable to a range of personal, cultural, and professional contexts. The principles explored in this chapter may support the spiritual seeker, the burned-out professional, the anxious student, or the overextended caregiver. Vedanta thus serves not as a metaphysical abstraction but as a set of psychological tools for navigating an increasingly unstable world.

Swami Vivekananda exemplified this integration of insight and action. His interpretation of Vedanta emphasized strength, clarity, and compassion, demonstrating that spiritual understanding is not a retreat from life but an engagement with it grounded in a deeper recognition of one's true nature. Vedanta contends that qualities such as strength, purity, and peace cannot be externally acquired because they are intrinsic to the self; the task is to uncover rather than import them.

In a cultural context where emotional fragility is widespread and psychological suffering is often concealed, Vedanta's message is both timely and therapeutic. It affirms that individuals are not defined by past events, present symptoms, or fluctuating emotions. The self, understood in Vedantic terms, stands beyond fear, failure, and even success. Although the path of self-realization requires sustained effort, it offers a meaningful way to meet life's inevitable challenges without losing inner equilibrium. Vedanta does not promise escape from adversity but provides a framework for remaining anchored and intact amid life's uncertainties. Such equanimity constitutes a form of freedom that is both psychologically grounded and existentially profound.

AI USE STATEMENT

To support the writing of this chapter, the authors, being non-native English speakers, used AI tools such as QuillBot and ChatGPT 5.1 for language enhancement, grammar refinement, and clarity of expression. These tools were employed to improve readability and ensure that complex philosophical ideas were communicated in clear and accessible English. All conceptual content, scholarly interpretation, and original insights remain the authors' own.

REFERENCES

Alpert, J. L. (2012). Loss of humanness: The ultimate trauma. *American Journal of Psychoanalysis*, *72*(2), 118–138. Advance online publication. DOI: 10.1057/ajp.2012.8 PMID: 22617097

Baier, K. (2019). Swami Vivekananda. Reform Hinduism, nationalism and scientistic yoga. *Interdisciplinary Journal for Religion and Transformation in Contemporary Society*, *5*(1), 230–257. DOI: 10.30965/23642807-00501012

Baka, E., Tan, Y., Wong, B. L. H., Xing, Z., & Yap, P. (2025). A scoping review of digital interventions for the promotion of mental health and prevention of mental health conditions for young people. *Oxford Open Digital Health*, *3*, oqaf005. Advance online publication. DOI: 10.1093/oodh/oqaf005 PMID: 40230873

Balcombe, L., & De Leo, D. (2020). Digital mental health challenges and the horizon ahead for solutions (Preprint). *JMIR Mental Health*. https://doi.org/DOI: 10.2196/preprints.26811

Berardi, C., Antonini, M., Jordan, Z., Wechtler, H., Paolucci, F., & Hinwood, M. (2024). Barriers and facilitators to the implementation of digital technologies in mental health systems: A qualitative systematic review to inform a policy framework. *BMC Health Services Research*, *24*(1), 243. DOI: 10.1186/s12913-023-10536-1 PMID: 38408938

Berne, E. (2013). *Transactional analysis in psychotherapy: A systematic individual and social psychiatry*. (Original work published 1961)

Bertelli, R. (2019). Does the cognitive-behavioural model of learning share features of Buddha's and Krishnamurti's teachings? Using the concept of automatic maladaptive thoughts as an example. *Advances in Social Sciences Research Journal*, *6*(2). Advance online publication. DOI: 10.14738/assrj.62.6222

Beshai, S. (2024). Mindfulness and CBT: A conceptual integration bridging ancient wisdom and modern cognitive theories of psychopathology. *Frontiers in Psychology*, *15*, 1489798. Advance online publication. DOI: 10.3389/fpsyg.2024.1489798 PMID: 39723397

Bhagabati, D., & Kumar, A. (2016). Evolving society and mental health. *Open Journal of Psychiatry & Allied Sciences*, *7*(2), 117. Advance online publication. DOI: 10.5958/2394-2061.2016.00018.5

Bhar, G. C. (2020). *Why things go wrong in life: Spiritual viewpoints*. Indian Science Cruiser., DOI: 10.24906/isc/2020/v34/i3/203784

Bhati, R., Mandal, M., & Singh, T. (2025). Ancient Indian perspectives and practices of mental well-being. *Frontiers in Psychology, 16*, 1616802. DOI: 10.3389/fpsyg.2025.1616802 PMID: 40528855

Bianco, S., Barilaro, P., & Palmieri, A. (2016). Traditional meditation, mindfulness and psychodynamic approach: An integrative perspective. *Frontiers in Psychology, 7*. Advance online publication. DOI: 10.3389/fpsyg.2016.00552 PMID: 27148153

Bijlenga, D., Kulcu, S., Van Gellecum, T., Eryigit, Z., & Kooij, J. S. (2017). Persistence and adherence to psychostimulants, and psychological well-being up to 3 years after specialized treatment of adult attention-deficit/hyperactivity disorder: A naturalistic follow-up study. *Journal of Clinical Psychopharmacology, 37*(6), 689–696. DOI: 10.1097/JCP.0000000000000787 PMID: 29049077

Binsale, L. J. (2017). *Self-concept clarity, trauma and psychopathology* (Doctoral dissertation). Lancaster University.

Brahmaprana, P. (2001). Vedanta: Death and the art of dying. *CrossCurrents.*

Canter, P. H. (2003). The therapeutic effects of meditation. *BMJ (Clinical Research Ed.), 326*(7398), 1049–1050. DOI: 10.1136/bmj.326.7398.1049 PMID: 12750183

Carter, M. J. (2017). How self-perceptions of identity change in person, role, and social identities relate to depression. *Identity, 17*(4), 242–257. DOI: 10.1080/15283488.2017.1379908

Carver, C. S., & Johnson, S. L. (2018). Impulsive reactivity to emotion and vulnerability to psychopathology. *The American Psychologist, 73*(9), 1067–1078. DOI: 10.1037/amp0000387 PMID: 30525782

Chattopadhyay, A., Gayen, M. T. K., & Sardar, M. C. (2025). *Yoga education and life skills*. Chyren Publication.

Chiappelli, F., Arora, R., Barkhordarian, B., & Ramchandani, M. (2012). Evidence-based clinical research: Toward a new conceptualization of the level and the quality of the evidence. *Annals of Ayurvedic Medicine, 1*(4), 60–64.

Chohan, S. K. (2010). Whispering selves and reflective transformations in the internal dialogue of teachers and students. *Journal of Invitational Theory and Practice.*

Clayton, M., Spaeth, P. E., Renna, M. E., Fresco, D. M., & Mennin, D. S. (2021). Optimizing cognitive behavioral therapy to reduce the burden of distress disorders within an emotion regulation framework. In *New directions in rational emotive behaviour therapy* (pp. 79–98). https://doi.org/DOI: 10.4324/9781003081593-6

Coelho, J., Pécune, F., Micoulaud-Franchi, J., Bioulac, B., & Philip, P. (2025). Promoting mental health in the age of new digital tools: Balancing challenges and opportunities of social media, chatbots, and wearables. *Frontiers in Digital Health, 7*, 1560580. DOI: 10.3389/fdgth.2025.1560580 PMID: 40182586

Cropley, M., Dijk, D. J., & Stanley, N. (2020). Job strain, work rumination, and sleep in school teachers. In *Work and rest: A topic for work and organizational psychology* (pp. 181–196). Psychology Press. DOI: 10.4324/9781003059714-4

de Lacey, S., Smith, C., & Paterson, C. (2009). Building resilience: A preliminary exploration of women's perceptions of the use of acupuncture as an adjunct to in vitro fertilisation. *BMC Complementary and Alternative Medicine, 9*(1), 50. DOI: 10.1186/1472-6882-9-50 PMID: 20003370

de Witt Huberts, J. C., Evers, C., & de Ridder, D. T. D. (2014). Because I am worth it: A theoretical framework and empirical review of a justification-based account of self-regulation failure. *Personality and Social Psychology Review, 18*(2), 119–138. DOI: 10.1177/1088868313507533 PMID: 24214148

Di Blasi, M., Cavani, P., Pavia, L., Lo Baido, R., La Grutta, S., & Schimmenti, A. (2015). The relationship between self-image and social anxiety in adolescence. *Child and Adolescent Mental Health, 20*(2), 74–80. DOI: 10.1111/camh.12071 PMID: 32680392

Dreyfus, H. L. (2007). Detachment, involvement, and rationality: Are we essentially rational animals? *Human Affairs, 17*(2), 101–109. DOI: 10.2478/v10023-007-0010-0

Dudeja, J. P. (2017). Scientific analysis of mantra-based meditation and its beneficial effects: An overview. *International Journal of Advanced Science. Technology and Engineering Management, 3*(6), 49101. Advance online publication. DOI: 10.22413/ijastems/2017/v3/i6/49101

Elices, M., Soler, J., Feliu-Soler, A., Carmona, C., Tiana, T., Pascual, J. C., & Álvarez, E. (2017). Combining emotion regulation and mindfulness skills for preventing depression relapse: A randomized controlled study. *Borderline Personality Disorder and Emotion Dysregulation, 4*(13), 13. Advance online publication. DOI: 10.1186/s40479-017-0064-6 PMID: 28690851

Espenes, K., Tørmoen, A. J., Rognstad, K., Nilsen, K. H., Waaler, P. M., Wentzel-Larsen, T., & Kjøbli, J. (2024). Effect of psychosocial interventions on children and youth emotion regulation: A meta-analysis. *Administration and Policy in Mental Health, 52*(5), 833–852. DOI: 10.1007/s10488-024-01373-3 PMID: 38717667

Farb, N. A. S., Segal, Z. V., Mayberg, H. S., Bean, J., McKeon, D., Fatima, Z., & Anderson, A. K. (2007). Attending to the present: Mindfulness meditation reveals distinct neural modes of self-reference. *Social Cognitive and Affective Neuroscience*, *2*(4), 313–322. DOI: 10.1093/scan/nsm030 PMID: 18985137

Fendt-Newlin, M., Jagannathan, A., & Webber, M. (2020). Cultural adaptation framework of social interventions in mental health: Evidence-based case studies from low- and middle-income countries. *The International Journal of Social Psychiatry*, *66*(1), 41–48. DOI: 10.1177/0020764019879943 PMID: 31580173

Fresco, D. M., & Mennin, D. S. (2018). All together now: Utilizing common functional change principles to unify cognitive behavioral and mindfulness-based therapies. *Current Opinion in Psychology*, *28*, 65–70. DOI: 10.1016/j.copsyc.2018.10.014 PMID: 30502664

Fresco, D. M., Mennin, D. S., Heimberg, R. G., & Ritter, M. (2013). Emotion regulation therapy for generalized anxiety disorder. *Cognitive and Behavioral Practice*, *20*(3), 282–300. DOI: 10.1016/j.cbpra.2013.02.001 PMID: 27499606

Gaur, V., & Jain, N. (2017). Spiritualizing inter-personal relationships: In view of Vedanta. *International Journal of Business Management & Research*, *7*(1), 33–44.

Ghista, D. N., Nandagopal, D., Ramamurthi, B., Das, A., Mukherji, A., & Srinivasan, T. M. (1976). Physiological characterisation of the meditative state during intuitional practice (the Ananda Marga system of meditation) and its therapeutic value. *Medical & Biological Engineering & Computing*, *14*(3), 209–214. DOI: 10.1007/BF02478750 PMID: 781406

Goldberg, S. B., Riordan, K. M., Sun, S., & Davidson, R. J. (2021). The empirical status of mindfulness-based interventions: A systematic review of 44 meta-analyses of randomized controlled trials. *Perspectives on Psychological Science*, *17*(1), 108–130. DOI: 10.1177/1745691620968771 PMID: 33593124

Gordon, K. (2003). The impermanence of being: Toward a psychology of uncertainty. *Journal of Humanistic Psychology*, *43*(1), 96–117. DOI: 10.1177/0022167802250731

Grossman, P. (2015). Mindfulness: Awareness informed by an embodied ethic. *Mindfulness*, *6*(1), 17–22. DOI: 10.1007/s12671-014-0372-5

Guendelman, S., Medeiros, S., & Rampes, H. (2017). Mindfulness and emotion regulation: Insights from neurobiological, psychological, and clinical studies. *Frontiers in Psychology*, *8*, 220. DOI: 10.3389/fpsyg.2017.00220 PMID: 28321194

Guha, D. (2005). Vivekananda's conception of normative ethics and resolution of ethical problems in business. *Management and Labour Studies*, *30*(2), 203–217. DOI: 10.1177/0258042X0503000204

Gundi, M., Kaikobad, R., & Sharma, S. (2025). Diversity in approaches in community-based mental health interventions in India: A narrative review and synthesis. *Global Mental Health (Cambridge, England)*, *12*, e89. DOI: 10.1017/gmh.2025.10046 PMID: 40895823

Gusha, K. Ç., Shala, I., & Kalo, R. (2017). Current problems in the mental health field. *European Journal of Social Sciences Education and Research*, *11*(1), 136–139. DOI: 10.26417/ejser.v11i1.p136-139

Hackett, J. D. (2014). Values anchoring: Strengthening the link between values and activist behaviors. *Social Influence*, *9*(4), 245–260. DOI: 10.1080/15534510.2013.787117

Hari, S. D. (2015). Concepts in Vedanta applicable to scientific explanation of consciousness. *Scientific GOD Journal*, *6*(4), 30–45.

Harris, R. (2023). Vivekananda: Indian swami and global guru. *Religions*, *14*(8), 1041. DOI: 10.3390/rel14081041

Hassan, M. ul, Shahnawaz, F., Imam, A., & Khan, J. (2012). Effect of yoga and exercise on job burnout and job satisfaction on doctors. *Indian Journal of Positive Psychology*, *3*(3), 309–313. DOI: 10.15614/ijpp/2012/v3i3/49751

Herrero de Jáuregui, M. (2015). The construction of inner religious space in wandering religion of classical Greece. *Numen*, *62*(3), 331–358. DOI: 10.1163/15685276-12341395

Hogan, C. (2013). Chronic stress: An approach to management in general practice. *Australian Family Physician*, *42*(3), 155–159. PMID: 23971061

Hollick, M. (2006). *The science of oneness: A worldview for the twenty-first century*. O Books.

Ji, M. (2023). *The origin of mindfulness revisited: A conceptual and historical review*. Lecture Notes in Education Psychology and Public Media., DOI: 10.54254/2753-7048/25/20230273

Jijina, P., Vasa, V., & Biswas, U. N. (2020). Construct description of Samatva from the Bhagavad Gita: Implications for holistic well-being. *Purushartha: A Journal of Management. Ethics and Spirituality*, *13*(2), 1–12.

Kapoor, S. (2002). *Encyclopaedia of Vedanta philosophy*. Concept Publishing Company.

Kariuki-Nyuthe, C., & Stein, D. J. (2015). Anxiety and related disorders and physical illness. In *Advances in Psychiatry*. DOI: 10.1159/000365538

Keshavan, M. S., & Bhargav, H. (2025). Dhyana yoga, the path of meditative being: Psychotherapeutic insights from the East. *Asian Journal of Psychiatry*, *108*, 104483. DOI: 10.1016/j.ajp.2025.104483 PMID: 40279762

King, A. P., & Fresco, D. M. (2019). A neurobehavioral account for decentering as the salve for the distressed mind. *Current Opinion in Psychology*, *28*, 280–286. DOI: 10.1016/j.copsyc.2019.02.009 PMID: 31059966

Kowall, J. (2014). The vicious cycle of self-identification. *Scientific GOD Journal*, *5*(2), 119–127.

Kuan, T. (2009). Rethinking non-self: A new perspective from the Ekottarika Āgama. *Buddhist Studies Review*, *26*(2), 155–166. DOI: 10.1558/bsrv.v26i2.155

Kumar, A., & Kumar, S. (2013). Karma Yoga: A path towards work in positive psychology. *Indian Journal of Psychiatry*, *55*(6, S2), 266–270. DOI: 10.4103/0019-5545.105511 PMID: 23858246

Kuzucu, Y. (2016). Do anger control and social problem-solving mediate relationships between difficulties in emotion regulation and aggression in adolescents? *Educational Sciences: Theory & Practice*, *16*(3), 915–933. DOI: 10.12738/estp.2016.3.0003

Lattie, E. G., Adkins, E. C., Winquist, N., Stiles-Shields, C., Wafford, Q. E., & Graham, A. K. (2019). Digital mental health interventions for depression, anxiety, and enhancement of psychological well-being among college students: Systematic review. *Journal of Medical Internet Research*, *21*(7), e12869. DOI: 10.2196/12869 PMID: 31333198

Lecercle, J.-J., & Riley, D. (2004). A voice without a mouth: Inner speech. In *The force of language* (pp. 19–35). Palgrave Macmillan., DOI: 10.1057/9780230503793_2

Lee, C.-H., & Park, S. R. (2023). Reviewing the concept of disidentification in the context of psychotherapy. *Culture and Convergence*, *45*(6), 427–445. DOI: 10.33645/cnc.2023.06.45.06.427

Lefebvre, V. A. (2001). Streams of consciousness and acts of awareness. In *Principia Cybernetica* (pp. 497–514). Springer., DOI: 10.1007/978-94-017-0691-9_36

Löchner, J., Carlbring, P., Schuller, B., Torous, J., & Sander, L. B. (2025). Digital interventions in mental health: An overview and future perspectives. *Internet Interventions : the Application of Information Technology in Mental and Behavioural Health*, *40*, 100824. DOI: 10.1016/j.invent.2025.100824 PMID: 40330743

Long, J. D. (2020). A complex ultimate reality: The metaphysics of the four yogas. *Religions, 11*(12), 655. DOI: 10.3390/rel11120655

Long, J. D. (2024). On Swami Vivekananda and caste prejudice: Ethical implications of the experience of non-duality. *Religions, 15*(8), 889. DOI: 10.3390/rel15080889

Madaio, J. (2017). Rethinking Neo-Vedānta: Swami Vivekananda and the selective historiography of Advaita Vedānta. *Religions, 8*(6), 101. DOI: 10.3390/rel8060101

Maharaj, A. (2017). Swami Vivekananda's Vedāntic critique of Schopenhauer's doctrine of the will. *Philosophy East & West, 67*(4), 1013–1031. DOI: 10.1353/pew.2017.0098

Maharaj, A. (2019). Śivajñāne jīver sevā: Reexamining Swami Vivekananda's practical Vedānta in the light of Sri Ramakrishna. *Journal of Dharma Studies, 2*(2), 175–187. DOI: 10.1007/s42240-019-00046-x

Maharaj, A. (2020). *Śivajñāne jīver sevā: Reexamining Swami Vivekananda's practical Vedānta in the light of Sri Ramakrishna*. Springer., DOI: 10.1007/s42240-019-00046-x

Marshall, J. E. (2012). Prophylactic effects of mindfulness: The role of mindfulness in the treatment of anxiety. [No DOI available]. *Journal of Clinical Psychology Practice, 3*(1), 22–31.

Matsumoto, N., & Mochizuki, S. (2018). Why do people overthink? A longitudinal investigation of a meta-cognitive model and uncontrollability of rumination. *Behavioural and Cognitive Psychotherapy, 46*(2), 129–143. DOI: 10.1017/S1352465818000103 PMID: 29510773

McKenna, J. F. (2006). The meaningfulness of mental health as being within a world of apparently meaningless being. In *New perspectives in psychotherapy* (pp. 233–249). Springer., DOI: 10.1007/1-4020-3737-6_20

Medhananda, S. (2022). *Swami Vivekananda's Vedāntic cosmopolitanism*. Oxford University Press., DOI: 10.1093/oso/9780197624463.001.0001

Mennin, D. S., Ellard, K. K., Fresco, D. M., & Gross, J. J. (2013). United we stand: Emphasizing commonalities across cognitive-behavioral therapies. *Behavior Therapy, 44*(2), 234–248. DOI: 10.1016/j.beth.2013.02.004 PMID: 23611074

Miehls, D. (2011). Surrender as a developmental achievement in couple systems. *Psychoanalytic Social Work, 18*(1), 34–49. DOI: 10.1080/15228878.2011.561706

Mishra, V. (2014). Ethical responsibility and the spectres of demonic sacralisation in Swami Vivekananda. In *The guru question* (pp. 199–214). Routledge., DOI: 10.4324/9781315819112-14

Mitra, S. (2000). The discourse vanishes: Revolution and resilience in Indian politics. *Contemporary South Asia*, *9*(3), 327–339. DOI: 10.1080/713658755

Montgomery, J. D. (2000). The self as a fuzzy set of roles, role theory as a fuzzy system. *Sociological Methodology*, *30*(1), 261–314. DOI: 10.1111/0081-1750.00081

Mrazek, M. D., Dow, B., Richelle, J., Pasch, A. M., Godderis, N., Pamensky, T. A., Rutila, B. A., & Mrazek, A. J. (2024). Aspects of acceptance: Building a shared conceptual understanding. *Frontiers in Psychology*, *15*, 1423976. DOI: 10.3389/fpsyg.2024.1423976 PMID: 38974104

Mulla, Z. R., & Krishnan, V. R. (2014). Karma-yoga: The Indian model of moral development. *Journal of Business Ethics*, *123*(2), 341–351. DOI: 10.1007/s10551-013-1842-8

Munns, L., Spark, N., Crossland, A., & Preston, C. (2024). The effects of yoga-based interventions on postnatal mental health and well-being: A systematic review. *Heliyon*, *10*(3), e25455. DOI: 10.1016/j.heliyon.2024.e25455 PMID: 38322903

Myers, M. W. (2000). *Brahman: A comparative theology*. Fordham University Press.

Nagar, P. (2024). Karma Yoga and management practice. *Gurugram University Business Review*, *1*, 1–12.

Nair, A. K., & Kutty, B. M. (2017). Meditation, cognitive reserve and the neural basis of consciousness. In *Meditation and Neuroscience* (pp. 37–56). https://doi.org/DOI: 10.1007/978-981-10-5777-9_3

National Institute of Mental Health. (2024). *Mental illness statistics*. https://www.nimh.nih.gov/health/statistics/mental-illness

National Institute of Mental Health and Neuro Sciences. (2016). *National Mental Health Survey of India, 2015–16: Prevalence, patterns and outcomes*. NIMHANS Publication.

Newman, M. G., Basterfield, C., Erickson, T. M., Caulley, E., Przeworski, A., & Llera, S. J. (2022). Psychotherapeutic treatments for generalized anxiety disorder: Cognitive and behavioral therapies, enhancement strategies, and emerging efforts. *Expert Review of Neurotherapeutics*, *22*(9), 751–770. DOI: 10.1080/14737175.2022.2125800 PMID: 36107159

Oei, N. Y. L., Veer, I. M., Wolf, O. T., Spinhoven, P., Rombouts, S. A. R. B., & Elzinga, B. M. (2012). Stress shifts brain activation towards ventral affective areas during emotional distraction. *Social Cognitive and Affective Neuroscience*, *7*(6), 653–662. DOI: 10.1093/scan/nsr024 PMID: 21498384

Pallathadka, H., & Roy, P. D. (2025). Transcendent unity and social transformation: A comprehensive analysis of Swami Vivekananda's philosophical legacy and contemporary relevance. *Stallion Journal for Multidisciplinary Associated Research Studies*, *4*(3), 91–109. DOI: 10.55544/sjmars.4.3.9

Palmieri, A., Fernandez, K. C., Cariolato, Y., Kleinbub, J. R., Salvatore, S., & Gross, J. J. (2022). Emotion regulation in psychodynamic and cognitive behaviour therapy: An integrative perspective. *Clinical*, 2022(2). https://doi.org/DOI: 10.36131/cnfioritieditore20220204

Pascoe, M. C., De Manincor, M. J., Hallgren, M., Baldwin, P. A., Tseberja, J., & Parker, A. G. (2021). Psychobiological mechanisms underlying the mental health benefits of yoga-based interventions: A narrative review. *Mindfulness*, *12*(12), 2877–2889. DOI: 10.1007/s12671-021-01736-z

Patla, I. (2025). *Addressing self-esteem in mental health: A systematic review* (Doctoral dissertation, California Southern University).

Permadhi, A. K., & Marhaeni, A. A. I. N. (2019). Effect of understanding the teaching of Karma Yoga and empowerment of poor family resource management. *International Journal of Sciences, Basic and Applied Research*, *45*(1), 256–269.

Phelps, J., & Manipod, V. (2012). Treating anxiety by discontinuing antidepressants: A case series. *Medical Hypotheses*, *79*(4), 477–479. DOI: 10.1016/j.mehy.2012.05.029 PMID: 22698959

Philippe, T. J., Sikder, N., Jackson, A., Koblanski, M. E., Liow, E., Pilarinos, A., & Vasarhelyi, K. (2022). Digital health interventions for delivery of mental health care: Systematic and comprehensive meta-review. *JMIR Mental Health*, *9*(5), e35159. DOI: 10.2196/35159 PMID: 35551058

Pillay, Y., Ziff, K., & Bhat, C. S. (2008). Vedānta personality development: A model to enhance the cultural competence of psychotherapists. *International Journal of Hindu Studies*, *12*(3), 273–291. DOI: 10.1007/s11407-008-9057-9

Powers, J., & LaBar, K. S. (2019). Regulating emotion through distancing: A taxonomy, neurocognitive model, and supporting meta-analysis. *Neuroscience and Biobehavioral Reviews*, *103*, 124–138. DOI: 10.1016/j.neubiorev.2018.04.023 PMID: 30502352

Prabhu, H. R. A., & Bhat, P. (2013). Mind and consciousness in Yoga–Vedanta: A comparative analysis with Western psychological concepts. *Indian Journal of Psychiatry*, *55*(6, S2), 338–342. DOI: 10.4103/0019-5545.105524 PMID: 23858252

Pradhan, B. (2019). *Yoga and mindfulness-based cognitive therapy*. Springer.

Rajneesh, B. S., & Neiman, S. C. (2001). *Awareness: The key to living in balance: Insights for a new way of living*. Osho International Foundation.

Ram-Prasad, C. (2002). *Advaita epistemology and metaphysics: An outline of Indian non-realism*. Routledge.

Rambachan, A. (2017). That from which all words return: The distinctive methods of language utilization in Advaita Vedānta. In *Language, cognition, and consciousness in Indian philosophy* (pp. 173–195). https://doi.org/DOI: 10.1007/978-3-319-64165-2_9

Ramsundarsingh, S. (2019). Vedanta and social work practice. *Social Thought*, *38*(1), 68–92.

Ross, D. S., & Vasantha, S. (2014). A conceptual study on impact of stress on work-life balance. *Sai Om Journal of Commerce & Management*, *1*(1), 1–8.

Santiago, P. N., & Gall, T. L. (2016). Acceptance and Commitment Therapy as a spiritually integrated psychotherapy. *Counseling and Values*, *61*(2), 239–255. DOI: 10.1002/cvj.12040

Saraswati, S. S., & Alston, A. J. (1997). *The method of the Vedanta: A critical account of the Advaita tradition*. State University of New York Press.

Sarkar, M. C. (2021). The concept of practical Vedanta philosophy of Swami Vivekananda and human development: An analytical study. *International Journal of Multidisciplinary Educational Research*, *1*(5), 17–20.

Shah, M. (2021). Acceptance-based therapies and Asian philosophical traditions: Similarities and differences in the concept of acceptance. *Journal of Rational-Emotive & Cognitive-Behavior Therapy*, *39*(3), 457–475. DOI: 10.1007/s10942-020-00355-2

Sharma, R. R., & Cooper, C. (2016). Indian approaches to coping with stress and burnout. In *Executive burnout* (pp. 163–220). Emerald Group Publishing. DOI: 10.1108/978-1-78635-286-620161010

Sharma, S. (2004). Vedanta as ved-ananta: A new unfolding of universal spiritual consciousness. *Social Science Research Network*. https://doi.org/DOI: 10.2139/ssrn.3188289

Sharratt, L. (2023). *Who I am and how I feel: The role of identity and self-concept in psychological distress* (Doctoral dissertation, Aston University).

Singh, B. D. (1999). Relevance of Nishkama Karma Yoga in today's business world. *Vision: The Journal of Business Perspective, 3*(2), 35–42. DOI: 10.1177/097226299900300205

Singh, R. K. (2015). To each his God: An Upanishadic approach to religion. *Journal of Indian Council of Philosophical Research, 32*(2), 221–232. DOI: 10.1007/s40961-015-0017-7

Singh, S. P. (2022). Sakshi and dhyana: The origin of mindfulness-based therapies. *BJPsych Bulletin, 46*(4), 216–220. DOI: 10.1192/bjb.2022.39 PMID: 35796539

Sousa, T., & Neves, P. (2021). Two tales of rumination and burnout: Examining the effects of boredom and overload. *Applied Psychology, 70*(3), 1018–1044. DOI: 10.1111/apps.12257

Southwick, S. M., & Charney, D. S. (2012). *Resilience: The science of mastering life's greatest challenges*. Cambridge University Press. DOI: 10.1017/CBO9781139013857

Spiteri, D. (2012). Does the adoption of an in-depth questioning approach promote self-reflexivity? Its application to the social work education context. *Social Work & Society, 10*(1), 1–14.

Steiner-Adair, C., & Barker, T. (2013). *The big disconnect: Protecting childhood and family relationships in the digital age*. HarperCollins.

Sukhsohale, N. D., Phatak, M. S., Sukhsohale, S. D., & Agrawal, S. B. (2012). Does Raja Yoga meditation bring out physiological and psychological general well-being among practitioners. *International Journal of Collaborative Research on Internal Medicine & Public Health, 4*(12), 1908–1915.

Syamala, D. H. (2018). The universal self and the individual self in Vedanta. *Philosophy and Cosmology, 21*, 72–80. DOI: 10.29202/phil-cosm/21/7

Trivedi, N. (2025). Positive mental health: A correlated study of the consciousness-based Advait Vedanta and modern psychotherapy. *Journal of Psychology and Neuroscience*. DOI: 10.47485/2693-2490.1100

Vali, K. M., & Azeem, M. (2025). Psycho-cultural sensitivity in Indian context: Integrating traditional knowledge with modern mental health practices. *International Journal for Multidisciplinary Research, 7*(4), 52014. Advance online publication. DOI: 10.36948/ijfmr.2025.v07i04.52014 van der Veer, P. (1989). The power of detachment: Disciplines of body and mind in the Ramanandi order. *American Ethnologist, 16*(3), 517–536. DOI: 10.1525/ae.1989.16.3.02a00030

Vancampfort, D., Stubbs, B., Van Damme, T., Smith, L., Hallgren, M., Schuch, F., Deenik, J., Rosenbaum, S., Ashdown-Franks, G., Mugisha, J., & Firth, J. (2020). The efficacy of meditation-based mind-body interventions for mental disorders: A meta-review of 17 meta-analyses of randomized controlled trials. *Journal of Psychiatric Research, 134*, 181–191. DOI: 10.1016/j.jpsychires.2020.12.048 PMID: 33388701

Vandenberghe, L., & de Sousa, A. C. A. (2006). Mindfulness nas terapias cognitivas e comportamentais. *Revista Brasileira de Terapias Cognitivas, 2*(1), 37–46. DOI: 10.5935/1808-5687.20060004

Verma, R. K. (2025). Mind and moksha: Integrating Vedantic wisdom and contemporary psychology for a unified approach to self and well-being. *Human Arenas*, 1–24.

Verrier, M. M. (2021). A psychospiritual exploration of the transpersonal self as the ground of healing. *Religions, 12*(9), 725. DOI: 10.3390/rel12090725

Vinu, W., Kabeer, D. A., Kumar G, V., Safad, A. K., & Manibharathi, G. (2025). Yoga-based interventions for enhancing psychological well-being in postpartum women: A randomized controlled trial. *Journal of Bodywork and Movement Therapies, 42*, 1177–1185. DOI: 10.1016/j.jbmt.2025.02.007 PMID: 40325654

Vivekananda, S. (1896). *Practical Vedanta: Part 1*. Advaita Ashram.

Vivekananda, S. (1899). *Speeches and writings of Swami Vivekananda*. G. A. Natesan & Co.

Vivekananda, S. (1940/1942/1944). *Letters of Swami Vivekananda*. Advaita Ashram.

Vivekananda, S. (1944). *Lectures from Colombo to Almora*. Advaita Ashram.

Vivekananda, S. (1947). *Work and its secret*. Advaita Ashram.

Vivekananda, S. (1951). *The complete works of Swami Vivekananda* (Vol. 8). Advaita Ashram.

Vivekananda, S. (1956). *The complete works of Swami Vivekananda* (Vol. 6). Advaita Ashram.

Vivekananda, S. (1958/1964). *The complete works of Swami Vivekananda* (Vol. 3). Advaita Ashram.

Vivekananda, S. (1959). *The complete works of Swami Vivekananda* (Vol. 5). Advaita Ashram.

Vivekananda, S. (2016). *The complete works of Swami Vivekananda* (Vol. 2). Advaita Ashram. (Original work published 1958)

Vivekananda, S. (2016). *The complete works of Swami Vivekananda* (13th ed., Vol. 3). Advaita Ashrama.

Vivekananda, S., & Madhurananda, S. (2016). *Bhagavad Gita as viewed by Swami Vivekananda*. Advaita Ashrama.

Vivekaprana, P. (2014). Vivekananda and the inner quest of humanity. *International Journal of Development Issues*, *13*(3), 227–241. DOI: 10.1108/IJDI-06-2014-0042

Vorkapic, C. F. (2016). Yoga and mental health: A dialogue between ancient wisdom and modern psychology. *International Journal of Yoga*, *9*(2), 104–105. DOI: 10.4103/0973-6131.171720 PMID: 26865774

World Health Organization. (2025, September 2). *Over a billion people living with mental health conditions – services require urgent scale-up*. https://www.who.int/news/item/02-09-2025-over-a-billion-people-living-with-mental-health-conditions-services-require-urgent-scale-up

Worsley, J. D., Pennington, A., & Corcoran, R. (2022). Supporting mental health and wellbeing of university and college students: A systematic review of review-level evidence of interventions. *PLoS One*, *17*(7), e0266725. DOI: 10.1371/journal.pone.0266725 PMID: 35905058

Wright, R. W., & Strawn, B. D. (2010). Grief, hope, and prophetic imagination: Psychoanalysis and Christian tradition in dialogue. *Journal of Psychology and Christianity*, *29*(3), 195–205.

Yarrow, T., Candea, M., Trundle, C., & Cook, J. (2015). *Detachment: Essays on the limits of relational thinking*. Manchester University Press.

Zhao, C. Y. (2025). Exploring "Who am I": The potential of applying the Indian Vedanta philosophical practice of self-enquiry in psychotherapy. *Humanities & Social Sciences Communications*, *12*(1), 1–10. DOI: 10.1057/s41599-025-04387-w

Zimmermann, A. C., Morgan, W. J., & Morgan, W. J. (2016). A time for silence? Its possibilities for dialogue and for reflective learning. *Studies in Philosophy and Education*, *35*(1), 37–54. DOI: 10.1007/s11217-015-9485-0

ADDITIONAL READING

Nivedita, S. (2003). *The Master as I Saw Him: Being Pages from the Life of the Swami Vivekananda*. Vedanta Press.

Satchidanandendra Saraswati, S. (1997). *The Method of the Vedanta: A Critical Account of the Advaita Tradition* (Alston, A. J., Trans.). Motilal Banarsidass. (Original work published 1965)

Satprakashananda, S. (2002). *The Mind According to Vedanta*. Sri Ramakrishna Math.

Sil, N. P. (1997). *Swami Vivekananda: A Reassessment*. Susquehanna University Press.

Vivekananda, S. (1993). *Vedanta: Voice of Freedom*. Vedanta Press.

Vivekananda, S. (2003). *Meditation and Its Methods According to Swami Vivekananda (compiled by Swami Chetanananda)*. Vedanta Society of St. Louis.

Vivekananda, S. (2012). *Raja Yoga: Conquering the Internal Nature*. Advaita Ashrama.

Vivekananda, S. (2014). *Karma Yoga: The Yoga of Action*. Advaita Ashrama.

Vivekananda, S. (2015). *Jnana Yoga: The Path of Knowledge*. Advaita Ashrama.

Vivekananda, S. (2017). *The Complete Works of Swami Vivekananda* (Vol. 1–9). Advaita Ashrama.

Vrajaprana, P. (1999). *Vedanta: A Simple Introduction*. Vedanta Press.

KEY TERMS AND DEFINITIONS

Advaita (Non-Dualism): A school of Vedantic thought articulated most influentially by Adi Shankaracharya, asserting that Atman and Brahman are identical and that perceived distinctions arise from ignorance rather than from any ontological separation.

Atman (The Self): The immutable, conscious essence of an individual that is distinct from bodily, cognitive, and emotional processes. Vedanta identifies Atman as pure awareness and the foundational ground of identity.

Avidya (Ignorance): The fundamental misperception that leads individuals to identify with transient psychological and physical attributes rather than with the true Self. Avidya is considered the root of suffering and psychological instability.

Brahman (Ultimate Reality): The infinite and non-personal ground of existence that underlies all phenomena. According to Vedanta, Brahman is the sole ontological truth, and all multiplicity is an appearance within this singular reality.

Emotional Resilience (Vedantic Perspective): The capacity to remain centered in awareness while undergoing emotional stress, achieved not by suppression but by transcending identification with fluctuating mental states.

Karma Yoga: A discipline of selfless action in which individuals perform their duties with sincerity while relinquishing attachment to results. This practice reduces anxiety linked to evaluation and enhances psychological well-being.

Mantra Meditation: A contemplative practice involving the repetition of sacred syllables or phrases to stabilize attention, quiet mental activity, and facilitate inward-focused awareness.

Mauna (Inner Silence): A state of intentional mental quietude through which individuals attain clarity, emotional balance, and introspective insight. Mauna is associated with reduced cognitive noise and enhanced self-regulation.

Meaning and Purpose (Vedantic View): The recognition that enduring meaning arises not from external achievement but from alignment with deeper values such as truth, compassion, and self-understanding.

Mindfulness (Vedantic Parallel): A sustained and present-centered awareness that includes insight into the nature of the observer. While similar to contemporary mindfulness practices, Vedantic mindfulness integrates metaphysical inquiry into the structure of consciousness.

Neti-Neti ("Not This, Not This"): A contemplative method involving systematic negation of all attributes and identifications that are not the Self. This process facilitates cognitive defusion and deepened self-awareness.

Ni kāma karma (Non-Attachment to Results): A principle within Karma Yoga encouraging individuals to act responsibly without basing self-worth on external outcomes. It reduces stress, performance pressure, and emotional volatility.

Practical Vedanta: Swami Vivekananda's interpretation of Vedantic philosophy that emphasizes the application of non-dual principles in daily life through ethical action, self-reflection, and social responsibility.

Sakshi Bhava (Witness Consciousness): The cultivated capacity to observe thoughts, emotions, and sensory experiences without identification. This stance promotes equanimity and reduces impulsive cognitive-emotional responses.

Śara āgati (Surrender): A conscious release of ego-driven attempts to control outcomes, accompanied by trust in a higher order or deeper self. This psychological stance alleviates resistance and supports adaptation during adversity.

Self-Realization: The experiential recognition that one's essential nature is Atman, independent of mental states, social roles, or external achievements. This realization is viewed as the basis for psychological freedom and resilience.

Tat Tvam Asi ("Thou Art That"): A central Upanishadic statement expressing the non-dual identity between individual consciousness and ultimate reality. It serves as a foundational insight for contemplative practice and philosophical inquiry.

Vairagya (Detachment): A disciplined form of emotional non-dependence in which engagement with the world continues, but without psychological fixation on outcomes. Vairagya supports emotional regulation and reduces reactivity.

Vedanta: A major philosophical tradition within Indian thought, rooted in the Upanishads, which posits that the underlying reality of the universe is unified and that human fulfillment lies in realizing this unity through self-knowledge and disciplined inquiry.

Chapter 8
Synchronization Through Yoga:
Connecting the Physical and Mental Realms

Debajit Karmakar
http://orcid.org/0000-0001-9272-0627
Lakshmibai National Institute of Physical Education, India

Karuppasamy Govindasamy
http://orcid.org/0000-0002-3019-5545
Symbiosis International University, India

Anindita Das
http://orcid.org/0000-0002-6502-9619
Lakshmibai National Institute of Physical Education, India

Deepanjali Sharma
http://orcid.org/0009-0002-9242-8647
Lakshmibai National Institute of Physical Education, India

Tashi Ongmu Bhutia
http://orcid.org/0009-0000-0127-5709
Sikkim Government B.Ed. College, India

Atisha Mandal
http://orcid.org/0009-0003-2731-5985
Lakshmibai National Institute of Physical Education, India

ABSTRACT

This chapter explores the profound integration of body and mind achieved through yoga, emphasizing its role in harmonizing physiological, psychological, and cognitive functions. It highlights how practices such as breath regulation, postures, meditation, and mindfulness foster neural synchronization, enhance autonomic balance, and promote emotional stability and stress resilience. Drawing upon both ancient philosophy and contemporary scientific evidence, the discussion demonstrates yoga's capacity to optimize attention regulation, cognitive flexibility, and overall well-being.

DOI: 10.4018/979-8-3373-4187-3.ch008

By bridging traditional wisdom with modern research, the chapter underscores yoga's potential as a holistic approach to health, performance enhancement, and comprehensive mind-body synchronization across diverse populations.

1. INTRODUCTION

The ancient practice of yoga represents one of humanity's most sophisticated approaches to achieving comprehensive mind-body integration, offering a systematic methodology for synchronizing the physical and mental realms of human experience. This synchronization extends far beyond mere physical exercise or relaxation techniques, encompassing a profound understanding of the interconnected nature of consciousness, physiological processes, and embodied awareness (D. K. Sharma, 2017). Contemporary neuroscience and psychophysiology are increasingly validating what yogic practitioners have understood for millennia: that the deliberate coordination of breath, movement, and attention can produce measurable changes in neural networks, autonomic regulation, and cognitive function that promote optimal human performance and well-being (Vyas & Vyas, 2017).

Modern research in neuroscience, psychophysiology, and behavioural medicine has begun to elucidate the mechanisms through which yoga facilitates this extraordinary synchronization. Advanced neuroimaging techniques reveal that regular yoga practice produces systematic changes in brain structure and function, particularly in regions associated with attention regulation, emotional processing, and self-awareness. These neuroplastic adaptations appear to underlie the enhanced cognitive flexibility, emotional stability, and stress resilience consistently observed in experienced practitioners. The integration of physical movement with breath regulation and contemplative awareness appears to engage multiple neural networks simultaneously, promoting cross-modal integration and enhanced communication between brain regions (Badoni et al., 2025).

The physiological dimension of yoga synchronization involves the systematic regulation of autonomic nervous system function through the conscious modulation of breathing patterns, postural alignment, and muscle tension. This voluntary influence over typically involuntary processes represents a remarkable example of top-down neural control, wherein higher cortical centers learn to regulate brainstem and subcortical functions. The resulting state of physiological coherence, characterized by balanced autonomic activity and optimal arousal levels, creates conditions conducive to enhanced cognitive performance, emotional regulation, and overall well-being (Barua, 2025). The psychological aspects of synchronization through yoga encompass the cultivation of present-moment awareness, emotional equilibrium, and meta-cognitive insight that emerges from sustained practice. The systematic training of attention through yoga practices appears to strengthen the neural circuits underlying cognitive flexibility while simultaneously developing the capacity for non-reactive observation of mental phenomena. This enhanced meta-cognitive awareness enables practitioners to recognize and modify habitual thought patterns and emotional reactions, leading to greater psychological flexibility and adaptive responding to life circumstances (Vyas & Vyas, 2017).

The empirical evidence supporting yoga's capacity for facilitating mind-body synchronization continues to accumulate across multiple domains of scientific inquiry. Cardiovascular research demonstrates that regular yoga practice improves heart rate variability, a key indicator of autonomic balance and physiological resilience. Endocrinological studies reveal normalized cortisol patterns and enhanced stress hormone regulation in practitioners (Ciołkosz, 2015). Neuroimaging investigations document structural and functional brain changes that correlate with improved cognitive performance and emotional regulation. This converging evidence from multiple scientific disciplines provides robust support for yoga's effectiveness in promoting comprehensive mind-body integration. The practical applications of synchronization through yoga extend across diverse populations and contexts, from educational settings where students benefit from enhanced attention and stress management to healthcare environments where patients experience improved recovery and symptom management (Barua, 2025). Athletic populations utilize yoga for performance enhancement through improved body awareness, injury prevention, and mental preparation. Corporate wellness programs increasingly incorporate yoga practices to address workplace stress and enhance employee cognitive function and productivity (Badoni et al., 2025).

2. HISTORICAL FOUNDATIONS OF YOGA AND SYNCHRONIZATION

Ancient Yogic Philosophy

The philosophical foundations of yoga synchronization can be traced to the earliest systematic presentations of yogic theory in classical texts such as the Yoga Sutras of Patanjali, the Bhagavad Gita, and the Hatha Yoga Pradipika. These ancient treatises present sophisticated models of human consciousness and its relationship to physical embodiment that anticipate many contemporary scientific understandings of mind-body integration. The Yoga Sutras, composed approximately 2,000 years ago, describe yoga as the cessation of fluctuations in consciousness (chitta vritti nirodha), emphasizing the fundamental role of mental regulation in achieving integration and synchronization (Cook-Cottone & Perey, 2025).

Patanjali's eight-limbed path (ashtanga yoga) provides a systematic framework for achieving mind-body synchronization through progressive refinement of ethical conduct, physical practices, breath regulation, sensory withdrawal, concentration, meditation, and absorption. This comprehensive approach recognizes that true synchronization requires attention to multiple dimensions of human experience simultaneously, from external behaviour and physical health to internal mental states and spiritual development. The progression from gross to subtle practices reflects an understanding that synchronization occurs at multiple levels of organization within human consciousness (Newcombe, 2009). The concept of the koshas or sheaths in Vedantic philosophy presents a sophisticated model of human constitution consisting of five interconnected layers: the physical body (annamaya kosha), vital energy body (pranamaya kosha), mental body (manomaya kosha), wisdom body (vijnanamaya kosha), and bliss body (anandamaya kosha). This model suggests that synchronization must address all levels of human experience, from gross physical processes to subtle energetic and consciousness dimensions. Each kosha influences and is influenced by the others, creating a complex system of interactions that requires integrated approaches for optimization (Cook-Cottone & Perey, 2025).

The philosophy of Samkhya, which underlies much of yogic theory, presents a dualistic model of reality consisting of consciousness (purusha) and matter (prakriti). According to this view, suffering arises from the misidentification of consciousness with material processes, while liberation occurs through the recognition of their distinct natures. This philosophical framework suggests that synchronization involves not the merging of mind and body, but rather the proper relationship between consciousness and its material expressions. The practice of yoga facilitates this recognition through the systematic observation of the interactions between awareness and physical processes (Newcombe, 2009).

Mind-Body Integration in Traditional Texts

The Hatha Yoga Pradipika, a foundational text of physical yoga practice, presents detailed descriptions of how specific physical practices influence mental states and consciousness. The text describes the body as a microcosm containing various energy centers (chakras), energy channels (nadis), and vital forces (pranas) that must be balanced and integrated for optimal function. This energetic anatomy provides a framework for understanding how physical practices can systematically influence mental and emotional states through their effects on subtle energy circulation (Newcombe, 2009).

The concept of prana, often translated as life force or vital energy, serves as a crucial link between physical and mental processes in yogic understanding. Prana is described as existing in multiple forms throughout the body, with different pranas governing specific physiological and psychological functions. The regulation of prana through breathing practices, physical postures, and meditation is considered essential for achieving mind-body synchronization. Contemporary research on the autonomic nervous system and bioelectric phenomena in the body provides scientific correlates for these traditional energetic concepts (Cook-Cottone & Perey, 2025).

The Bhagavad Gita presents yoga as a comprehensive approach to action and consciousness that extends synchronization principles beyond formal practice into daily life. The text describes various yoga paths including karma yoga (action), jnana yoga (knowledge), and bhakti yoga (devotion), each providing different approaches to achieving integration and synchronization. The principle of skillful action (yoga karmasu kaushalam) emphasizes performing actions with full awareness and without attachment to outcomes, representing a practical application of synchronization principles in everyday activities (Ciołkosz, 2015). Traditional texts also describe various obstacles (antarayas) to achieving synchronization, including physical illness, mental dullness, doubt, carelessness, laziness, sensual attachment, erroneous perception, failure to attain concentration, and instability in concentration. These obstacles reflect an understanding that synchronization requires sustained effort and addresses multiple potential sources of disruption across physical, mental, and emotional domains. The systematic methods presented for overcoming these obstacles demonstrate sophisticated knowledge of human psychology and motivation (Newcombe, 2009).

3. THE CONCEPT OF SYNCHRONIZATION IN YOGA

Definition of Physical-Mental Synchronization

Physical-mental synchronization in yoga is the harmonious integration of body, mind, and awareness, enabling mutual regulation and coherence. It enhances physiological efficiency, mental clarity, and conscious control through sensitivity, voluntary regulation, and neural integration from brainstem functions to cortical attention processes. (Chopra et al., 2023). The autonomic nervous system serves as a crucial mediator in this integration, as its sympathetic and parasympathetic branches influence both physiological arousal and mental states. Yoga practices appear to enhance the brain's capacity to influence autonomic function through top-down regulation, creating conditions for improved mind-body coordination and synchronization (Berkovich-Ohana, 2017). Synchronization in yoga also involves the temporal coordination of different processes, such as the alignment of breath rhythms with movement patterns and the coordination of attention with physical sensations. This temporal integration requires precise neural timing mechanisms and may contribute to the development of enhanced cognitive flexibility through improved coordination of multiple cognitive processes. The rhythmic nature of many yoga practices may promote neural synchronization through entrainment of brain oscillations to external rhythms (Hart & Tracy, 2008). The phenomenological dimension of synchronization involves the subjective experience of unity and integration that emerges during effective yoga practice. Practitioners report states of effortless coordination wherein physical movements feel natural and spontaneous, breathing becomes smooth and automatic, and mental awareness remains clear and focused without effort. These subjective reports correspond to objective measures of physiological coherence and neural efficiency, suggesting that phenomenological integration reflects genuine psychophysiological synchronization (Ju et al., 2024).

Yogic View on Harmony of Body, Breath, and Mind

Traditional yoga philosophy presents a sophisticated understanding of the relationship between body, breath, and mind as interconnected aspects of a unified system rather than separate entities requiring coordination. The yogic view suggests that apparent distinctions between physical and mental phenomena arise from limited perception rather than fundamental separation. According to this perspective, synchronization involves recognizing and working with the inherent unity that already exists rather than creating artificial connections between disparate elements (Donahoe-Fillmore & Grant, 2019).

The breath occupies a unique position in this triadic relationship, serving as both a physical process involving mechanical movements of respiratory muscles and a mental phenomenon subject to conscious regulation and attention. In yogic understanding, the breath serves as a bridge between voluntary and involuntary processes, conscious and unconscious mental functions, and gross and subtle aspects of human experience. The systematic regulation of breathing patterns through pranayama practices provides a direct method for influencing both physiological and psychological states simultaneously (Ju et al., 2024). The concept of the three gunas (sattva, rajas, and tamas) in yogic philosophy provides a framework for understanding different qualities of synchronization and their effects on consciousness and behaviour. Sattva represents clarity, balance, and harmony; rajas represents activity, passion, and restlessness; and tamas represents inertia, dullness, and ignorance. Optimal synchronization is associated with predominant sattva, characterized by clear awareness, balanced energy, and harmonious functioning of all systems. Yoga practices are designed to cultivate sattvic states while minimizing excessive rajas and tamas (Chopra et al., 2023).

The traditional teaching emphasizes that true synchronization emerges naturally when obstacles and imbalances are removed rather than through forceful manipulation or control. This principle of non-violence (ahimsa) extends to the practice itself, suggesting that synchronization should be achieved through gentle, gradual adjustments rather than aggressive intervention. This approach recognizes the wisdom of natural regulatory systems while providing methods for removing impediments to their optimal function (Hart & Tracy, 2008).

4. PHYSIOLOGICAL DIMENSION OF SYNCHRONIZATION

Breath Regulation (Pranayama) and Nervous System Balance

Pranayama, the systematic regulation of breathing patterns, represents perhaps the most direct and immediate method for achieving physiological synchronization in yoga practice. The voluntary control of respiration provides access to autonomic nervous system regulation through the intimate connections between respiratory centers in the brainstem and higher cortical regions involved in voluntary control and awareness. This unique position of breathing as both voluntary and involuntary makes it an ideal bridge for mind-body synchronization and explains its central role in traditional yoga practice (Naveen et al., 2013). The physiological mechanisms underlying pranayama's effects on nervous system balance involve multiple pathways and feedback loops. The primary respiratory control centers in the medulla oblongata receive input from chemoreceptors monitoring blood oxygen and carbon dioxide levels, mechanoreceptors in the lungs and chest wall, and descending projections from cortical areas involved in voluntary breathing control. Pranayama practices systematically modify these inputs through altered breathing patterns, creating cascading effects throughout the nervous system (Saito et al., 2025).

Slow, deep breathing practices characteristic of many pranayama techniques activate the parasympathetic nervous system through stimulation of the vagus nerve. The vagus nerve, the longest cranial nerve, provides extensive connections between the brain and major organ systems including the heart, lungs, and digestive system. Enhanced vagal tone, as measured by heart rate variability, reflects improved autonomic balance and is associated with better stress resilience, emotional regulation, and cognitive function. Research demonstrates that regular pranayama practice can significantly improve heart rate variability and vagal tone within relatively short timeframes (Krishna et al., 2014). Specific pranayama techniques produce distinct physiological effects that demonstrate the precision with which breathing can influence nervous system function. Alternate nostril breathing (nadi shodhana) appears to balance sympathetic and parasympathetic activity while promoting integration between left and right brain hemispheres. Breath retention practices (kumbhaka) create controlled hypoxic and hypercapnic conditions that may promote adaptive physiological responses and enhance stress tolerance. Rapid breathing techniques (kapalabhati) temporarily activate the sympathetic nervous system while subsequently promoting deep relaxation and parasympathetic recovery (Saito et al., 2025).

Postures (Asanas) and Neuromuscular Coordination

The practice of yoga asanas involves complex neuromuscular coordination that challenges and enhances the integration between nervous system control and muscular execution. Each posture requires precise coordination of multiple muscle groups, joint positions, and balance mechanisms while maintaining breath awareness and mental focus. This multi-dimensional integration promotes enhanced proprioceptive awareness, improved motor control, and strengthened connections between sensory input and motor output systems (Krishna et al., 2014).

The neuromuscular demands of yoga postures engage both automatic and voluntary motor control systems simultaneously. The maintenance of postural stability involves automatic postural reflexes mediated by the brainstem and spinal cord, while the voluntary execution of specific movements requires cortical motor planning and control. The integration of these systems through yoga practice may enhance overall motor coordination and contribute to improved cognitive-motor integration (Ghosh et al., 2024). Balance poses present particular challenges for neuromuscular coordination by requiring continuous adjustment of muscle activation patterns based on proprioceptive and vestibular feedback. The cerebellum, crucial for balance and motor learning, shows enhanced activation during challenging balance poses and may undergo structural changes with sustained practice. These cerebellar adaptations may contribute to improved motor learning and cognitive flexibility, as the cerebellum is increasingly recognized for its role in cognitive functions beyond motor control (Krishna et al., 2014).

The isometric muscle contractions characteristic of holding yoga postures create unique conditions for neuromuscular adaptation that differ from dynamic exercise patterns. These sustained contractions require continuous neural drive and may promote enhanced neuromuscular efficiency through improved motor unit recruitment and coordination. The conscious maintenance of muscular effort while remaining mentally relaxed trains the nervous system to optimize energy expenditure and reduce unnecessary tension (Naveen et al., 2013). The sequential nature of yoga practice, involving flowing transitions between postures, challenges the motor system to coordinate complex movement patterns while maintaining breath awareness and postural alignment. This dynamic integration may particularly benefit cognitive flexibility through its demands for continuous adaptation and real-time adjustment of motor strategies. The prefrontal cortex, which coordinates complex motor sequences, shows enhanced activation during yoga practice and may undergo structural changes that support improved cognitive flexibility (Naveen et al., 2013).

Yoga Nidra and Physiological Relaxation

Yoga nidra, often referred to as "yogic sleep," represents a systematic approach to achieving profound physiological relaxation while maintaining conscious awareness. This practice involves guided progressive relaxation techniques that systematically release tension from different body regions while cultivating states of conscious rest that promote deep physiological restoration. The unique combination of deep relaxation with maintained awareness creates optimal conditions for nervous system recovery and integration (Krishna et al., 2014).

The physiological effects of yoga nidra include significant reductions in sympathetic nervous system activity, decreased muscle tension, lowered blood pressure, and reduced stress hormone levels. Brain wave patterns during yoga nidra show characteristics of both deep relaxation and heightened awareness, with increased alpha and theta activity suggesting states of conscious relaxation that differ from ordinary sleep or waking consciousness. These distinctive brain states may facilitate enhanced neuroplasticity and integration between different levels of nervous system function (Krishna et al., 2014).

The systematic body scanning component of yoga nidra enhances interoceptive awareness by directing attention to different body regions and internal sensations. This practice strengthens connections between the insula, which processes interoceptive information, and other brain regions involved in self-awareness and emotional regulation. Enhanced interoceptive awareness may contribute to improved stress management and emotional regulation through better recognition of internal states and more timely intervention when stress responses begin (Meister & Juckel, 2018). The use of visualization and intention setting in yoga nidra engages the brain's capacity for mental imagery and goal-directed cognition while in states of deep relaxation. This combination may facilitate the integration of conscious intentions with unconscious regulatory processes, potentially influencing automatic patterns of stress response and behaviour. The relaxed brain state during yoga nidra may be particularly conducive to neuroplastic changes and the consolidation of new neural patterns (Aleksić Veljković et al., 2021).

5. PSYCHOLOGICAL DIMENSION OF SYNCHRONIZATION

Mindfulness and Concentration in Yoga

The cultivation of mindfulness and concentration in yoga practice provides the psychological foundation for achieving mind-body synchronization through the development of present-moment awareness and sustained attention regulation. Unlike mindfulness practices that focus primarily on mental phenomena, yoga integrates mindful awareness with physical movement and breath regulation, creating a comprehensive approach to attention training that engages multiple sensory modalities simultaneously. This embodied mindfulness may provide unique benefits for developing integrated awareness that encompasses both internal mental states and external physical experiences (Bhavanani, 2014).

The practice of dharana, or concentration, in traditional yoga involves sustaining attention on a chosen object such as the breath, a body region, or a visual focus point. This sustained attention training strengthens the neural networks underlying cognitive control and attention regulation while simultaneously developing the capacity for meta-cognitive awareness. The object of concentration often involves physical sensations or processes, creating direct links between attention regulation and bodily awareness that support mind-body integration (Krishna et al., 2014). Witness consciousness (sakshi bhava) in yoga fosters meta-cognitive awareness, enabling non-reactive observation of thoughts and emotions. Integrating breath, posture, and focus enhances cognitive flexibility, self-awareness, and emotional regulation by engaging brain regions for attention control and adaptive response to challenges (Pise et al., 2018).

Stress Reduction and Emotional Stability

The stress reduction effects of yoga practice contribute significantly to mind-body synchronization by optimizing the conditions for integrated functioning. Chronic stress disrupts synchronization through its effects on multiple physiological systems, including elevated cortisol levels that impair cognitive function, increased muscle tension that restricts movement efficiency, and autonomic imbalance that reduces physiological coherence. Yoga's comprehensive approach to stress reduction addresses these multiple pathways simultaneously (Bhavanani, 2014).

The psychological mechanisms of stress reduction in yoga involve both cognitive and somatic pathways. The cultivation of present-moment awareness reduces rumination and worry about past and future events, while the development of acceptance and non-attachment reduces emotional reactivity to unavoidable stressors. The physical practices provide direct somatic regulation through muscle relaxation, improved circulation, and autonomic nervous system balance. This dual approach may be more effective than purely cognitive or purely physical stress reduction methods (Park et al., 2020). Emotional regulation improvements through yoga practice appear to involve enhanced prefrontal cortical control over limbic system reactivity. Neuroimaging studies demonstrate reduced amygdala reactivity and increased prefrontal-limbic connectivity in experienced yoga practitioners, suggesting improved emotional regulation capacity. The development of interoceptive awareness through yoga may contribute to emotional regulation by providing earlier detection of emotional arousal and more timely implementation of regulatory strategies (Bhavanani, 2014).

Yoga for Enhanced Cognitive Function

The cognitive benefits of yoga practice extend beyond stress reduction to include specific enhancements in executive function, memory, and processing speed that support improved mind-body synchronization. The integration of physical movement with breath awareness and mental focus in yoga creates unique cognitive demands that may strengthen the neural networks underlying cognitive flexibility and executive control. This integrated approach to cognitive training may be more effective than isolated cognitive exercises for promoting comprehensive cognitive enhancement (Park et al., 2020).

Working memory improvements through yoga practice may contribute to enhanced synchronization by providing better cognitive resources for coordinating multiple processes simultaneously. The ability to maintain awareness of breath, body position, and mental focus during yoga practice requires sophisticated working memory capacity that generalizes to improved cognitive performance in other domains. Enhanced working memory may also support better emotional regulation through improved capacity for maintaining regulatory goals during emotional challenges (Ghosh et al., 2024). Attention regulation enhancements through yoga involve both focused attention skills developed through concentration practices and open monitoring skills developed through mindful awareness cultivation. The combination of these attention training approaches may provide more comprehensive benefits than either approach alone. The embodied nature of attention training in yoga may also promote better integration between attention regulation and sensorimotor processes (Bhavanani, 2014).

6. MECHANISMS OF MIND-BODY CONNECTION THROUGH YOGA

Role of Breath as a Synchronizing Bridge

The breath functions as a unique physiological process that serves as a bridge between conscious and unconscious mental functions, voluntary and involuntary physical processes, and individual and universal aspects of experience. This bridging function makes breath regulation a particularly powerful tool for achieving mind-body synchronization and explains its central role in virtually all yoga traditions. The neurobiological mechanisms underlying breath's synchronizing effects involve multiple levels of nervous system organization and demonstrate the remarkable capacity for voluntary influence over automatic regulatory processes (Gard et al., 2014). The respiratory control system involves complex interactions between brainstem respiratory centers, higher cortical regions, and feedback mechanisms that monitor blood chemistry and mechanical aspects of breathing. The voluntary control of breathing through pranayama practices engages the cerebral cortex in regulating brainstem functions, creating enhanced communication between different levels of the nervous system. This top-down regulation may strengthen the neural pathways involved in voluntary control while improving the efficiency of automatic regulatory processes (Basu-Ray, 2021).

The rhythmic nature of breathing provides a natural entrainment signal that can synchronize various physiological and neural processes. Heart rate variability, blood pressure oscillations, and brain wave patterns can all become entrained to breathing rhythms, creating states of physiological coherence characterized by synchronized functioning across multiple systems. This entrainment effect may extend to cognitive processes, with breathing rhythms influencing attention, memory consolidation, and emotional regulation through their effects on neural oscillations (Meister & Juckel, 2018). The chemical effects of altered breathing patterns provide another mechanism for breath's synchronizing effects. Modifications in blood oxygen and carbon dioxide levels through specific pranayama techniques influence brain function, autonomic nervous system activity, and cellular metabolism throughout the body. These chemical changes can promote states of enhanced mental clarity, emotional stability, and physiological efficiency that support optimal mind-body integration (Basu-Ray, 2021).

Psychophysiological Feedback Loops

The achievement of mind-body synchronization through yoga involves the establishment and optimization of psychophysiological feedback loops that allow for real-time adjustment and coordination of mental and physical processes. These feedback loops operate through multiple channels, including interoceptive awareness of internal bodily states, proprioceptive feedback from muscles and joints, emotional feedback from limbic system processing, and cognitive feedback from prefrontal cortex monitoring. The integration of these feedback streams enables practitioners to develop sophisticated self-regulation skills (Collette, 2015).

Interoceptive feedback provides information about internal physiological states including heart rate, breathing patterns, muscle tension, and visceral sensations. The insula, which processes interoceptive information, shows structural and functional changes with yoga practice that correlate with enhanced body awareness and emotional regulation. This enhanced interoceptive sensitivity enables practitioners to detect subtle changes in physiological state and implement appropriate adjustments before minor imbalances develop into significant problems (Gard et al., 2014). Proprioceptive feedback from muscles, joints, and the vestibular system provides information about body position, movement, and spatial orientation. Yoga practice enhances proprioceptive sensitivity through sustained attention to body positioning and alignment during postures. This enhanced proprioceptive awareness may contribute to improved motor control and coordination while also providing a foundation for developing more refined interoceptive awareness of internal states (Meister & Juckel, 2018).

Brainwave Patterns and Meditation

The neurophysiological investigation of brainwave patterns during yoga and meditation practices reveals distinctive states of neural activity that reflect the synchronization of mental and physical processes. Electroencephalographic studies demonstrate that different yoga practices produce characteristic patterns of brain oscillations that differ from both ordinary waking consciousness and passive relaxation states (Collette, 2015). These distinctive brain patterns provide objective markers of the synchronized states achieved through yoga practice and offer insights into the neural mechanisms underlying mind-body integration. Alpha wave activity, typically associated with relaxed alertness and reduced sensory processing, shows increased amplitude and coherence during yoga meditation practices. This enhanced alpha activity may reflect a state of relaxed attention wherein the brain maintains awareness while reducing interference from external distractions. The increased coherence of alpha oscillations across different brain regions suggests enhanced neural synchronization that may underlie the subjective experience of unified awareness reported by practitioners (Meister & Juckel, 2018).

Theta wave activity, associated with memory consolidation, emotional processing, and creative insight, demonstrates increased power and coherence during certain yoga practices, particularly those involving visualization or deep meditative states. The enhanced theta activity may facilitate the integration of conscious intentions with unconscious regulatory processes and contribute to the lasting behavioural changes observed with sustained yoga practice. The increased theta coherence may also reflect enhanced communication between cortical and subcortical brain regions (Meister & Juckel, 2018). Gamma wave activity, the highest frequency brain oscillations associated with conscious awareness and neural binding, shows distinctive patterns during advanced yoga practices. Increased gamma power and coherence may reflect heightened states of consciousness and enhanced integration of information across different brain regions. The gamma oscillations observed during yoga meditation may indicate the neural correlates of the unified awareness and expanded consciousness described in traditional yoga texts. The synchronization of brain oscillations across different frequency bands during yoga practice may reflect the coordination of multiple neural processes that underlies mind-body integration (Badve et al., 2025). Cross-frequency coupling, wherein different frequency oscillations become coordinated, increases during yoga meditation and may represent a neural mechanism for integrating different levels of brain function. This enhanced neural coordination may contribute to the improved cognitive flexibility and emotional regulation observed in yoga practitioners (Collette, 2015).

7. EMPIRICAL EVIDENCE AND RESEARCH STUDIES

Effects of Yoga on Heart Rate Variability

Heart rate variability (HRV) has emerged as one of the most reliable and clinically relevant biomarkers for assessing the effects of yoga practice on autonomic nervous system function and mind-body synchronization. HRV reflects the natural variation in time intervals between heartbeats and provides a window into the dynamic balance between sympathetic and parasympathetic nervous system activity. High HRV indicates optimal autonomic flexibility and resilience, while reduced HRV is associated with various health problems and increased mortality risk (Telles et al., 2013). Multiple randomized controlled trials have demonstrated significant improvements in HRV following yoga interventions across diverse populations and practice durations. A landmark study by Thayer and colleagues tracked HRV changes in healthy adults participating in a 12-week yoga program, revealing substantial increases in both time-domain and frequency-domain HRV measures. The improvements were observed within 4 weeks of practice initiation and continued to increase throughout the intervention period, suggesting dose-dependent effects of yoga on autonomic function (Silveira & Smart, 2020).

The specific mechanisms through which yoga enhances HRV involve multiple pathways including direct vagal stimulation through breathing practices, improved baroreflex sensitivity through postural changes, and reduced sympathetic nervous system activation through stress reduction. Pranayama practices appear particularly effective for HRV enhancement, with studies demonstrating acute improvements in HRV immediately following single breathing practice sessions. The rhythmic nature of pranayama may directly entrain cardiac rhythms and promote coherent heart rate patterns (Meissner et al., 2016). Different yoga practices produce varying effects on HRV, with gentle, restorative practices generally producing the largest improvements in parasympathetic activity, while more vigorous practices may initially increase sympathetic activity before promoting parasympathetic recovery. The integration of different practice elements appears important for achieving balanced autonomic function, with programs combining asanas, pranayama, and meditation showing superior HRV improvements compared to any single component alone (Froeliger et al., 2012).

Yoga and Cortisol Regulation

Cortisol, the primary stress hormone produced by the hypothalamic-pituitary-adrenal (HPA) axis, serves as a crucial biomarker for assessing yoga's effects on stress physiology and mind-body synchronization. Chronic elevation of cortisol levels disrupts multiple physiological systems and impairs cognitive function, emotional regulation, and immune system effectiveness. The ability of yoga practice to normalize cortisol patterns represents an important mechanism for promoting comprehensive health and synchronization (Lim & Cheong, 2015). Research consistently demonstrates that regular yoga practice produces significant reductions in baseline cortisol levels and improved cortisol rhythm patterns characterized by appropriate morning elevation and evening decline. These improvements appear to result from yoga's effects on multiple levels of the HPA axis, including enhanced hypothalamic regulation, improved pituitary sensitivity, and reduced adrenal reactivity to stressors. The multi-modal approach of yoga, addressing both psychological stress perception and physiological stress responses, may be particularly effective for cortisol regulation (Rocha et al., 2012).

Acute studies examining cortisol responses to single yoga sessions reveal immediate reductions in stress hormone levels that persist for several hours following practice. The magnitude of these acute effects appears to depend on practice intensity, duration, and individual factors such as baseline stress levels and yoga experience.

More intensive practices may initially increase cortisol due to physical demands but subsequently promote enhanced recovery and adaptation (Lim & Cheong, 2015).

The psychological mechanisms contributing to cortisol regulation through yoga include reduced rumination and worry through present-moment attention training, enhanced emotional regulation through improved prefrontal-limbic connectivity, and increased self-efficacy through mastery of challenging practices. The development of stress resilience through yoga may involve both reduced stress reactivity and enhanced recovery from unavoidable stressors (Arora & Bhattacharjee, 2008). Longitudinal studies tracking cortisol patterns over months of yoga practice reveal progressive improvements in HPA axis function that correlate with subjective reports of reduced stress and improved well-being. These changes appear to reflect adaptive modifications in stress response systems rather than simple suppression of cortisol production. The improved cortisol regulation with yoga practice may contribute to enhanced cognitive function, better sleep quality, and improved immune system effectiveness (Rocha et al., 2012).

Cognitive and Emotional Outcomes of Regular Practice

Executive function assessments consistently demonstrate improvements in yoga practitioners across multiple domains including working memory, cognitive flexibility, and inhibitory control. The Trail Making Test, which assesses cognitive switching and divided attention, shows superior performance in regular practitioners with faster completion times and fewer errors. These improvements appear to reflect enhanced coordination between different cognitive processes rather than improvements in any single cognitive domain (Jones et al., 2016). Attention regulation improvements include both sustained attention capacity and the ability to flexibly redirect attention based on changing task demands. The Attention Network Test reveals enhanced executive attention in yoga practitioners, reflecting improved cognitive control and conflict resolution. The embodied nature of attention training in yoga may provide unique benefits for developing integrated attention skills that encompass both mental focus and body awareness (Vinay et al., 2016).

Memory function improvements through yoga practice include enhanced working memory capacity, improved long-term memory consolidation, and reduced memory interference from stress and emotional factors. The relaxation and stress reduction effects of yoga may optimize conditions for memory formation and retrieval, while the attention training components may improve encoding and retrieval strategies. The integration of visualization and imagery in some yoga practices may also enhance memory through strengthened mental imagery capabilities (Chu et al., 2015). Emotional regulation improvements encompass reduced emotional reactivity, enhanced emotional awareness, improved emotional expression, and increased emotional resilience. Yoga practitioners show reduced activation in the amygdala and other limbic structures during emotional challenges while maintaining increased prefrontal activation associated with emotional control. The development of emotional intelligence through yoga involves both cognitive understanding of emotional processes and somatic awareness of emotional manifestations in the body (Chu et al., 2015).

8. PRACTICAL APPROACHES TO ACHIEVE SYNCHRONIZATION

The establishment of a consistent daily yoga routine represents the foundation for achieving sustained mind-body synchronization through the cumulative effects of regular practice. The design of an effective daily routine must balance multiple considerations including time constraints, individual needs and limitations, seasonal variations, and the progressive development of skills and awareness. Traditional yoga teachings emphasize the importance of regularity over intensity, suggesting that consistent daily practice, even if brief, produces more significant benefits than sporadic intensive sessions (Upadhya, 2025).

A balanced daily yoga routine typically incorporates elements from multiple practice categories to address different aspects of synchronization comprehensively. Morning practices often emphasize energizing and awakening sequences that prepare the nervous system for daily activities while establishing present-moment awareness and intention setting. These might include gentle movement sequences, activating breathing practices, and concentration techniques that promote alertness and mental clarity (Sengupta, 2012). The morning routine serves to establish synchronization at the beginning of each day and may influence the quality of attention and awareness throughout subsequent activities. Evening practices generally focus on relaxation, integration, and preparation for restorative sleep. These routines often include gentle stretching sequences, calming breathing practices, and meditation techniques that promote nervous system recovery and consolidation of the day's experiences. The evening practice serves to restore synchronization after the challenges and disruptions of daily life while promoting optimal conditions for sleep and recovery. The transition from active daily engagement to restorative rest requires careful attention to nervous system regulation and gradual downregulation of arousal (Varne & A, 2023).

The sequencing of practices within daily routines follows traditional principles that optimize physiological and psychological effects while minimizing potential contraindications or adverse reactions. The typical sequence progresses from centering and breath awareness through physical warm-up, main posture practice, breathing exercises, and concluding meditation or relaxation (Balaji et al., 2012).

This progression respects the natural warming and cooling cycles of the body while systematically engaging different aspects of mind-body integration. Individual adaptation of daily routines requires careful assessment of constitutional factors, current health status, life circumstances, and personal goals. Ayurvedic principles suggest that different body types (doshas) may benefit from different practice emphases, with some individuals requiring more calming practices while others need more energizing approaches. Seasonal adjustments may also be beneficial, with more warming practices during cold periods and more cooling practices during hot seasons (Sengupta, 2012).

9. APPLICATIONS OF SYNCHRONIZATION THROUGH YOGA

Yoga for Students and Academic Performance

The application of yoga practices for enhancing academic performance and supporting student well-being represents a growing area of research and implementation with significant implications for educational success and lifelong learning skills. Students at all educational levels face increasing academic pressures, social challenges, and technological distractions that can disrupt mind-body synchronization and impair learning capacity. Yoga's comprehensive approach to attention training, stress management, and cognitive enhancement offers valuable tools for addressing these challenges while promoting optimal conditions for learning and development (Badve et al., 2025). The cognitive benefits of yoga practice particularly relevant to academic performance include enhanced attention regulation, improved working memory capacity, reduced test anxiety, and increased cognitive flexibility. Attention regulation improvements enable students to maintain focus during lectures, reading, and study sessions while reducing susceptibility to distractions from internal thoughts or external stimuli. The development of sustained attention through yoga practice may be particularly beneficial in contemporary educational environments characterized by frequent attention switching and digital distractions (Govindasamy et al., 2024).

Working memory enhancements through yoga practice provide students with improved capacity for holding and manipulating information during complex cognitive tasks such as problem-solving, reading comprehension, and mathematical reasoning. The integration of physical movement with cognitive demands in yoga may strengthen the neural networks underlying working memory through enhanced coordination between motor and cognitive systems. These improvements may be particularly beneficial for students with attention difficulties or learning disabilities (Berkovich-Ohana, 2017).

Stress reduction effects of yoga practice contribute to academic performance through multiple pathways including improved sleep quality, enhanced immune function, reduced test anxiety, and better emotional regulation during academic challenges. Chronic stress impairs memory consolidation, reduces cognitive flexibility, and interferes with creative problem-solving, making stress management crucial for optimal academic performance (D. Sharma & Sharma, 2024). The comprehensive stress reduction achieved through yoga practice may be more effective than isolated stress management techniques due to its integration of cognitive, emotional, and physiological approaches. The social and emotional learning benefits of yoga practice support academic success through improved interpersonal relationships, enhanced self-awareness, and better emotional regulation during social challenges.

Yoga in Sports and Performance Enhancement

The application of yoga practices for athletic performance enhancement represents a sophisticated approach to optimizing the mind-body coordination, mental resilience, and recovery capacity essential for peak athletic performance. Elite athletes increasingly recognize that physical training alone is insufficient for achieving optimal performance, and that mental training, stress management, and recovery optimization are equally important components of comprehensive athletic development. Yoga's integration of physical conditioning with mental training provides a unique approach to addressing these multiple performance factors simultaneously (Berkovich-Ohana, 2017). The biomechanical benefits of yoga for athletic performance include improved flexibility, enhanced proprioceptive awareness, better movement efficiency, and reduced injury risk. The systematic stretching and strengthening components of asana practice address muscle imbalances and movement restrictions that commonly develop through sport-specific training. The emphasis on postural alignment and movement quality in yoga may help athletes develop more efficient movement patterns that enhance performance while reducing wear and tear on joints and tissues (D. Sharma & Sharma, 2024).

Balance and coordination improvements through yoga practice benefit virtually all athletic activities through enhanced proprioceptive awareness and neuromuscular control. The challenging balance poses in yoga require continuous adjustment of muscle activation patterns based on sensory feedback, training the nervous system to make rapid, precise adjustments that translate to improved athletic performance. The cerebellum, crucial for balance and motor learning, shows enhanced function with yoga practice that may contribute to improved motor skills across different sports. The mental training aspects of yoga provide athletes with valuable tools for managing competition stress, maintaining focus during performance, and recovering from setbacks or poor performances (Govindasamy et al., 2024). The attention regulation skills developed through yoga practice enable athletes to maintain optimal focus during competition while avoiding either excessive tension or inadequate arousal. The development of present-moment awareness helps athletes perform in "flow states" characterized by effortless execution and peak performance.

Breathing regulation techniques from pranayama provide athletes with practical tools for managing arousal levels, optimizing oxygenation, and enhancing recovery between training sessions or competitive events. Specific breathing practices can be used to increase alertness and energy before competition, maintain calm focus during performance, or promote relaxation and recovery following intense training (Ganpat et al., 2013). The conscious control of breathing may also help athletes manage performance anxiety and maintain optimal psychological states under pressure. Recovery and regeneration benefits of yoga include enhanced sleep quality, reduced inflammation, improved circulation, and accelerated tissue repair processes. The relaxation and stress reduction effects of yoga promote optimal conditions for physiological recovery while the gentle movement and stretching components enhance circulation and lymphatic drainage. The integration of relaxation with gentle movement may be more effective for recovery than either passive rest or active recovery alone (Govindasamy et al., 2024).

Yoga for Stress Management in Professionals

Professional environments across diverse industries increasingly recognize the need for effective stress management interventions that can address the complex psychological and physiological demands of modern work. Chronic workplace stress contributes to decreased productivity, increased healthcare costs, higher turnover rates, and reduced job satisfaction, making effective stress management both a personal health issue and an organizational imperative. Yoga's comprehensive approach to stress management offers valuable tools for addressing these challenges while promoting enhanced performance and well-being (Yoshihara et al., 2011).

The physiological stress reduction effects of yoga practice address the immediate health consequences of chronic workplace stress including elevated blood pressure, muscle tension, sleep disruption, and compromised immune function. Regular yoga practice normalizes stress hormone patterns, improves autonomic nervous system balance, and enhances physiological resilience to stress exposure. These improvements contribute to better physical health while also supporting cognitive function and emotional stability necessary for optimal work performance (D. Sharma & Sharma, 2024).

Cognitive benefits of yoga practice particularly relevant to professional performance include enhanced attention regulation, improved decision-making under pressure, increased creativity and problem-solving capacity, and better working memory function. The attention training components of yoga help professionals maintain focus during complex tasks while reducing susceptibility to distractions and interruptions. The stress reduction effects optimize cognitive function by reducing the interference from anxiety and worry that commonly impairs workplace performance. Emotional regulation improvements through yoga practice enable professionals to maintain composure during challenging interpersonal interactions, manage frustration and disappointment more effectively, and maintain positive relationships with colleagues and clients. The development of equanimity and present-moment awareness through yoga may be particularly valuable for professionals in high-stress occupations such as healthcare, emergency services, and executive leadership roles (Ciołkosz, 2015).

Yoga for Health and Disease Prevention

The application of yoga practices for health promotion and disease prevention represents one of the most extensively researched areas of yoga therapeutics, with mounting evidence supporting its effectiveness for addressing both specific medical conditions and general health optimization. The mind-body synchronization achieved through yoga practice appears to influence fundamental health processes including immune function, inflammation regulation, cardiovascular health, and mental health resilience that contribute to disease prevention and health promotion across diverse populations (Ciołkosz, 2015). Cardiovascular health benefits of yoga practice include reduced blood pressure, improved cholesterol profiles, enhanced endothelial function, and decreased risk of coronary artery disease. The combination of physical activity, stress reduction, and breathing regulation in yoga provides multiple mechanisms for cardiovascular protection that may be more comprehensive than any single intervention alone. The meditation components of yoga may provide additional cardiovascular benefits through their effects on stress reactivity and autonomic nervous system balance (Ganpat et al., 2013).

Immune system enhancement through yoga practice involves multiple pathways including reduced chronic inflammation, improved lymphocyte function, enhanced natural killer cell activity, and better vaccine responses. The stress reduction effects of yoga play a crucial role in immune enhancement, as chronic stress suppresses immune function through cortisol-mediated mechanisms (D. Sharma & Sharma, 2024). The physical movements in yoga may also promote lymphatic circulation and immune system activation through mechanical effects on lymph flow and tissue circulation. Mental health benefits of yoga practice include reduced symptoms of depression and anxiety, improved mood regulation, enhanced self-esteem, and better stress resilience. The comprehensive approach of yoga addresses mental health through multiple mechanisms including neurotransmitter regulation, stress hormone normalization, enhanced social connection, and the development of coping skills and psychological resilience. The integration of physical activity with mindfulness and breathing practices may provide superior mental health benefits compared to any single approach alone (Ganpat et al., 2013).

10. FUTURE DIRECTIONS IN YOGA SYNCHRONIZATION RESEARCH

The future of research into yoga's effects on mind-body synchronization promises to advance our understanding of these ancient practices while developing more precise and personalized approaches to implementation. Emerging technologies, refined research methodologies, and interdisciplinary collaboration offer unprecedented opportunities for investigating the mechanisms underlying yoga's effects while optimizing intervention design for specific populations and applications (D. K. Pal et al., 2017).

Advanced neuroimaging techniques including ultra-high field magnetic resonance imaging, multi-modal brain imaging, and real-time neurofeedback provide increasingly detailed insights into the neural mechanisms underlying mind-body synchronization through yoga practice (Gururaja et al., 2020). These technologies enable researchers to observe brain changes with greater spatial and temporal resolution while providing practitioners with immediate feedback about their neural states during practice. The integration of neurofeedback with traditional yoga instruction may accelerate learning and enhance the precision of practice. Physiological monitoring technologies including continuous heart rate variability monitoring, stress hormone tracking, and sleep quality assessment provide objective measures of synchronization that can guide practice adaptation and optimization (Gururaja et al., 2020). Wearable devices and mobile applications offer opportunities for continuous monitoring and personalized feedback that could enhance the effectiveness of yoga interventions while providing valuable data for research purposes. Genetic and epigenetic research investigating individual differences in responsiveness to yoga practice may reveal biomarkers that predict optimal practice approaches for different individuals. Understanding how genetic variations in neurotransmitter systems, stress response pathways, and neuroplasticity mechanisms influence yoga practice effects could guide personalized intervention design and optimization. Epigenetic research examining gene expression changes following yoga practice may illuminate molecular mechanisms underlying synchronization and identify optimal practice parameters for inducing beneficial genetic adaptations (D. K. Pal et al., 2017).

Artificial intelligence and machine learning approaches offer potential for analyzing complex patterns in physiological and behavioural data to identify optimal practice sequences, timing, and adaptations for individual practitioners. These technologies could integrate multiple sources of data including genetic information, physiological monitoring, subjective reports, and practice history to provide personalized recommendations for achieving optimal synchronization (Curtis et al., 2012). The development of AI-assisted yoga instruction could make high-quality, personalized guidance more widely accessible. Mechanistic research focusing on the specific neural circuits and physiological pathways underlying yoga's effects on synchronization will continue to refine our understanding of how these practices work and how they can be optimized. This research includes investigation of neurotransmitter systems, inflammatory pathways, autonomic nervous system regulation, and brain network connectivity changes that mediate the benefits of practice. Understanding these mechanisms may enable the development of targeted interventions for specific conditions or populations (Chawla et al., 2023).

Longitudinal studies tracking practitioners over decades of practice will provide insights into the long-term effects of sustained yoga practice on health, cognitive function, and quality of life. These studies may reveal critical periods for practice initiation, optimal practice patterns for different life stages, and the cumulative effects of sustained practice on aging and disease prevention. Long-term studies may also identify factors that support sustained practice adherence and optimal outcomes. Cross-cultural research investigating how different cultural contexts influence yoga practice effects and synchronization outcomes will inform adaptation strategies for diverse populations (R. Pal et al., 2023). Understanding how cultural values, social support systems, and environmental factors influence practice effectiveness may guide culturally sensitive implementation approaches. This research may also reveal universal principles of mind-body synchronization that transcend cultural boundaries. Integration with other therapeutic modalities including psychotherapy, physical therapy, and medical treatment represents an important direction for expanding the applications of yoga for synchronization (Curtis et al., 2012). Research investigating the synergistic effects of combining yoga with other interventions may reveal optimal integration strategies while identifying potential contraindications or interactions. This research may also inform the development of yoga-informed approaches to conventional therapies.

11. CONCLUSION

The systematic study of synchronization through yoga highlights a profound integration of mind and body, bridging ancient wisdom with modern scientific understanding. Evidence shows that yoga produces measurable improvements in brain function, autonomic regulation, stress hormones, and cognitive performance, reflecting genuine mind-body harmony. These outcomes arise from multiple mechanisms, including heightened attention, enhanced interoceptive awareness, reduced stress, and improved physiological coordination through breath control and mindful movement. The combined use of meditation, asana, and pranayama generates synergistic benefits beyond those of individual practices, with breath functioning as a key link between mental and physical processes. Practically, yoga synchronization supports learning, recovery, and overall well-being across diverse populations. Its adaptability allows meaningful application across ages, abilities, and settings. However, challenges such as over-physicalization, cultural appropriation concerns, and limited access to holistic instruction emphasize the need for inclusive, comprehensive education. Future research will refine mechanisms and develop personalized pathways to optimal integration.

REFERENCES

Aleksić Veljković, A., Katanić, B., & Masanovic, B. (2021). Effects of a 12-Weeks Yoga Intervention on Motor and Cognitive Abilities of Preschool Children. *Frontiers in Pediatrics*, *9*, 799226. Advance online publication. DOI: 10.3389/fped.2021.799226 PMID: 34926359

Arora, S., & Bhattacharjee, J. (2008). Modulation of immune responses in stress by Yoga. *International Journal of Yoga*, *1*(2), 45. DOI: 10.4103/0973-6131.43541 PMID: 21829284

Badoni, P., Kumar, N., Singh, R., Gupta, K., Kalra, P., & Arora, V. (2025). Exploring the synergy of yoga and ayurveda in metaverse. In *Exploring the Metaverse* (pp. 165–187). Elsevier., https://www.sciencedirect.com/science/article/pii/B9780443241321000119 DOI: 10.1016/B978-0-443-24132-1.00011-9

Badve, R., Varadharajan, E., Govindasamy, K., Dongre, S., Velusamy, S., Kambitta Valappil, I. N., Karmakar, D., Çitozi, R., & Geantă, V. A. (2025). Considering the Impact of Yoga on Psychological Well-being and Quality of Life in Perimenopausal Women: A Randomized Controlled Trial. *Physical Education Theory and Methodology*, *25*(2), 331–339. DOI: 10.17309/tmfv.2025.2.14

Balaji, P. A., Varne, S. R., & Ali, S. S. (2012). Physiological effects of yogic practices and transcendental meditation in health and disease. *North American Journal of Medical Sciences*, *4*(10), 442. https://www.ncbi.nlm.nih.gov/pmc/articles/PMC3482773/. DOI: 10.4103/1947-2714.101980 PMID: 23112963

Barua, R. (2025). Harmonizing Body and Mind: Investigating the Combined Impact of Yoga and Mindfulness Meditation on Depression, Anxiety, Stress. In *Global Innovations in Physical Education and Health* (pp. 203–232). IGI Global Scientific Publishing. https://www.igi-global.com/chapter/harmonizing-body-and-mind/361163

Basu-Ray, I. (2021). A Mechanistic Model for Yoga as a Preventive and Therapeutic Modality. *International Journal of Yoga*, *14*(2), 152–157. DOI: 10.4103/ijoy.IJOY_136_20 PMID: 34188388

Berkovich-Ohana, A. (2017). A case study of a meditation-induced altered state: Increased overall gamma synchronization. *Phenomenology and the Cognitive Sciences*, *16*(1), 91–106. DOI: 10.1007/s11097-015-9435-x

Bhavanani, A. B. (2014). Diverse dimensions of Yoga. *Yoga Mimamsa*, *46*(1–2), 3–8. DOI: 10.4103/0044-0507.137846

Chawla, V., Brems, C., Freeman, H., Ravindran, A., & Noordsy, D. L. (2023). The Future of Yoga for Mental Health Care. *International Journal of Yoga, 16*(1), 38–41. DOI: 10.4103/ijoy.ijoy_25_23 PMID: 37583539

Chopra, D., Stern, E., Bushell, W. C., & Castle, R. D. (2023). Yoga and pain: A mind-body complex system. *Frontiers in Pain Research (Lausanne, Switzerland), 4*, 1075866. Advance online publication. DOI: 10.3389/fpain.2023.1075866 PMID: 36910253

Chu, I.-H., Lin, Y.-J., Wu, W.-L., Chang, Y.-K., & Lin, I.-M. (2015). Effects of Yoga on Heart Rate Variability and Mood in Women: A Randomized Controlled Trial. *Journal of Alternative and Complementary Medicine (New York, N.Y.), 21*(12), 789–795. DOI: 10.1089/acm.2015.0138 PMID: 26505201

Ciołkosz, M. (2015). The Possible Significance of Sensorimotor Synchronisation in Modern Postural Yoga Practice. *Studia Religiologica. Zeszyty Naukowe Uniwersytetu Jagiellońskiego, 48*(4), 327–340. https://www.ceeol.com/search/article-detail?id=477117

Collette, A. (2015). The Felt Sense of Interconnectedness: A qualitative analysis of perceptions on finding resilience in the aftermath of trauma using the mind-body connections of Yoga. *Theses and Dissertations (Comprehensive)*. https://scholars.wlu.ca/etd/1735

Cook-Cottone, C., & Perey, I. (2025). Defining Embodiment, Yoga, and Yoga as Embodied Mindfulness. In Cook-Cottone, C., & Tylka, T. L. (Eds.), *Yoga as Embodied Mindfulness: Integrating Research and Practice* (pp. 11–31). Springer Nature Switzerland., DOI: 10.1007/978-3-031-83418-9_2

Curtis, K., Weinrib, A., & Katz, J. (2012). Systematic Review of Yoga for Pregnant Women: Current Status and Future Directions. *Evidence-Based Complementary and Alternative Medicine : eCAM, 2012*(1), 715942. DOI: 10.1155/2012/715942 PMID: 22927881

Donahoe-Fillmore, B., & Grant, E. (2019). The effects of yoga practice on balance, strength, coordination and flexibility in healthy children aged 10–12 years. *Journal of Bodywork and Movement Therapies, 23*(4), 708–712. DOI: 10.1016/j.jbmt.2019.02.007 PMID: 31733751

Froeliger, B. E., Garland, E. L., Modlin, L. A., & McClernon, F. J. (2012). Neurocognitive correlates of the effects of yoga meditation practice on emotion and cognition: A pilot study. *Frontiers in Integrative Neuroscience, 6*, 48. https://www.frontiersin.org/journals/integrative-neuroscience/articles/10.3389/fnint.2012.00048/full. DOI: 10.3389/fnint.2012.00048 PMID: 22855674

Ganpat, T. S., Nagendra, H. R., & Selvi, V. (2013). Efficacy of yoga for mental performance in university students. *Indian Journal of Psychiatry*, *55*(4), 349. DOI: 10.4103/0019-5545.120550 PMID: 24459305

Gard, T., Noggle, J. J., Park, C. L., Vago, D. R., & Wilson, A. (2014). Potential self-regulatory mechanisms of yoga for psychological health. *Frontiers in Human Neuroscience*, *8*, 770. DOI: 10.3389/fnhum.2014.00770 PMID: 25368562

Ghosh, T., Duraipandian, C., Joseph, S., Kumasi, B., Salvi, N. M., Elayaraja, M., Astuti, Y., Orhan, B. E., Karmakar, D., & Govindasamy, K. (2024). Effects of Yoga and Combined Yoga with Neuro-Linguistic Programming on Psychological Management in Mothers of Adolescents: A Randomized Controlled Trial. *Sport Mont, 22*(3), 99–105. http://www.sportmont.ucg.ac.me/?sekcija=article&artid=2071

Govindasamy, K., Kaur, D., Elayaraja, M., Sethi, D., Kalidas, S., Karmakar, D., Orhan, B. E., Astuti, Y., & Parpa, K. (2024). Immediate Effect of Uddiyana Bandha on Heart Rate Variability in Patients with Hypertension: A Randomised Controlled Study. *Annals of Neurosciences*, *09727531241299258*, 09727531241299258. Advance online publication. DOI: 10.1177/09727531241299258 PMID: 39678718

Gururaja, C., Rangaprakash, D., & Deshpande, G. (2020). Research Trends in the Application of Yoga to Human Health: A Data Science Approach. *International Journal of Public Mental Health and Neurosciences*, *7*(1), 8–13. https://www.ncbi.nlm.nih.gov/pmc/articles/PMC8455111/ PMID: 34553079

Hart, C. E., & Tracy, B. L. (2008). Yoga as Steadiness Training: Effects on Motor Variability in Young Adults. *Journal of Strength and Conditioning Research*, *22*(5), 1659–1669. DOI: 10.1519/JSC.0b013e31818200dd PMID: 18714217

Jones, S. M. W., Guthrie, K. A., Reed, S. D., Landis, C. A., Sternfeld, B., LaCroix, A. Z., Dunn, A., Burr, R. L., & Newton, K. M. (2016). A yoga & exercise randomized controlled trial for vasomotor symptoms: Effects on heart rate variability. *Complementary Therapies in Medicine*, *26*, 66–71. DOI: 10.1016/j.ctim.2016.03.001 PMID: 27261984

Ju, X., Liu, H., Xu, J., Hu, B., Jin, Y., & Lu, C. (2024). Effect of Yoga Intervention on Problem Behavior and Motor Coordination in Children with Autism. *Behavioral Sciences (Basel, Switzerland)*, *14*(2), 116. DOI: 10.3390/bs14020116 PMID: 38392469

Krishna, B. H., Pal, P., Pal, G. K., Balachander, J., Jayasettiaseelon, E., Sreekanth, Y., Sridhar, M. G., & Gaur, G. S. (2014). Effect of yoga therapy on heart rate, blood pressure and cardiac autonomic function in heart failure. *Journal of Clinical and Diagnostic Research : JCDR, 8*(1), 14. https://www.ncbi.nlm.nih.gov/pmc/articles/PMC3939525/ PMID: 24596712

Lim, S.-A., & Cheong, K.-J. (2015). Regular Yoga Practice Improves Antioxidant Status, Immune Function, and Stress Hormone Releases in Young Healthy People: A Randomized, Double-Blind, Controlled Pilot Study. *Journal of Alternative and Complementary Medicine (New York, N.Y.), 21*(9), 530–538. DOI: 10.1089/acm.2014.0044 PMID: 26181573

Meissner, M., Cantell, M. H., Steiner, R., & Sanchez, X. (2016). Evaluating Emotional Well-Being after a Short-Term Traditional Yoga Practice Approach in Yoga Practitioners with an Existing Western-Type Yoga Practice. *Evidence-Based Complementary and Alternative Medicine : eCAM, 2016*(1), 7216982. DOI: 10.1155/2016/7216982 PMID: 27123033

Meister, K., & Juckel, G. (2018). A Systematic Review of Mechanisms of Change in Body-Oriented Yoga in Major Depressive Disorders. *Pharmacopsychiatry, 51*(3), 73–81. DOI: 10.1055/s-0043-111013 PMID: 28571077

Naveen, G. H., Thirthalli, J., Rao, M. G., Varambally, S., Christopher, R., & Gangadhar, B. N. (2013). Positive therapeutic and neurotropic effects of yoga in depression: A comparative study. *Indian Journal of Psychiatry, 55*(7, Suppl 3), S400–S404. https://journals.lww.com/indianjpsychiatry/fulltext/2013/55003/positive_therapeutic_and_neurotropic_effects_of.17.aspx. DOI: 10.4103/0019-5545.116313 PMID: 24049208

Newcombe, S. (2009). The Development of Modern Yoga: A Survey of the Field. *Religion Compass, 3*(6), 6. Advance online publication. DOI: 10.1111/j.1749-8171.2009.00171.x

Pal, D. K., Bhalla, A., Bammidi, S., Telles, S., Kohli, A., Kumar, S., Devi, P., Kaur, N., Sharma, K., Kumar, R., Malik, N., Thakur, V., Bhargava, G. G., Goyal, A. K., Devi, G., Chauhan, S., Singh, G., Ahmad, S., Joshi, M., & Anand, A. (2017). Can Yoga-Based Diabetes Management Studies Facilitate Integrative Medicine in India Current Status and Future Directions. *Integrative Medicine International, 4*(3–4), 125–141. DOI: 10.1159/000479816

Pal, R., Adhikari, D., Heyat, M. B. B., Ullah, I., & You, Z. (2023). Yoga Meets Intelligent Internet of Things: Recent Challenges and Future Directions. *Bioengineering (Basel, Switzerland), 10*(4), 459. DOI: 10.3390/bioengineering10040459 PMID: 37106646

Park, C. L., Finkelstein-Fox, L., Groessl, E., Elwy, A. R., & Lee, S. Y. (2020). Exploring How Different Types of Yoga Change Psychological Resources and Emotional Well-Being across a Single Session. *Complementary Therapies in Medicine*, *49*, 102354. DOI: 10.1016/j.ctim.2020.102354 PMID: 32147083

Pise, V., Pradhan, B., & Gharote, M. (2018). Effect of yoga practices on psycho-motor abilities among intellectually disabled children. *Journal of Exercise Rehabilitation*, *14*(4), 581–585. DOI: 10.12965/jer.1836290.145 PMID: 30276177

Rocha, K. K. F., Ribeiro, A. M., Rocha, K. C. F., Sousa, M. B. C., Albuquerque, F. S., Ribeiro, S., & Silva, R. H. (2012). Improvement in physiological and psychological parameters after 6 months of yoga practice. *Consciousness and Cognition*, *21*(2), 843–850. DOI: 10.1016/j.concog.2012.01.014 PMID: 22342535

Saito, H., Iwai, Y., Yamano, A., Matsushita, K., Yokoyama, H., Nakazawa, K., & Ito, S. (2025). Comparing muscle coordination patterns in yoga-focused exercises with those in standard stabilization exercises. *Journal of Bodywork and Movement Therapies*, *44*, 245–250. DOI: 10.1016/j.jbmt.2025.05.059 PMID: 40954586

Sengupta, P. (2012). Health Impacts of Yoga and Pranayama: A State-of-the-Art Review. *International Journal of Preventive Medicine*, *3*(7), 444–458. https://www.ncbi.nlm.nih.gov/pmc/articles/PMC3415184/ PMID: 22891145

Sharma, D., & Sharma, B. R. (2024). The Impact of Yoga and Meditation on Mental and Physical Well-being. *Journal of Ayurveda and Integrated Medical Sciences*, *9*(5), 144–153. DOI: 10.21760/jaims.9.5.23

Sharma, D. K. (2017). Yoga and meditation: Integral correlation is a bit of mystery. *Journal of Applied Consciousness Studies*, *5*(2), 42–47. https://journals.lww.com/joacs/fulltext/2017/05020/yoga_and_meditation__integral_correlation_is_a_bit.4.aspx

Silveira, K., & Smart, C. M. (2020). Cognitive, physical, and psychological benefits of yoga for acquired brain injuries: A systematic review of recent findings. *Neuropsychological Rehabilitation*, *30*(7), 1388–1407. DOI: 10.1080/09602011.2019.1583114 PMID: 30789008

Telles, S., Singh, N., Bhardwaj, A. K., Kumar, A., & Balkrishna, A. (2013). Effect of yoga or physical exercise on physical, cognitive and emotional measures in children: A randomized controlled trial. *Child and Adolescent Psychiatry and Mental Health*, *7*(1), 37. DOI: 10.1186/1753-2000-7-37 PMID: 24199742

Upadhya, Y. (2025). A Comprehensive Exploration of the Holistic Healing Power of Yoga. *Journal of Rapti Babai Campus*, *5*(1), 152–163. DOI: 10.3126/jrbc.v5i1.78102

Varne, S. R., & A, B. P. (2023). A systematic review on molecular, bio-chemical, and pathophysiological mechanisms of yoga, pranayama and meditation causing beneficial effects in various health disorders. *Indian Journal of Integrative Medicine, 3*(4), 87–96. https://www.mansapublishers.com/ijim/article/view/4284

Vinay, A. V., Venkatesh, D., & Ambarish, V. (2016). Impact of short-term practice of yoga on heart rate variability. *International Journal of Yoga*, *9*(1), 62. DOI: 10.4103/0973-6131.171714 PMID: 26865773

Vyas, B., & Vyas, R. (2017). *Contemporizing Raj Yoga: Neuroscience and Practices*. Dr. Bhaskar Vyas. https://books.google.com/books?hl=en&lr=&id=SY3vDwAAQBAJ&oi=fnd&pg=PR1&dq=Synchronization+through+Yoga:+Connecting+the+Physical+and+Mental+Realms&ots=Y3xKy8uG7R&sig=cOoP0g8Y9sxJezNoN8ZCjrUCP_s

Yoshihara, K., Hiramoto, T., Sudo, N., & Kubo, C. (2011). Profile of mood states and stress-related biochemical indices in long-term yoga practitioners. *BioPsychoSocial Medicine*, *5*(1), 6. DOI: 10.1186/1751-0759-5-6 PMID: 21635790

Chapter 9
The Triad of Transformation:
Exploring the Synergistic Landscape of Mindfulness, Meditation, and Yoga in Contemporary Mental Health Enhancement

Sohom Saha
http://orcid.org/0009-0006-9438-1554
Lakshmibai National Institute of Physical Education, India

Mahendra Kumar Singh
http://orcid.org/0000-0001-9989-9420
Lakshmibai National Institute of Physical Education, India

Simran Obhrai
http://orcid.org/0009-0007-5227-9364
Guru Nanak Dev University, India

ABSTRACT

The global mental health crisis, characterized by escalating rates of anxiety, depression, and existential distress, has exposed the limitations of conventional biomedical approaches. This chapter explores the integrative potential of mindfulness, meditation, and yoga as a synergistic triad for promoting comprehensive mental well-being. Grounded in both ancient contemplative traditions and contemporary empirical research, the triad fosters emotional regulation, neuroplastic adaptability, embodied awareness, and a deeper sense of meaning. Rather than focusing solely

DOI: 10.4018/979-8-3373-4187-3.ch009

on symptom reduction, these practices support psychological resilience and spiritual growth. The chapter further investigates their increasing application across therapeutic, educational, and occupational domains, highlighting their adaptability, scientific credibility, and cross-cultural relevance. It calls for a paradigm shift toward person-centered, developmental models of care that recognize contemplative practices as foundational tools for long-term healing and flourishing.

INTRODUCTION: THE LANDSCAPE OF MODERN MENTAL HEALTH

The modern psyche world introduces a paradox of the most unconditional level that undermines our universal concepts of mental soundness and treatment. Notwithstanding stunning progress in psychological investigation, neurobiological comprehension, and the production of evidence-based clinical interventions, rates of anxiety, depression, and psychological trouble are rising all through the world at an alarming rate (Santomauro et al., 2021; World Health Organization, 2022). Such a confusing trend has generated what most researchers and clinicians have seen as a global mental health crisis of an extent and dimension that has never been witnessed before, a crisis that not only requires urgent responses but also unique and radical solutions that go beyond the paradigm of conventional treatment interventions. The newly released global health statistics of the World Health Organization create a gloomy picture of what is happening in the world today in terms of mental health epidemic. Due to its current status as a disease causing the greatest disability in the world, depression impacts more than 280 million individuals of all demographic lines and accounts to around 3.8 percent of the total global population (World Health Organization, 2017). Simultaneously, anxiety disorders impact an estimated 301 million individuals worldwide, with women being disproportionately affected at nearly twice the rate of men (GBD 2019 Mental Disorders Collaborators, 2022). These figures, while staggering in their scope, represent only the documented cases and likely underestimate the true prevalence of psychological distress, particularly in regions with limited mental health infrastructure and significant cultural barriers to seeking psychological care (Vigo et al., 2016).

The COVID-19 pandemic has further exacerbated this crisis, serving as a global catalyst that has intensified existing mental health challenges while creating new forms of psychological distress. Meta-analytic evidence indicates that the pandemic resulted in a 25% increase in anxiety and depression worldwide, with young people and women being disproportionately affected (Santomauro et al., 2021). The prevalence of the pandemic was not limited to acute psychological symptoms and affected the social network, financial security, and underlying historical principles of security and certainty that the basis of psychological well-being relies on (Xiong et al., 2020). This growing epidemic has also spurred a paradigm shift regarding how mental health professionals, researchers and policymakers think about and treat mental health care. It has become increasingly understood that although traditional biomedical models have their utility in their use, they might not be able to cope with the complexity and high-dimensionality of current psychological distress (Engel, 1977; Ghaemi, 2009). Such recognition has led to the movement in a more integrative and holistic paradigm that complies with the connectedness of mind, body, spirit and the social environment in shaping and sustaining mental wellbeing (Suls & Rothman, 2004).

The shortcomings of purely biomedical approach are also especially visible when it comes to reviewing the treatment outcomes and long-term recovery rates connected with traditional methods of treatment. Although the efficacy of psychopharmacological interventions and standard psychotherapies was proved in clinical trials, the results in practice do not always match the research results, and considerable percentages of patients show partial response rates, treatment resistance, or relapse (Cuijpers et al., 2014; Rush et al., 2006). More importantly, such level of reductionist practice in treating symptoms alone does not normally correct the underlying patterns of thought, feeling, and relating that maintain the psychological distress (Hayes et al., 2006a). In this context of increasing rates of psychological complaints and known shortcomings of traditional treatment methods, ancient contemplation methods, namely mindfulness, meditation, and yoga, have been found to be empowering therapeutic interventions, which not only provide short-term symptom relief but also provide long-term transformative capabilities (Cramer et al., 2013a; Goyal et al., 2014; Khoury et al., 2015). In this context of increasing rates of psychological complaints and known shortcomings of traditional treatment methods, ancient contemplation methods, namely mindfulness, meditation, and yoga, have been found to be empowering therapeutic interventions, which not only provide short-term symptom relief but also provide long-term transformative capabilities

This scientific validation of contemplative practices is one of the most important trends in mental health research of the 21st century. Mindfulness-based interventions have repeatedly shown to effectuate the symptoms of depression, anxiety, chronic pain, and stress-related disorder through systematic reviews and meta-analyses (Hofmann et al., 2010; Khoury et al., 2015). Likewise, the emotional control, attention, and overall psychological health have been found to significantly improve via meditation exercises (Goyal et al., 2014; Sedlmeier et al., 2012). Being a complex mind-body therapy approach, yoga has proven to be a successful treatment of depression, anxiety, post-traumatic stress disorder, and several other chronic conditions (Cramer et al., 2013a; Uebelacker et al., 2010). However, the legitimization of these mindfulness practices by the mainstream mental health care will be an important paradigm shift beyond the symptom-oriented treatment toward an approach focused on enabling core skills in mindfulness, emotional control, and psychological resilience (Vago & Silbersweig, 2012). This transition recognizes that attainment of sustainable mental health goes beyond merely eliminating the symptoms but involves voyage into the development of the positive states of mind, effective coping skills and the overall spiritual equation wherein individuals change their ways of dealing with the mind, emotions and incidents (Keyes, 2002).

The alienation of the modern lifestyle, the lack of connection to our own bodies, our breath, our current experience, and our deeper sense of purpose and meaning, has given rise to new psychological misery on a scale never before seen in human history that traditional solutions can frequently not overcome in their entirety (Baumeister et al., 2013; Williams, 2020). This disintegration takes different interrelated forms that culminate into the mental health epidemic. The continual state of physiological and psychological arousal caused by the acute stress of high-intensity living has produced an endemic condition of accelerated existence that plagues the capacity of the human system to automatically regulate itself (Schneiderman et al., 2005). It is the fear of being always connected enabled by digital technologies and social media platforms that has essentially changed the way people think, build relationships and shape their identity (Twenge & Campbell, 2018). Studies have revealed that over-uses of social media are coupled with high prevalence rates of depression, anxiety, and loneliness, specifically in adolescents and young adults (Primack et al., 2017). This has threatened the ability to think deeply, form real social links and remain in the present due to the phenomenon of continuous partial attention whereby people experience divided mental attention amongst various digital sources (Stone, 2008).

The melancholy of social isolation is one more serious aspect of modern fragmentation. Regardless of soaring connectivity begotten by the digital world, the epidemic of loneliness and social isolation has become the defining issue of physical and mental health (Cacioppo & Cacioppo, 2018). Declining traditional community, the family chain, and the significant social practices have deprived a lot of them the appropriate social service system, leading to a feeling of isolation and that is why there is a feeling of meaningless existence (Putnam, 2000). Existential emptiness that frequently goes hand-in-hand with material wealth in the developed countries is a very specific kind of psychological distress, which also becomes problematic in terms of traditional treatment strategies (Baumeister et al., 2013). The existence of this phenomenon which manifests itself in the form of feelings of meaninglessness, purposelessness, and spiritual emptiness even when material success is achieved, suggests that symptom-oriented treatment alone is not sufficient and that interventions that can help people answer some of the most basic existential questions such as the meaning of life and the right purpose and the worth of existence should be sought (Frankl, 1963). Such traditional mental health treatment methods, although useful in that they can reduce symptoms and help during times of crisis, nevertheless tend to focus on the superficial forms of the problem rather than on the patterns of consciousness and embodiment that underlie the development of psychological distress (Hayes et al., 2006b). An example of this type of treatment is cognitive-behavioral approaches, which are subject centered in their primary areas (i.e. identifying and changing dysfunctional thought patterns) and may not fully deal with the underlying somatic, emotional and spiritual layers of psychological suffering (Mahoney, 2003).

The emergence of contemplative practices in mainstream mental health care represents a recognition that authentic healing requires more than cognitive restructuring or pharmacological intervention, it demands a fundamental transformation in how individuals relate to their thoughts, emotions, bodily sensations, and life experiences (Vago & Silbersweig, 2012). This transformation is not merely therapeutic in the traditional sense of symptom reduction, but developmental, inviting individuals into greater self-awareness, emotional regulation, authentic well-being, and a more integrated way of being in the world. The integration of mindfulness, meditation, and yoga into contemporary mental health practice offers a unique opportunity to address the multidimensional nature of psychological distress while cultivating positive psychological capacities that extend far beyond symptom management (Segal et al., 2002). These practices work synergistically to promote what researchers have termed "positive mental health", a state characterized not merely by the absence of psychological symptoms, but by the presence of emotional well-being, life satisfaction, optimism, and psychological flourishing (Keyes, 2002).

The scientific body of evidence that underlies contemplative practices is swiftly expanding, as neuroimaging techniques are demonstrating the neuroplastic transformations that are a result of routine meditation and mindfulness practice (Davidson & Lutz, 2008; Lutz et al., 2008a). The results indicate that contemplative practices operate on the most basic levels of brain composition and functions, aiding adaptive changes in brain circuits connected with attention, emotional self-control, self-awareness, and stress resilience (Tang et al., 2015). At this pivotal moment in the development of mental health care, unification of ancient wisdom traditions and modern scientific knowledge provides unprecedented access to healing, growth and change. The intersection of mindfulness, meditation and yoga is not simply an extension of current treatment capabilities, but a complete reinvention of what psychological health care even looks like in the 21st century.

PART I: THE INDIVIDUAL VOICES - UNDERSTANDING EACH PRACTICE

Mindfulness: The Art of Present-Moment Awareness

The practice of being aware in the moment with an open mind, taking curiosity and acceptance is known as mindfulness, and is essentially the most recognized form of contemplative practice in mental health nowadays (Kabat-Zinn, 2003). Mindfulness has its roots in Buddhist meditation practices, and especially the Vipassana or insight meditation tradition, and has been effectively incorporated into a secular therapeutic tradition in ways that preserve its seeds of transformational potential. Phenomenology of mindfulness awareness suggests that there is a paradigm shift in the consciousness that changes the automaticity of the reactive patterns of thinking and feeling into a more spacious response approach of awareness (Chessick, 2007). This shift is characterized by what researchers call "metacognitive awareness", the capacity to observe one's thoughts and emotions without being overwhelmed or controlled by them (Wells, 2000). This metacognitive ability is an essential treatment process that enables human beings to be aware of adverse thinking habit, emotional hyper-responsiveness, and repetitive patterns of behavior that lead to psychological discomposure.

Jon Kabat-Zinn's pioneering work in developing Mindfulness-Based Stress Reduction (MBSR) demonstrated that mindfulness training could significantly reduce symptoms of anxiety, depression, and chronic pain while improving overall quality of life (Kabat-Zinn, 1994). Later studies have confirmed these results in all kinds of population and settings, and mindfulness has become an evidence-based tool used in response to a considerable variety of mental health issues (Goyal et al., 2014). The therapeutic mechanisms of mindfulness operate through several interconnected pathways. To begin with, mindfulness builds the ability to be in the present moments, which breaks the circle of ruminating and worrying that is observed in anxiety and depressive disorders (Watkins & Teasdale, 2004). Second, mindfulness strengthens skills in emotional regulation that tend to put space between stimulus and response which lets the individual make more conscientious decisions in relating to tough experiences (Gross, 2002). Third, mindfulness promotes self-compassion and acceptance, reducing the self-criticism and judgment that often exacerbate psychological suffering (Neff, 2011). Neuroimaging research has revealed that mindfulness practice produces measurable changes in brain structure and function, including increased gray matter density in areas associated with learning, memory, and emotional regulation, and decreased activity in the default mode network associated with rumination and self-referential thinking (Tang et al., 2015). These neuroplastic changes provide a biological foundation for the psychological benefits of mindfulness practice. The integration of mindfulness into daily life transforms not only how individuals relate to their thoughts and emotions but also how they engage with relationships, work, and life challenges. Mindful awareness becomes a foundation for authentic living, characterized by greater presence, compassion, and wisdom (Kornfield, 2008).

Meditation: The Journey Inward

Meditation encompasses a diverse family of practices designed to train attention, cultivate specific mental states, and develop insight into the nature of consciousness itself. Although it is often confused with mindfulness, meditation is more generically defined as part of a family of contemplative practices encompassing other techniques of concentration, loving-kindness meditation, visualization exercises, and other types of insight meditation (Lutz et al., 2008b). Meditation practices are numerous and diverse, including intensely concentrated forms of concentration that cultivate sustained attention to objects one focuses on, to more open uncensored monitoring practices that cultivate choiceless awareness of all that appears in consciousness (Lutz et al., 2008b). All forms of meditation are beneficial and have their own specific advantages, focusing on various particular issues in mental training and improvement. The practice of concentration meditation which includes breath awareness or single pointed attention develops the quality of enduring attention and stability of mind. This kind of practice is especially helpful to those, who have anxiety or ADHD or other difficulties with attention (Zylowska et al., 2008). The practice of focused attention forms a basis of all other meditation activities and leads to better mental performance, emotional efficiency as well as better thinking in general. Loving-kindness meditation, a practice that entails developing attitudes of kindness and compassion toward self and others has been found to augment positive emotions, decrease implicit prejudice and reinforce bonds among people (Hofmann et al., 2011). It is especially helpful to people who have issues with depression, social anxiety, and problems in their interpersonal communication because it breaks the pattern of loneliness and internal criticism that such issues tend to produce. The contemplative traditions of insight meditation that entail witnessing the coming and going of thoughts, emotion, feelings, and sensations without just clinging or repelling aim to develop wisdom and insight concerning the actual nature of experience itself. Such practices have the potential of creating radical personal transformations and reducing the magnitude of psychological suffering by acknowledging the impermanent and interdependent nature of everything (Goldstein, 2013).

Neuroscience of meditation shows that various forms of practice result in varied patterns of brain activity and structural transformations. Among long-term meditators, cortical thickness increases in the regions related to attention and sensory processing, and the amygdala undergoes alteration, which is related to less emotional responsiveness (Luders et al., 2009). These discoveries indicate that meditation physically transforms the brain in a manner that facilitates improved health and strength. Incorporation of the meditative states into everyday life is another important factor of contemplative progress. Instead of having to stay restricted to a formal practice of sitting, the understanding and abilities acquired during the practice of meditation gradually enter every realm of life, resulting in a much more harmonious and conscious manner of existence (Teasdale et al., 2002).

Yoga: The Union of Body, Mind, and Spirit

Yoga, literally meaning "union" or "to yoke," represents perhaps the most comprehensive system of mind-body integration within contemplative traditions. Yoga originated in ancient India more than 5,000 years ago and comprises of physical postures (asanas), breathing exercises (pranayama), ethical standards (yamas and niyamas), and philosophical rules all of which help in supporting the growth of proper physical health, mental clarity, and spiritual awareness (Feuerstein, 2008). The embodied wisdom of yogic practices recognizes that the body is not merely a vehicle for the mind but an integral aspect of consciousness itself. This understanding challenges the Western dualistic separation of mind and body, offering instead a unified vision of human beings as integrated psychosomatic systems (Mehta, 2011). Through the practice of yoga, individuals develop a more intimate and compassionate relationship with their physical form while simultaneously cultivating mental and emotional well-being. The therapeutic applications of yoga for mental health have been extensively documented in research literature. Studies have shown that regular yoga practice can significantly reduce symptoms of anxiety, depression, PTSD, and chronic stress while improving sleep quality, self-esteem, and overall quality of life (Cramer et al., 2013b). The mechanisms underlying these benefits are multifaceted, involving physiological changes in the nervous system, hormonal regulation, and neurotransmitter balance. Breath awareness, or pranayama, represents a central component of yogic practice that serves as a bridge between conscious and unconscious processes. Through specific breathing techniques, practitioners can directly influence their autonomic nervous system, shifting from sympathetic (stress) activation to parasympathetic (relaxation) dominance (Brown & Gerbarg, 2005). This capacity to consciously regulate the nervous system through breath provides a powerful tool for managing anxiety, depression, and trauma-related symptoms.

Table 1. Comparative Framework of the Three Core Contemplative Practices

Dimension	Mindfulness	Meditation	Yoga
Primary Focus	Present-moment awareness; non-judgmental observation	Attention training, insight, emotional regulation	Body-mind integration through movement, breath, and awareness
Core Components	Awareness of thoughts, emotions, sensations	Focused attention, open monitoring, loving-kindness	Asanas (postures), pranayama (breathing), relaxation
Psychological Mechanisms	Reduces rumination, increases metacognition	Strengthens attention networks, reduces emotional reactivity	Enhances interoception, regulates autonomic nervous system
Neurobiological Effects	Lowers default mode network activity	Increases prefrontal cortex thickness; reduces amygdala volume	Improves vagal tone; balances sympathetic-parasympathetic activity
Evidence-Based Benefits	Decreases anxiety, stress, and negative affect	Improves emotional stability, clarity, and well-being	Reduces depression, PTSD symptoms, and physiological stress markers
Practical Application	Daily awareness practices, MBSR	Seated practice, MBCT, compassion training	Therapeutic yoga, trauma-sensitive yoga, mind-body therapy
Ideal For	Overthinking, stress reactivity	Emotional regulation, cognitive clarity	Somatic distress, tension, trauma stored in the body

The physical yoga positions though often considered a kind of exercise are in fact a highly elaborate psychosomatic integration. All the poses are made to cause particular effects on body and mind, some energize and keep the mind alert whilst others cause relaxation and contemplation (Iyengar, 1995). Mindful awareness when practiced in holding poses fosters not only the physical strengths of power, and flexibility but also fosters mental strengths of patience, acceptance and equanimity. Yoga philosophy, as outlined in classical texts such as Patanjali's Yoga Sutras, provides a comprehensive framework for understanding the nature of human suffering and the path to liberation. The eight-limbed path also incorporates a system of ethics, movement of the body, breathing, withdrawal of the senses, concentration, meditation and finally the condition of union or samadhi (Satchidananda, 1990). This scientific method of human development also provides a road map on how to attend not only the symptoms of the human psyche but also the essential root causes of human ills. The trauma-informed applications of yoga have gained particular attention in recent years, as researchers and clinicians recognize yoga's unique capacity to address trauma stored in the body (van der Kolk, 2014). In contrast to conventional forms of talk therapy, which only focus on involving the mind cognitive process, yoga offers a clear route towards being able to tap into and experience trauma and heal it through body awareness and smooth movements. This approach is particularly valuable for individuals whose trauma is too overwhelming to process through verbal means alone.

PART II: THE HARMONIOUS BLEND - INTEGRATION THEMES

The Synergy of Practice

The integration of mindfulness, meditation, and yoga creates synergistic effects that transcend the sum of their individual benefits. This synergy emerges from the complementary ways these practices address different aspects of human experience while reinforcing common underlying principles of awareness, acceptance, and transformation (Philippot et al., 2002). When practiced together, these modalities create a comprehensive system of mental training that addresses cognitive, emotional, physical, and spiritual dimensions of well-being. Mindfulness provides the foundation of present-moment awareness that enhances both meditative concentration and yogic embodiment. Meditation develops the capacity for sustained attention and emotional regulation that deepens mindful awareness and supports the mental focus required for yoga practice. Yoga cultivates the physical and energetic foundation that supports both sitting meditation and mindful living. The cross-pollination effects between practices are numerous and profound

Figure 1. **The Triad of Transformation Model**

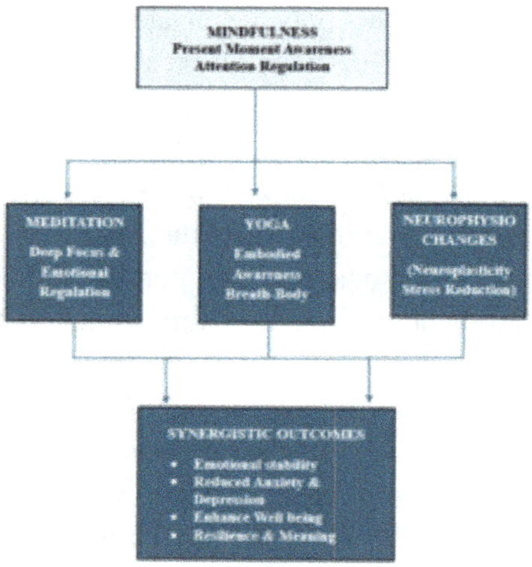

Studies have started to examine the increased advantages of integrated practice strategies. Meta-analysis comparing multi-component mindfulness-yoga interventions with one component interventions have revealed better outcomes in regard to anxiety, depression and general well-being when practices are integrated and exercised instead of when they are in practice in isolation (Sharma et al., 2017). The results can be explained by the fact that the synergistic effect of contemplative practices adds new properties to the ones they have had, which can improve the results of therapy. The integration of consciousness should be considered one of the main results of collective practice. As opposed to cultivating various aspects of awareness separately, a coherent practice cultivates a single continuum of consciousness that brings the cognitive, emotional, and somatic domains of awareness together at once. This combined consciousness turns out to be the source of genuine health and permanent change. It takes both insight and ability to develop coherent series of practice that respect the specific offerings of each modality, and at the same time makes effective use of their synergetic possibilities. Effective integration could start with soft yoga movement to warm up the muscles, followed by the breathing techniques to balance the nervous system, then sitting meditation to stabilise focused awareness, and, finally, mindful movement to bring together mental insights into a living practice.

Pathways to Healing

Mindfulness, meditation, and yoga are integrated practices, which provide several routes of healing that combine the multidimensional nature of psychological suffering. This experience is accomplished systemically, as opposed to the treatment of symptoms one at a time, and aims to change the patterns of consciousness and embodiment that cause mental problems (Pascoe et al., 2017). Itinerary of fragmentation to wholeness is one primary route of healing by contemplative practice. Psychological distress these days is usually based on the fact that we are disconnected with our bodies and our own emotions, as well as our own values and our true self. Each of these disconnections can be addressed in an elaborate, long-term way by experiencing integrated mindfulness, meditation, and yoga, which establishes a route to wholeness and integration. Embodiment Awareness as a means of healing trauma is another important pathway especially since trauma is widespread in mental conditions. The prevalent methods of dealing with traumas usually include a cognitive processing and narrative reconstruction, which is overwhelming to the individuals whose trauma is retained in the body (van der Kolk, 2014). The kind, incarnated process of the integrated contemplative practice is safe journey of discovering and healing trauma through somatic experiencing, mindful movement, and breath awareness.

Resilience and emotional regulation cultivated through contemplative practice work similarly to the formation of what researchers term "emotional granularity", the capacity to differentiate between various emotional states and to react to each of them appropriately (Barrett, 2017). This ability can be cultivated by observing the emotional experience conscientiously through meditation, the awareness of the emotional expression in yoga, and the moment-to- moment management of the emotional reactivity through mindfulness. Self-compassion and acceptance represent fundamental healing factors that are cultivated through all three practices. Mindfulness develops acceptance of present-moment experience without judgment. Meditation cultivates loving-kindness and compassion toward oneself and others. Yoga promotes self-care and acceptance of one's physical limitations and capacities. Together, these practices create a foundation of self-compassion that transforms the inner critic and supports authentic self-acceptance.

The development of meaning and purpose often emerges naturally from sustained contemplative practice as individuals develop greater clarity about their values, priorities, and authentic aspirations. This existential dimension of healing is particularly important for addressing depression and anxiety that stem from a sense of meaninglessness or disconnection from purpose. Neuroplasticity research has revealed that contemplative practices literally reshape the brain in ways that support these healing pathways. Regular practice increases gray matter density in areas associated with learning, memory, and emotional regulation while decreasing activity in networks associated with rumination and self-referential thinking (Luders et al., 2013). These neurological changes provide a biological foundation for the psychological transformation that occurs through contemplative practice.

Table 2. The Triad of Transformation Protocol: A Structured Integrative Model

Stage	Practice Component	Duration	Neuro-Psychological Purpose	Expected Outcomes
1. Grounding	Mindful Breathing	3-5 minutes	Activates prefrontal cortex; reduces arousal	Increased present-moment awareness
2. Embodied Regulation	Gentle Yoga Flow	8-12 minutes	Regulates autonomic nervous system; enhances interoception	Reduced physiological stress; improved body awareness
3. Emotional Stabilization	Focused Attention Meditation	8-10 minutes	Strengthens attention networks; reduces rumination	Greater emotional regulation and calm

Stage	Practice Component	Duration	Neuro-Psychological Purpose	Expected Outcomes
4. Compassion & Integration	Loving-Kindness Meditation	3-5 minutes	Activates compassion circuits; decreases self-criticism	Higher self-acceptance and interpersonal connectedness
5. Daily Real-Life Practice	Informal Mindfulness Activities	Throughout day	Reinforces habit formation; builds resilience	Enhanced well-being, reduced stress response

PART III: LIVING INTEGRATION - CONTEMPORARY APPLICATIONS

Therapeutic Landscapes

Mindfulness, meditation and yoga are emerging in modern therapeutic practice as a paradigm of how to be more holistic and client-centered in considering mental health care. This change signifies the result of an increased appreciation that healing cannot solely be individualized towards reducing symptoms, but it must address the complete person, mind, body and spirit (Siegel, 2010). There is a growing use of contemplative practices in the therapeutic toolbox of mental health professionals resulting in the development of new mixed methods of therapy that integrate conventional therapies with mindfulness-based treatment, meditation training, and yoga therapy. Such integrative models have been especially successful with such matters as anxiety, depression, PTSD, addiction, and persistent pain (Roemer & Orsillo, 2009). The therapeutic evolution has specifically been due to the development of mindfulness-based interventions (MBIs). Mindfulness-Based Stress Reduction (MBSR), Mindfulness-Based Cognitive Therapy (MBCT), and Acceptance and Commitment Therapy (ACT) programs have worked in a manner that has projected contemplative practices as evidence-based interventions to treat a variety of mental health conditions (Hayes et al., 2011). These programs show that ancient practices of wisdom can be effectively transferred into modern treatment settings with preservation of their most important transformative nature.

Yoga therapy has since become a field in itself that keenly involves applying yogic practices and principles toward the wellness of body, mind, and soul. In contrast to yoga classes in general, the yoga therapy is personal and targeted at overcoming particular mental health issues and frequently delivered by experienced yoga practitioners, who are also educated in psychological healing. Studies have revealed yoga therapy to be efficient in management of anxiety, depression, PTSD and other mental disorders. Incorporation of sacred space into clinics is a significant element of the process of contemplative practices in treatment. It includes both the physical environment and the therapeutic relationship, itself, to form a container where thoughts are safe to explore, and vulnerability can be practiced, and change can take place. Many therapists who have begun implementing the contemplative practices have observed that their personal meditation and mindfulness skill may help in boosting their therapeutic presence and efficacy (Germer & Siegel, 2012).

This integration has a very important dimension which is the therapist as contemplative practitioner. What many therapists discover is that not only is their contemplative practice a solid source of support to their own well-being, but it contributes substantively to the development of their clinical abilities, such as their presence, empathy and capacity to hold space of client suffering. This understanding has brought with it more focus on contemplative education to mental health professionals. Mental health training programs are more often beginning to include contemplative elements as mental health professionals begin to understand that effective integration of such practices needs personal experience and understanding. Institutions like the Institute for Meditation and Psychotherapy or the Mindfulness-Based Resilience Training (MBRT), are courses specifically designed in which one can train in contemplative practice and work in the field as a therapist.

Educational Transformation

Institutions of learning at every level are realizing the promise of contemplative practices to counteract the stress levels of students, improve learning as well as emotional intelligence. This acknowledgment has seen the creation of mindfulness-based contemplative educational programs where components of mindfulness, meditation, and yoga are incorporated in educational programs and campus life (Barbezat & Bush, 2014). Stress is an epidemic among students that is becoming a crisis situation as the prevalence of anxiety and depression in college students has skyrocketed during the last ten years (Lederer & Hoban, 2022). Classical academic paradigms that target cognitive development as the only way of learning end up leaving out the emotional and somatic layer of learning, ahead of causing burnout and notable psyche-related issues among the students. Contemplative pedagogy is one of the major transitions in the philosophy of education, addressing the fact that cognitive engagement is not the only aspect of successful learning, as it can all be supported by emotional regulation, somatic knowing, and reflection. This model develops learning climate that helps to nurture the entire student; the mind, body and the soul as opposed to solely concentrating on the mind (Palmer, 2010).

The schools with mindfulness programs have demonstrated great success in enhancing students with more attention, emotional control, better grades and at the same time less anxiety and behavioral disorders (Zenner et al., 2014). There are also programs like Mindful Schools and Learning to BREATHE which have been used in thousands of schools across the world and offer evidence-based strategies of introducing mindfulness in classrooms. Educational yoga programs have also revealed great gains on the well-being and academic performance of the students. Yoga in schools has been proved to enhance attention and decrease anxiety and assist emotional management in students of any age group (Butzer et al., 2015). The programs usually incorporate physical postures along with breathing exercises and relaxation, and allow students to develop practical mechanisms of stress management and promotion of well-being. One of the most innovative developments has been in the expression of contemplative practices at the college level as universities increasingly create courses, programs and even majors in contemplative studies. The Association for Contemplative Mind in Higher Education supports faculty and administrators in integrating contemplative practices into academic life, providing resources and training for effective implementation.

The idea of creating mindful learning environments implies but cannot be reduced to introducing contemplative practices into existing curricula, or to a conceptual re-framing/reenvisaging learning as such. In contemplative education we understand learning to be, essentially, transformation and provide learning environments conducive to a profound inner reflection, real inquiry, and personal development. The empirical studies on contemplative education revealed that those students who engaged into mindfulness and meditation programs exhibit higher academic achievements, lower levels of stress and increased levels of emotional well-being (Shapiro et al., 2011). Such advantages are not confined to the academic environment but the students learn skills in life that help them become successful in general.

Workplace Wellness Revolution

Utilization of contemplative practices in the workplace is probably one of the greatest breakthroughs in modern-day wellness programs. Companies all around the world are finding that mindfulness training, meditation, and yoga classes in the workplace are improving employee health and effectiveness, to the point where people are now referring to the trend as a "workplace wellness revolution" (Gelles, 2015). There is a strong business reason to include contemplative programs in the workplace, as the studies revealed that such programs have the potential to help decrease the number of healthcare expenditures, reduce the level of sick days, increase employee engagement, and boost productivity (Virgili, 2015). Major corporations like Google, Intel, and Salesforce have introduced full-scale mindfulness programs that have become the paradigm to other organizations that want to take care of their employees. Workplace stress has become epidemic, with surveys showing that most workers cite high levels of stress that has impacted their health and relationships and work performance.

The mindfulness-based systems at the workplace usually consist of meditation teaching, stress-management training, and mindful communication training. The programs assist the employees to develop a greater level of emotional control, enhanced focus, and resilience to manage the challenges at the workplace. A study has determined that workers engaged in use of mindfulness programs at work have noted minimized stress levels, job pleasure, and enhanced work-life balance (Jamieson & Tuckey, 2017). Yoga in the work places has also become popular with organizations realizing the importance of giving their employees a chance to stretch their muscles and relieve themselves of stress in the course of the day through exercises. Such programs usually contain some kind of gentle stretching, breathing programs, and relaxation exercises that may be done in the office. The research has indicated that yoga sessions in the workplace can lead to the decrease in workplace stress, promotion of good physical health as well as well-being (Hartfiel et al., 2011).

The development of leadership on the basis of the contemplative practices has been a hot topic in the field of organizational studies since the organizations realized that mindfulness can support their leaderships in making decisions in benefit of the organizations and can also improve their communication and build better organizational cultures. Combined traditional leadership training and contemplative practices have been found promising where leaders can become more present, authentic, and effective through such programs (Boyatzis & McKee, 2005). The role of economics of employee well-being has gained prominence as institutions are now appreciating the financial advantage of employee mental health investment. In some studies, it has been indicated that wellness programs such as contemplative practice at the workplace may have a high payback with lowered medical expenses, minimized workforce turnover, and higher availability (Baicker et al., 2010).

PART IV: THE EXPANDING HORIZON - FUTURE LANDSCAPES

Cultural Integration and Global Adaptation

Spreading contemplative practices across the globe offers uniquely potential and challenging opportunities as the traditionally Eastern practice needs to be changed to fit to various cultural setting, keeping its fundamental integrity intact. In this process of cultural integration, issues of authenticity, appropriation and adaptation have to be pursued keenly (Hickey, 2010). Adhering to the old traditions and moving towards the innovation is the main conflict of the modern contemplative movement. As much as one would want to retain wisdom and integrity of traditional practices, it would be a great fault not to keep such practices open, applicable and inclusive to various populations and modern settings. Such a balance needs continuous communication between the traditional teachers and the modern practitioners, researchers, and clinicians. Such a process demands profound respect of the traditional teachings combined with the understanding of the necessity of cultural translation and adaptations. (Purser et al., 2013). The concept of structuring wisdom traditions bridges is an opportunity to make more inclusive and holistic of contemplative methods. Instead of considering the various traditions as mutually exclusive, there is an increasing awareness that different traditions of contemplation can be seen as complimentary and compatible such that they can be respectfully and effectively combined.

Culturally adapted contemplative interventions development has emerged as an active research and development subject. To illustrate, scholars have created programs about mindfulness specifically targeted to Latino populations, African American populations, and other cultural groups because interventions have to be culturally appropriate and relevant (Dutton et al., 2013). To make contemplative spaces more inclusive through the creation of inclusive contemplative communities, concerns relating to issues of diversity, equity, and inclusion should be addressed continuously. This involves overcoming access barriers, including price and cultural representation, and opening up friendly places to the persons of diverse backgrounds and identities. The issues of cultural humility around contemplative practice is the understanding that Western-based practitioners and teachers have little or no insights into the cultural background where the practices are established. Such a modesty can lead to the development of more respectful and natural interaction with contemplative traditions as well as promote true learning and change.

Technology and Transformation

The nexus of technology and contemplative practice is among the most vibrant fields of modern development presenting not only new unprecedented opportunities in access and delivery, but also posing essential questions to the traditional ways of practice implementation (Berthon & Pitt, 2019). Online channels have become a game-changer when it comes to exposure and availability of practices based in contemplation, and about one in every four people all around the world utilizes smartphone applications to aid the process of meditation with products like Headspace, Calm, and Insight Timer standing out as the most dominant. These platforms have democratized access to contemplative practices, making them available to individuals who might not otherwise have access to in-person instruction or community support. Most of the research studies have evaluated the effectiveness of the use of digital contemplative interventions, and especially the app-based mindfulness programs have been found to have great advantages in the reduction of anxiety, depression, and stress (Flett et al., 2019). Nevertheless, it is unclear how effective digital interventions are in the long term in comparison with face-to-face instructions and in community-based practice.

The virtual reality (VR) technology has expanded the horizons of contemplative practice, providing the immersive environments which are capable of facilitating the processes of meditation and mindfulness training. VR meditation experiences may allow giving the user a peaceful natural setting or visualization which can increase and sharpen the depth and quality of practice. The area of VR-based contemplative interventions is still new and demonstrates positive outcomes of research (Navarro-Haro et al., 2017). Artificial intelligence (AI) and machine learning technologies are at the stage of just being applied to contemplative practices where the content of the contemplative practice may be personified with respect to the needs, preferences, and improvement of the individual. Meditation apps that utilize AI can learn the behavior and would be able to deliver personalized lessons that grow along with the training of the practitioner. The issue of technological authenticity in delivery has been an impeding issue in the contemplative community. Although technology can offer great support to the practice, it is feared that digital provision might erode deepness and transformative capacity found in the ancient contemplation courses. Creating solutions that will keep a necessary essence of contemplative practice and take advantage of technological possibilities is still a challenge.

Research and Understanding

Billions of religious believers have experienced significant changes in the contemplative science over the last few decades, as scholars have used scientific techniques rigorously to study how and why contemplative practices work. The study has confirmed numerous historical assertions regarding the positive effects of meditation, mindfulness and yoga in addition to unearthing some fresh knowledge regarding their transformative properties (Davidson & Lutz, 2008). The neuroplasticity studies have been of key use to determine scientific validity of the contemplative practices. Studies using neuroimaging techniques have shown that meditation and mindfulness practice produce measurable changes in brain structure and function. This includes increased gray matter density in areas associated with attention, emotional regulation, and self-awareness (Luders et al., 2013).

Measurement of contemplative practices and effects has been a substantial obstacle in the domain since reliable and valid scales are yet to be developed. The conventional science metrics might fail to measure the perceptual and the intriguing impacts of contemplative practice, prompting scientists to come up with new evaluation processes that are more attuned to the contemplation effects (Baer et al., 2008). Study of the mechanisms of contemplative practices has identified several routes by which such practices result in well-being, such as altering the quality of attention, emotional processing, self-awareness, and compassion. These mechanisms may play a vital role in the interpretation of how the therapeutic use of contemplative practices works and how interventions can be improved. Investigations into exceptional contemplative practitioners, including long term meditators and advanced yoga practitioners, has offered clues into the pinnacle of the contemplative development. The study on such people has uncovered extraordinary abilities in terms of attention, emotional control and pain tolerance, which points to the profound power of long-term contemplative training (Lutz et al., 2004).

The future directions in contemplative research are the exploration of the dosage and timing of the contemplative interventions, personal differences in the reactions to the contemplative practices and the use of contemplative practices in special populations and conditions. There is also growing interest in studying the social and cultural dimensions of contemplative practice and their relationship to individual outcomes. The integration of contemplative practice and scientific inquiry represents a unique collaboration between ancient wisdom traditions and modern scientific methods. This partnership can enhance our knowledge of human consciousness, wellbeing, potential and confirm and conserve previous contemplative knowledge.

Synthesis and Future Directions

The study of mindfulness, meditation, and yoga as holistic practices of contemplation demonstrate that they have great potential in managing the mental health challenges of our era. These practices are synergistically combined to develop the holistic model of well-being, which focuses on cognitive, emotional, physical, and spiritual levels of human experience. The data provided in the present chapter proves that contemplative practice provides appropriate, accessible, and sustainable methods of mental health improvement. The introduction of these practices to therapeutic, educative and working environments creates a major paradigm shift towards the more holistic, prevention-focused mindset of approaching mental care. The future of contemplative practices in mental health enhancement lies in continued integration across multiple domains, including healthcare, education, workplace wellness, and community programs. Such inclusion needs continued cooperation among traditional contemplative teachers, modern practitioners, scholars and medical workers.

Technologically advanced and culturally sensitive methods of contemplative practice development will be essential to accessing a wide range of people and making it as accessible as possible. This involves developing programs, which respect classical knowledge but meet modern needs as well as realities. Research will remain crucial in confirming and improving the contemplative approaches to the improvement of mental health. Research in the future needs to aim at comprehending ideal implementation plans, discovering individual variation in reaction to contemplative practices, and examining long-run consequences of compound contemplative intervention.

Limitations and Future Considerations

Although the triad of mindfulness, meditation, and yoga offers a powerful integrative framework for mental health enhancement, certain limitations must be acknowledged. Individual differences in readiness, trauma history, and physical capacity may influence outcomes. Some individuals may experience emotional discomfort when confronting internal experiences during meditation or may be at risk of injury during yoga without proper instruction. Cultural sensitivity is also essential, as these practices originate from rich philosophical traditions that must be respectfully represented in contemporary applications. Despite these considerations, the triad remains a promising, adaptable, and evidence-supported model. Future research should refine standardized protocols, explore long-term effects, and examine culturally tailored adaptations.

CONCLUSION

Mindfulness, meditation, yoga the three-part golden standard of ancient wisdom carried out with modern knowledge is at the service of human flourishing. These practices do not just alleviate symptoms, they also represent means of gaining access to radical change in our relations with ourselves, with others and the surrounding world. Contemplative practices in the modern mental health care system bring us full circle by rediscovering the wholeness of human beings instead of looking at them as a combination of symptoms to eliminate. This comprehensive model acknowledges the fact that true healing needs to be holistic in nature and sustainable well-being can be achieved through the development of a conscious mind and awareness, compassion and wisdom. The wisdom of contemplative practice provides the tools that we need to encounter the uncertainty and difficulties that lie ahead, and to strategize the approach to them, as well as the resilience needed to be ready to do that. Further popularization of mindfulness, meditation, and yoga in the field of mainstream healthcare, education, and the wider society is a tremendous potential to deal with the root causes of human suffering as well as enhancing authentic thriving.

The change that this contemplative practice yields is bigger than personal healing as it goes further to the communal level and the building of more conscious, compassionate societies. This holistic method of psychological well-being has given us a chance to not only heal psychological suffering, but also develop the intelligence, and open hearts we need to build a happier and kinder world. Contemplative practice is eventually a gradual path to wholeness, genuineness, and relationality. The more people and groups pursue these practices, the faster we advance toward attaining the vision of the world in which human beings will live more consciously, empathically, and much wiser. Such a change is not only a therapeutic process; it is also a radical reorganization of human consciousness that can solve the most serious problems of modern life.

REFERENCES

Baer, R. A., Smith, G. T., Lykins, E., Button, D., Krietemeyer, J., Sauer, S., Walsh, E., Duggan, D., & Williams, J. M. G. (2008). Construct validity of the five-facet mindfulness questionnaire in meditating and nonmeditating samples. *Assessment, 15*(3), 329–342. DOI: 10.1177/1073191107313003 PMID: 18310597

Baicker, K., Cutler, D., & Song, Z. (2010). Workplace wellness programs can generate savings. *Health Affairs (Project Hope), 29*(2), 304–311. DOI: 10.1377/hlthaff.2009.0626 PMID: 20075081

Barbezat, D. P., & Bush, M. (2014). *Contemplative practices in higher education: Powerful methods to transform teaching and learning* (pp. xxiii, 231). Jossey-Bass/Wiley.

Barrett, L. F. (2017). *How emotions are made: The secret life of the brain* (pp. xv, 425). Houghton Mifflin Harcourt.

Baumeister, R. F., Vohs, K. D., Aaker, J. L., & Garbinsky, E. N. (2013). Some key differences between a happy life and a meaningful life. *The Journal of Positive Psychology, 8*(6), 505–516. DOI: 10.1080/17439760.2013.830764

Berthon, P. R., & Pitt, L. F. (2019). Types of mindfulness in an age of digital distraction. *Business Horizons, 62*(2), 131–137. DOI: 10.1016/j.bushor.2018.10.003

Boyatzis, R., & McKee, A. (2005). *Resonant Leadership: Renewing Yourself and Connecting with Others Through Mindfulness, Hope and CompassionCompassion.* Harvard Business Press.

Brown, R. P., & Gerbarg, P. L. (2005). Sudarshan Kriya yogic breathing in the treatment of stress, anxiety, and depression: Part I-neurophysiologic model. *Journal of Alternative and Complementary Medicine (New York, N.Y.), 11*(1), 189–201. DOI: 10.1089/acm.2005.11.189 PMID: 15750381

Butzer, B., Ebert, M., Telles, S., & Khalsa, S. B. S. (2015). School-based Yoga Programs in the United States: A Survey. *Advances in Mind-Body Medicine, 29*(4), 18–26. PMID: 26535474

Cacioppo, J. T., & Cacioppo, S. (2018). The growing problem of loneliness. *Lancet, 391*(10119), 426. DOI: 10.1016/S0140-6736(18)30142-9 PMID: 29407030

Chessick, C. (2007). The Mindful Brain: Reflection and Attunement in the Cultivation of Well-Being. *The American Journal of Psychiatry, 164*(10), 1619–1620. DOI: 10.1176/appi.ajp.2007.07081292 PMID: 22688157

Cramer, H., Lauche, R., Langhorst, J., & Dobos, G. (2013a). Yoga for depression: A systematic review and meta-analysis. *Depression and Anxiety*, *30*(11), 1068–1083. DOI: 10.1002/da.22166 PMID: 23922209

Cramer, H., Lauche, R., Langhorst, J., & Dobos, G. (2013b). Yoga for depression: A systematic review and meta-analysis. *Depression and Anxiety*, *30*(11), 1068–1083. DOI: 10.1002/da.22166 PMID: 23922209

Cuijpers, P., Karyotaki, E., Weitz, E., Andersson, G., Hollon, S. D., & van Straten, A. (2014). The effects of psychotherapies for major depression in adults on remission, recovery and improvement: A meta-analysis. *Journal of Affective Disorders*, *159*, 118–126. DOI: 10.1016/j.jad.2014.02.026 PMID: 24679399

Davidson, R. J., & Lutz, A. (2008). Buddha's Brain: Neuroplasticity and Meditation. *IEEE Signal Processing Magazine*, *25*(1), 176–174. DOI: 10.1109/MSP.2008.4431873 PMID: 20871742

Dutton, M. A., Bermudez, D., Matas, A., Majid, H., & Myers, N. L. (2013). Mindfulness-Based Stress Reduction for Low-Income, Predominantly African American Women With PTSD and a History of Intimate Partner Violence. *Cognitive and Behavioral Practice*, *20*(1), 23–32. DOI: 10.1016/j.cbpra.2011.08.003 PMID: 24043922

Engel, G. L. (1977). The need for a new medical model: A challenge for biomedicine. *Science*, *196*(4286), 129–136. DOI: 10.1126/science.847460 PMID: 847460

Feuerstein, G. (2008). *The Yoga Tradition: Its History, Literature, Philosophy, and Practice*. Hohm Press.

Flett, J. A. M., Hayne, H., Riordan, B. C., Thompson, L. M., & Conner, T. S. (2019). Mobile mindfulness meditation: A randomised controlled trial of the effect of two popular apps on mental health. *Mindfulness*, *10*(5), 863–876. DOI: 10.1007/s12671-018-1050-9

Frankl, V. E. (1963). *Man's search for meaning: An introduction to logotherapy*. Washington Square Press.

GBD 2019 Mental Disorders Collaborators. (2022). Global, regional, and national burden of 12 mental disorders in 204 countries and territories, 1990-2019: A systematic analysis for the Global Burden of Disease Study 2019. *The Lancet Psychiatry*, *9*(2), 137-150. DOI: 10.1016/S2215-0366(21)00395-3

Gelles, D. (2015). *Mindful work: How meditation is changing business from the inside out*. Houghton Mifflin Harcourt.

Germer, C. K., & Siegel, R. D. (2012). *Wisdom and Compassion in Psychotherapy: Deepening Mindfulness in Clinical Practice*. Guilford Press.

Ghaemi, S. N. (2009). The rise and fall of the biopsychosocial model. *The British Journal of Psychiatry, 195*(1), 3–4. DOI: 10.1192/bjp.bp.109.063859 PMID: 19567886

Goldstein, J. (2013). *Mindfulness: A Practical Guide to Awakening*. Sounds True.

Goyal, M., Singh, S., Sibinga, E. M. S., Gould, N. F., Rowland-Seymour, A., Sharma, R., Berger, Z., Sleicher, D., Maron, D. D., Shihab, H. M., Ranasinghe, P. D., Linn, S., Saha, S., Bass, E. B., & Haythornthwaite, J. A. (2014). Meditation programs for psychological stress and well-being: A systematic review and meta-analysis. *JAMA Internal Medicine, 174*(3), 357–368. DOI: 10.1001/jamainternmed.2013.13018 PMID: 24395196

Gross, J. J. (2002). Emotion regulation: Affective, cognitive, and social consequences. *Psychophysiology, 39*(3), 281–291. DOI: 10.1017/S0048577201393198 PMID: 12212647

Hartfiel, N., Havenhand, J., Khalsa, S. B., Clarke, G., & Krayer, A. (2011). The effectiveness of yoga for the improvement of well-being and resilience to stress in the workplace. *Scandinavian Journal of Work, Environment & Health, 37*(1), 70–76. DOI: 10.5271/sjweh.2916 PMID: 20369218

Hayes, S. C., Luoma, J. B., Bond, F. W., Masuda, A., & Lillis, J. (2006a). Acceptance and commitment therapy: Model, processes and outcomes. *Behaviour Research and Therapy, 44*(1), 1–25. DOI: 10.1016/j.brat.2005.06.006 PMID: 16300724

Hayes, S. C., Luoma, J. B., Bond, F. W., Masuda, A., & Lillis, J. (2006b). Acceptance and commitment therapy: Model, processes and outcomes. *Behaviour Research and Therapy, 44*(1), 1–25. DOI: 10.1016/j.brat.2005.06.006 PMID: 16300724

Hayes, S. C., Villatte, M., Levin, M., & Hildebrandt, M. (2011). Open, aware, and active: Contextual approaches as an emerging trend in the behavioral and cognitive therapies. *Annual Review of Clinical Psychology, 7*(1), 141–168. DOI: 10.1146/annurev-clinpsy-032210-104449 PMID: 21219193

Hickey, W. S. (2010). Meditation as Medicine: A Critique. *Cross Currents, 60*(2), 168–184. DOI: 10.1111/j.1939-3881.2010.00118.x

Hofmann, S. G., Grossman, P., & Hinton, D. E. (2011). Loving-kindness and compassion meditation: Potential for psychological interventions. *Clinical Psychology Review, 31*(7), 1126–1132. DOI: 10.1016/j.cpr.2011.07.003 PMID: 21840289

Hofmann, S. G., Sawyer, A. T., Witt, A. A., & Oh, D. (2010). The effect of mindfulness-based therapy on anxiety and depression: A meta-analytic review. *Journal of Consulting and Clinical Psychology, 78*(2), 169–183. DOI: 10.1037/a0018555 PMID: 20350028

Iyengar, B. K. S. (1995). *Light on Yoga: The Bible of Modern Yoga - Its Philosophy and Practice - By the World's Foremost Teacher*. Knopf Doubleday Publishing Group.

Jamieson, S. D., & Tuckey, M. R. (2017). Mindfulness interventions in the workplace: A critique of the current state of the literature. *Journal of Occupational Health Psychology, 22*(2), 180–193. DOI: 10.1037/ocp0000048 PMID: 27643606

Kabat-Zinn, J. (1994). *Wherever You Go, There You Are: Mindfulness Meditation in Everyday Life*. Hachette Books.

Kabat-Zinn, J. (2003). Mindfulness-Based Interventions in Context: Past, Present, and Future. *Clinical Psychology : a Publication of the Division of Clinical Psychology of the American Psychological Association, 10*(2), 144–156. DOI: 10.1093/clipsy.bpg016

Keyes, C. L. M. (2002). The mental health continuum: From languishing to flourishing in life. *Journal of Health and Social Behavior, 43*(2), 207–222. DOI: 10.2307/3090197 PMID: 12096700

Khoury, B., Sharma, M., Rush, S. E., & Fournier, C. (2015). Mindfulness-based stress reduction for healthy individuals: A meta-analysis. *Journal of Psychosomatic Research, 78*(6), 519–528. DOI: 10.1016/j.jpsychores.2015.03.009 PMID: 25818837

Kornfield, J. (with Internet Archive). (2008). *The wise heart: A guide to the universal teachings of Buddhist psychology*. New York : Bantam Books. http://archive.org/details/wiseheartguideto0000korn_q5q7

Lederer, A. M., & Hoban, M. T. (2022). The development of the American College Health Association-National College Health Assessment III: An improved tool to assess and enhance the health and well-being of college students. *Journal of American College Health, 70*(6), 1606–1610. DOI: 10.1080/07448481.2020.1834401 PMID: 33400616

Luders, E., Thompson, P. M., Kurth, F., Hong, J.-Y., Phillips, O. R., Wang, Y., Gutman, B. A., Chou, Y.-Y., Narr, K. L., & Toga, A. W. (2013). Global and regional alterations of hippocampal anatomy in long-term meditation practitioners. *Human Brain Mapping, 34*(12), 3369–3375. DOI: 10.1002/hbm.22153 PMID: 22815233

Luders, E., Toga, A. W., Lepore, N., & Gaser, C. (2009). The underlying anatomical correlates of long-term meditation: Larger hippocampal and frontal volumes of gray matter. *NeuroImage*, *45*(3), 672–678. DOI: 10.1016/j.neuroimage.2008.12.061 PMID: 19280691

Lutz, A., Greischar, L. L., Rawlings, N. B., Ricard, M., & Davidson, R. J. (2004). Long-term meditators self-induce high-amplitude gamma synchrony during mental practice. *Proceedings of the National Academy of Sciences of the United States of America*, *101*(46), 16369–16373. DOI: 10.1073/pnas.0407401101 PMID: 15534199

Lutz, A., Slagter, H. A., Dunne, J. D., & Davidson, R. J. (2008a). Attention regulation and monitoring in meditation. *Trends in Cognitive Sciences*, *12*(4), 163–169. DOI: 10.1016/j.tics.2008.01.005 PMID: 18329323

Lutz, A., Slagter, H. A., Dunne, J. D., & Davidson, R. J. (2008b). Attention regulation and monitoring in meditation. *Trends in Cognitive Sciences*, *12*(4), 163–169. DOI: 10.1016/j.tics.2008.01.005 PMID: 18329323

Mahoney, M. J. (2003). *Constructive Psychotherapy: A Practical Guide*. Guilford Press.

Mehta, N. (2011). Mind-body Dualism: A critique from a Health Perspective. *Mens Sana Monographs*, *9*(1), 202–209. DOI: 10.4103/0973-1229.77436 PMID: 21694971

Navarro-Haro, M. V., López-Del-Hoyo, Y., Campos, D., Linehan, M. M., Hoffman, H. G., García-Palacios, A., Modrego-Alarcón, M., Borao, L., & García-Campayo, J. (2017). Meditation experts try Virtual Reality Mindfulness: A pilot study evaluation of the feasibility and acceptability of Virtual Reality to facilitate mindfulness practice in people attending a Mindfulness conference. *PLoS One*, *12*(11), e0187777. DOI: 10.1371/journal.pone.0187777 PMID: 29166665

Neff, K. (with Internet Archive). (2011). *Self-compassion: The proven power of being kind to yourself*. New York : William Morrow. http://archive.org/details/selfcompassionpr0000neff

Palmer, P. J. (with Internet Archive). (2010). *The heart of higher education: A call to renewal : transforming the academy through collegial conversations*. San Francisco : Jossey-Bass. http://archive.org/details/heartofhigheredu0000palm

Pascoe, M. C., Thompson, D. R., & Ski, C. F. (2017). Yoga, mindfulness-based stress reduction and stress-related physiological measures: A meta-analysis. *Psychoneuroendocrinology*, *86*, 152–168. DOI: 10.1016/j.psyneuen.2017.08.008 PMID: 28963884

Philippot, P., Chapelle, G., & Blairy, S. (2002). Respiratory feedback in the generation of emotion. *Cognition and Emotion, 16*(5), 605–627. DOI: 10.1080/02699930143000392

Primack, B. A., Shensa, A., Sidani, J. E., Whaite, E. O., Lin, L. Y., Rosen, D., Colditz, J. B., Radovic, A., & Miller, E. (2017). Social Media Use and Perceived Social Isolation Among Young Adults in the U.S. *American Journal of Preventive Medicine, 53*(1), 1–8. DOI: 10.1016/j.amepre.2017.01.010 PMID: 28279545

Purser, R., & Order, C. P. is a professor of management at S. F. S. U. H. is an ordained teacher in the K. B. T., Cranks, co-host of the podcast T. M., Loy, D., & Teacher, C. (2013, July 1). *Beyond McMindfulness*. HuffPost. https://www.huffpost.com/entry/beyond-mcmindfulness_b_3519289

Putnam, R. D. (2000). *Bowling alone: The collapse and revival of American community*. Touchstone Books/Simon & Schuster., DOI: 10.1145/358916.361990

Roemer, L., & Orsillo, S. M. (2009). *Mindfulness- and acceptance-based behavioral therapies in practice* (pp. xii, 244). The Guilford Press.

Rush, A. J., Trivedi, M. H., Wisniewski, S. R., Nierenberg, A. A., Stewart, J. W., Warden, D., Niederehe, G., Thase, M. E., Lavori, P. W., Lebowitz, B. D., McGrath, P. J., Rosenbaum, J. F., Sackeim, H. A., Kupfer, D. J., Luther, J., & Fava, M. (2006). Acute and longer-term outcomes in depressed outpatients requiring one or several treatment steps: A STAR*D report. *The American Journal of Psychiatry, 163*(11), 1905–1917. DOI: 10.1176/ajp.2006.163.11.1905 PMID: 17074942

Santomauro, D. F., Mantilla Herrera, A. M., Shadid, J., Zheng, P., Ashbaugh, C., Pigott, D. M., Abbafati, C., Adolph, C., Amlag, J. O., Aravkin, A. Y., Bang-Jensen, B. L., Bertolacci, G. J., Bloom, S. S., Castellano, R., Castro, E., Chakrabarti, S., Chattopadhyay, J., Cogen, R. M., Collins, J. K., & Ferrari, A. J. (2021). Global prevalence and burden of depressive and anxiety disorders in 204 countries and territories in 2020 due to the COVID-19 pandemic. *Lancet, 398*(10312), 1700–1712. DOI: 10.1016/S0140-6736(21)02143-7 PMID: 34634250

Satchidananda, S. (with Internet Archive). (1990). *The yoga sutras of Patanjali*. Yogaville, Va.: Integral Yoga Publications. http://archive.org/details/yogasutrasofpata0000satc

Schneiderman, N., Ironson, G., & Siegel, S. D. (2005). STRESS AND HEALTH: Psychological, Behavioral, and Biological Determinants. *Annual Review of Clinical Psychology, 1*(1), 607–628. DOI: 10.1146/annurev.clinpsy.1.102803.144141 PMID: 17716101

Sedlmeier, P., Eberth, J., Schwarz, M., Zimmermann, D., Haarig, F., Jaeger, S., & Kunze, S. (2012). The psychological effects of meditation: A meta-analysis. *Psychological Bulletin, 138*(6), 1139–1171. DOI: 10.1037/a0028168 PMID: 22582738

Segal, Z. V., Williams, J. M. G., & Teasdale, J. D. (2002). *Mindfulness-based cognitive therapy for depression: A new approach to preventing relapse* (pp. xiv, 351). Guilford Press.

Shapiro, S. L., Brown, K. W., & Astin, J. (2011). Toward the integration of meditation into higher education: A review of research evidence. *Teachers College Record, 113*(3), 493–528. DOI: 10.1177/016146811111300306

Sharma, A., Barrett, M. S., Cucchiara, A. J., Gooneratne, N. S., & Thase, M. E. (2017). A Breathing-Based Meditation Intervention for Patients With Major Depressive Disorder Following Inadequate Response to Antidepressants: A Randomized Pilot Study. *The Journal of Clinical Psychiatry, 78*(1), e59–e63. DOI: 10.4088/JCP.16m10819 PMID: 27898207

Siegel, D. J. (2010). *Mindsight: The new science of personal transformation* (pp. xviii, 314). Bantam Books.

Stone, L. (2008, July 24). Continuous Partial Attention—Not the Same as Multi-Tasking. *Bloomberg.Com*. https://www.bloomberg.com/news/articles/2008-07-23/continuous-partial-attention-not-the-same-as-multi-tasking

Suls, J., & Rothman, A. (2004). Evolution of the biopsychosocial model: Prospects and challenges for health psychology. *Health Psychology: Official Journal of the Division of Health Psychology, American Psychological Association, 23*(2), 119–125. DOI: 10.1037/0278-6133.23.2.119 PMID: 15008654

Tang, Y.-Y., Hölzel, B. K., & Posner, M. I. (2015). The neuroscience of mindfulness meditation. *Nature Reviews. Neuroscience, 16*(4), 213–225. DOI: 10.1038/nrn3916 PMID: 25783612

Teasdale, J. D., Moore, R. G., Hayhurst, H., Pope, M., Williams, S., & Segal, Z. V. (2002). Metacognitive awareness and prevention of relapse in depression: Empirical evidence. *Journal of Consulting and Clinical Psychology, 70*(2), 275–287. DOI: 10.1037/0022-006X.70.2.275 PMID: 11952186

Twenge, J. M., & Campbell, W. K. (2018). Associations between screen time and lower psychological well-being among children and adolescents: Evidence from a population-based study. *Preventive Medicine Reports, 12*, 271–283. DOI: 10.1016/j.pmedr.2018.10.003 PMID: 30406005

Uebelacker, L. A., Epstein-Lubow, G., Gaudiano, B. A., Tremont, G., Battle, C. L., & Miller, I. W. (2010). Hatha yoga for depression: Critical review of the evidence for efficacy, plausible mechanisms of action, and directions for future research. *Journal of Psychiatric Practice, 16*(1), 22–33. DOI: 10.1097/01.pra.0000367775.88388.96 PMID: 20098228

Vago, D. R., & Silbersweig, D. A. (2012). Self-awareness, self-regulation, and self-transcendence (S-ART): A framework for understanding the neurobiological mechanisms of mindfulness. *Frontiers in Human Neuroscience, 6*, 296. DOI: 10.3389/fnhum.2012.00296 PMID: 23112770

van der Kolk, B. A. (2014). *The body keeps the score: Brain, mind, and body in the healing of trauma* (pp. xvi, 443). Viking.

Vigo, D., Thornicroft, G., & Atun, R. (2016). Estimating the true global burden of mental illness. *The Lancet. Psychiatry, 3*(2), 171–178. DOI: 10.1016/S2215-0366(15)00505-2 PMID: 26851330

Virgili, M. (2015). Mindfulness-Based Interventions Reduce Psychological Distress in Working Adults: A Meta-Analysis of Intervention Studies. *Mindfulness, 6*(2), 326–337. DOI: 10.1007/s12671-013-0264-0

Watkins, E., & Teasdale, J. D. (2004). Adaptive and maladaptive self-focus in depression. *Journal of Affective Disorders, 82*(1), 1–8. DOI: 10.1016/j.jad.2003.10.006 PMID: 15465571

Wells, A. (2000). *Emotional disorders and metacognition: Innovative cognitive therapy* (pp. ix, 236). John Wiley & Sons Ltd.

Williams, A. (2020). Twenge, J. M. (2017). iGen: Why Today's Super-Connected Kids Are Growing Up Less Rebellious, More Tolerant, Less Happy and Completely Unprepared for Adulthood. New York, NY: Atria. ISBN: 978-1-5011-5201-6 paperback. 342 pp. *Family and Consumer Sciences Research Journal, 48*(3), 290–293. DOI: 10.1111/fcsr.12345

World Health Organization. (2017). *Depression and Other Common Mental Disorders.* https://www.who.int/publications/i/item/depression-global-health-estimates

World Health Organization. (2022). *World mental health report: Transforming mental health for all.* https://www.who.int/publications/i/item/9789240049338

Xiong, J., Lipsitz, O., Nasri, F., Lui, L. M. W., Gill, H., Phan, L., Chen-Li, D., Iacobucci, M., Ho, R., Majeed, A., & McIntyre, R. S. (2020). Impact of COVID-19 pandemic on mental health in the general population: A systematic review. *Journal of Affective Disorders, 277*, 55–64. DOI: 10.1016/j.jad.2020.08.001 PMID: 32799105

Zenner, C., Herrnleben-Kurz, S., & Walach, H. (2014). Mindfulness-based interventions in schools-a systematic review and meta-analysis. *Frontiers in Psychology*, *5*, 603. DOI: 10.3389/fpsyg.2014.00603 PMID: 25071620

Zylowska, L., Ackerman, D. L., Yang, M. H., Futrell, J. L., Horton, N. L., Hale, T. S., Pataki, C., & Smalley, S. L. (2008). Mindfulness meditation training in adults and adolescents with ADHD: A feasibility study. *Journal of Attention Disorders*, *11*(6), 737–746. DOI: 10.1177/1087054707308502 PMID: 18025249

Chapter 10
Undulations:
The Flow of Breath and Emotions

Shreya Bakshi
http://orcid.org/0009-0009-8365-8177
Amity University, Noida, India

ABSTRACT

Breath and emotion are intricately connected, forming continuous waves that shape our inner experiences and outward expressions. This chapter explores the physiological, psychological, and cultural ties between breathing patterns and emotional states, demonstrating how breath acts as both a mirror and a regulator of emotion. Insights from neuroscience, somatic psychology, and cultural traditions reveal that conscious breath practices—such as mindfulness, breathwork, and pranayama—enhance emotional resilience, interoceptive awareness, and self-regulation. Breath also holds symbolic significance in art, literature, and spiritual traditions, where it serves as a non-verbal language of expression and transformation. By developing breath literacy—the awareness and intentional modulation of breathing—we gain tools not only for personal well-being but also for fostering presence, connection, and adaptability in a fast-paced world. Ultimately, breath emerges as a tide, guiding us back to equilibrium amidst life's emotional undulations.

1. INTRODUCTION – THE PULSE OF BEING

When asked about the meaning of life, we often find ourselves caught in a timeless existential warp. How does one define life? Is it the body? Is it the mind? Family? Job? Accomplishment? Or, is it a combination of everything and yet nothing? We find ourselves in this corollary, not realizing that the very act of pondering, is evidence of life in its fundamental sense. All movements and functions that symbolize life

DOI: 10.4018/979-8-3373-4187-3.ch010

are dynamic in nature. This dynamism is sustained by energy and all human energy is transformed and consumed by the very vital process of breathing.

Breath is the first and the last wave of our existence — the subtle undulation that marks the rhythm of life itself. It is a tide within, flowing in and out, invisible yet felt, shaping the contours of our physical being and the landscapes of our emotions. To breathe is to be alive, and to be alive is to move through shifting currents of feeling. These undulations—between inhale and exhale, between tension and release, between fear and calm—form an intimate dance that threads through our body and mind.

In this chapter, the intertwined rhythms of breath and emotion are explored, delving into how these flows are not separate streams but reciprocal waves that inform, modulate, and sometimes disrupt each other. "Undulations" serves as a metaphor that captures both the physiological oscillations of breath and the mercurial tides of emotional experience.

Breath is not merely a mechanical function sustaining life; it is a living dialogue between our autonomic systems and conscious awareness, between biology and spirit, between movement and stillness.

Breath has long been a focal point in many cultural, philosophical, and spiritual traditions, recognized as the vital life force—*prana*, *qi*, *pneuma*, *ruach*—that animates the human form. Modern science echoes these ancient insights, revealing the neurobiological pathways that connect breath to emotional regulation. At the same time, clinical practice shows us how disrupted breathing patterns both reflect and shape psychological distress. Through this interdisciplinary lens, we can appreciate breath not only as a physiological necessity but also as a profound site of emotional presence and transformation. This acknowledgment is vital to integrate multiple perspectives on breathing so that a nuanced understanding of the same can assist a diverse spectrum from clinical psychology to pulmonary rehabilitation.

The chapter will begin with a survey of the neurobiological foundations of breathing and emotion, then explore physiological patterns linked to emotional states. It will examine how dysfunctional breathing patterns emerge in distress and trauma, followed by an integrated biopsychosocial perspective. Later sections will delve into cultural meanings and practices of breath, the poetics of emotional flow, and practical ways breath awareness can support emotional wellbeing. Ultimately, this chapter invites a deeper listening—to the undulations of breath as a guide through the shifting seas of feeling.

2. THE NEUROBIOLOGY OF BREATHING AND EMOTION

Breathing Patterns and Emotional States: A Neurobiological Perspective

The connection between respiratory patterns and emotional states has been a subject of significant interest across disciplines such as psychophysiology, neuroscience, and affective science. Breathing, typically perceived as a mere physiological necessity, is profoundly intertwined with the regulation and expression of emotions. Decades of research have elucidated substantiated this. Philippot et al., (2002), found that specific respiratory patterns correspond with distinct emotional experiences such as joy, anger, fear, and sadness. For example, emotions like fear and anxiety are often characterized by rapid, shallow breathing, while states of relaxation and contentment are associated with slower and deeper respiratory cycles. Interestingly, these patterns are not merely reflective but also causative; consciously adopting certain breathing styles can evoke corresponding emotional states, suggesting a dynamic bidirectionality in the emotion-breathing nexus (Philippot et al., 2002).

Among the various features of breathing, respiratory variability, including phenomena such as sighing, plays a crucial role in emotional regulation. Sighing, characterized by a deep, often involuntary inhalation followed by a prolonged exhalation, has been proposed to serve as a physiological 'reset' mechanism for the respiratory system, potentially recalibrating both somatic and affective states (Vlemincx et al., 2013). This adaptive mechanism may provide relief from psychological tension and facilitate emotional homeostasis, particularly during periods of stress or cognitive overload.

The neurobiological substrates underpinning these interactions are complex and involve coordinated processes between the brainstem, limbic system, and cortical regions (Homma & Masaoka, 2008a). The brainstem, particularly the medulla oblongata, houses the primary respiratory centers, including the pre-Bötzinger complex, which generates the rhythmic patterns of breathing. Simultaneously, the limbic system—encompassing structures such as the amygdala, hippocampus, and hypothalamus—integrates emotional and autonomic responses. Cortical regions, especially the prefrontal cortex and anterior cingulate cortex, contribute to the conscious modulation of breathing and the appraisal of emotional stimuli.

Moreover, respiratory patterns reflect broader dimensions of emotional response beyond discrete emotions. Boiten, Frijda, and Wientjes (1994) proposed that variations in respiration correspond to general affective dimensions such as calmness versus excitement, relaxation versus tenseness, and active versus passive coping strategies. Despite significant advancements, much of the existing research has predominantly focused on basic respiratory parameters like rate, amplitude, and tidal volume. Boiten et al. (1994) argue for a more nuanced investigation into the morphology of the respiratory cycle—such as inspiratory and expiratory phases—which could yield finer distinctions in the psychophysiological mapping of emotions.

The Neurobiology of Breathing: Advances and Gaps

The neurobiology of breathing has been a central concern within neuroscience for nearly a century, contributing valuable insights into the fundamental mechanisms that sustain life.

Historical as well as contemporary scholarship has examined multiple dimensions of how breathing is regulated and sustained across the lifespan. For instance, early work traced the developmental emergence of respiratory control, highlighting how neural and physiological mechanisms mature to support stable ventilatory patterns from infancy onward (Haddad & Farber, 1991). Subsequent research has focused on the neurochemical processes that generate and modulate respiratory rhythms, identifying the intricate interactions among neurotransmitters and neural circuits that allow for adaptive adjustments to internal and external demands (McCrimmon et al., 2008). Complementing these perspectives, studies at the cellular level have mapped the activity of specific neuronal populations responsible for shaping the tempo and variability of breathing, thereby illuminating the micro-level dynamics that underpin the broader respiratory system (Berger, 1990). Together, these lines of inquiry reveal the multilayered nature of respiratory regulation, spanning developmental, neurochemical, and cellular domains.

The development of specialized in vitro preparations, such as isolated brainstem-spinal cord mounts, has significantly advanced our understanding by enabling precise manipulation of the extracellular and intracellular milieu. These preparations have been instrumental in dissecting the electrophysiological properties of respiratory neurons, the synaptic circuits involved in rhythm generation, and the sensitivity of these systems to chemical stimuli like carbon dioxide (Berger, 1990; McCrimmon et al., 2008). Additionally, research has examined how environmental stressors, such as hypoxia and hypercapnia, impact the adaptability of the respiratory network, particularly across sleep-wake states and developmental stages.

Nevertheless, despite these advancements, recent years have seen a noticeable decline in studies focused on the synaptic and cellular foundations of breathing (Dick et al., 2018). This decline is concerning given that a deeper understanding of these processes is critical not only for basic science but also for clinical interventions in disorders involving respiratory dysfunctions, such as sleep apnea, sudden infant death syndrome (SIDS), and panic disorders.

Interactions Between Respiratory Control and Emotional Processing

Neurobiology explains how the interface between breathing and emotions is mediated by intricate neuroanatomical and neurochemical pathways. Among other structures, the lateral parabrachial nucleus (LPB) within the brainstem has emerged as a key structure in this context. Recent studies have highlighted the role of μ-opioid receptor-expressing neurons in the LPB, which are essential for integrating affective pain and breathing regulation through their projections to the central amygdala and the pre-Bötzinger complex (Liu et al., 2021). These pathways exemplify how nociceptive (pain-related) signals and affective states can directly modulate respiratory rhythms, influencing both the experience of pain and the corresponding emotional responses.

The pre-Bötzinger complex, widely recognized as the core respiratory pattern generator, exhibits highly sophisticated rhythmogenic capacities that allow it to maintain both stability and adaptability in respiratory output (Ashhad et al., 2022). This intrinsic flexibility is essential for modulating breathing in response to shifting internal and external conditions. Physiologically, the system must adjust ventilation to accommodate variations in metabolic demand, such as those triggered by acute fear, where activation of the sympathetic nervous system accelerates respiratory rate as part of the broader 'fight or flight' cascade. Conversely, intentional practices such as slow, deliberate breathing during meditative or contemplative states can downregulate arousal by enhancing parasympathetic tone, thereby promoting relaxation and emotional regulation. These contrasting examples illustrate how the rhythmic properties of the pre-Bötzinger complex support a dynamic interplay between neurophysiological mechanisms and affective states, enabling breathing to function as both a reflexive and an experientially modifiable process.

This bidirectional relationship extends into cognitive domains as well. Slow, deliberate breathing has been shown to enhance attentional control, modulate emotional reactivity, and improve stress resilience—effects that are mediated by top-down cortical regulation (Homma & Masaoka, 2008a; Ashhad et al., 2022). Such findings have profound implications for therapeutic interventions. Techniques like mindfulness-based stress reduction (MBSR), pranayama, and biofeedback leverage these principles to promote psychological well-being by harnessing the body's innate capacity to regulate emotions through the breath.

The Dual Control of Breathing: A Neurophysiological Bridge Between Body and Emotion

Breathing occupies a distinctive position among physiological processes due to its dual regulatory capacity—it is both an involuntary, automatic function and a consciously modifiable action. At its most fundamental level, respiration is controlled by neural networks within the brainstem, particularly the medulla oblongata and the pons, which orchestrate the rhythmic contraction and relaxation of respiratory muscles to sustain life (Homma & Masaoka, 2008a; Feldman & Del Negro, 2006). These centers generate an intrinsic respiratory rhythm, ensuring continuous ventilation even in the absence of conscious intervention.

Unlike other autonomic functions such as digestion or cardiac activity, however, respiration can be voluntarily modulated. Humans can consciously alter the pace, depth, and pattern of their breathing—an ability that provides a rare window for top-down influence over autonomic states (Homma & Masaoka, 2008b). This capacity positions breath as a potent interface between the body and mind, offering a channel through which cognitive and emotional processes can be intentionally regulated.

Emotional states inherently modulate breathing patterns, forming an integrated feedback system between affective experience and respiratory control. For instance, episodes of acute anxiety or fear often manifest as rapid, shallow breathing, a hallmark of sympathetic nervous system activation that prepares the body for fight-or-flight responses (Boiten, Frijda, & Wientjes, 1994). Conversely, states of relaxation, tranquility, or focused attention tend to be accompanied by slow, deep breathing that aligns with parasympathetic dominance and vagal activation (Porges, 2007). This reciprocal relationship underscores the embodied nature of emotional experiences—whereby bodily sensations, particularly those related to breath, both reflect and shape affective states.

The limbic system, notably the amygdala and hippocampus, plays a central role in this process. These structures are pivotal in emotional processing, memory encoding, and stress responses, and they maintain robust connections with the brainstem's respiratory centers (Homma & Masaoka, 2008b). The amygdala, for instance, amplifies sympathetic arousal during fear or threat perception, which can elevate respiratory rate and alter breathing depth. In contrast, conscious regulation of breathing—such as through slow, diaphragmatic breathing—can engage the prefrontal cortex, enabling top-down modulation of limbic reactivity, thereby dampening emotional intensity and fostering cognitive-emotional integration.

Central to this mind-body dialogue is the vagus nerve, the tenth cranial nerve, which constitutes a primary component of the parasympathetic nervous system. The vagus nerve's influence extends across cardiac function, gastrointestinal activity, and respiration. According to Polyvagal Theory, proposed by Stephen Porges (2007), the myelinated branch of the vagus—termed the ventral vagal complex—facilitates social engagement and emotional regulation by promoting physiological states of calm and safety. Slow, rhythmic breathing stimulates vagal afferents, thereby enhancing parasympathetic tone, reducing heart rate, and fostering psychological resilience (Porges, 2007). This mechanism provides a neurophysiological basis for practices such as pranayama, mindfulness meditation, and biofeedback therapies that harness breath control to alleviate stress and modulate emotional responses.

Interoception, the brain's capacity to perceive and interpret internal bodily signals, is intimately connected with breath awareness. The insular cortex, along with the anterior cingulate cortex, serves as a critical hub for integrating interoceptive information derived from pulmonary stretch receptors, chemoreceptors monitoring blood gas levels, and cardiovascular inputs. This integration yields a conscious sense of the body's internal milieu, contributing not only to homeostatic regulation but also to the subjective experience of emotion (Critchley & Harrison, 2013). Enhancing interoceptive awareness through breath-focused mindfulness practices has been associated with improved emotional regulation, greater resilience to stress, and reductions in anxiety and depressive symptoms (Farb et al., 2015).

Thus, by cultivating deliberate control over breath, individuals can access a tangible method to navigate the turbulence of emotional fluctuations. The practice of mindful breathing acts as an anchor, translating physiological rhythms into tools of psychological steadiness and presence. As empirical research continues to illuminate these interconnections, breath emerges not merely as a life-sustaining function but as a transformative medium for embodied self-regulation and mental well-being.

3. THE PHYSIOLOGY OF BREATH AND EMOTION

Breathing as the Embodied Language of Emotion

Breathing represents the body's most immediate and primal expression of emotion—a somatic language that often precedes and transcends verbal articulation. The rhythm, depth, and cadence of breath not only mirror the shifting landscape of affective states but also actively participate in shaping emotional experiences. When fear or anxiety surfaces, the breath instinctively becomes rapid and shallow, a physiological preparation aligned with the 'fight or flight' response orchestrated by the sympathetic nervous system (Homma & Masaoka, 2008b). In moments of grief, respiration may slow, punctuated by deep sighs that seem to carry the weight of sorrow with each exhalation. Conversely, the lightness of joy is often accompanied by fuller, more expansive breathing, reflecting an embodied sense of openness and vitality.

These respiratory patterns are intricately regulated by the autonomic nervous system (ANS), particularly its two primary branches: the sympathetic nervous system (SNS) and the parasympathetic nervous system (PNS). The SNS, often characterized as the body's accelerator, mobilizes energy in response to perceived threats by increasing heart rate, diverting blood flow to muscles, and accelerating breathing to enhance oxygen delivery (Thayer & Lane, 2000). This state is marked by decreased respiratory variability and heightened vigilance. In contrast, the PNS, with the vagus nerve as its principal conduit, functions as the body's brake, promoting states of rest, digestion, and recovery. Vagal activation slows both the heart rate and respiratory rhythm, fostering a sense of calm and physiological restoration (Porges, 2007).

Empirical studies have consistently validated the close coupling between emotional states and distinct respiratory patterns. Research by Philippot et. al. (2002), demonstrated that individuals exhibit recognizable breathing signatures when experiencing emotions such as joy, sadness, anger, and fear. These patterns are not merely reflexive but are orchestrated through complex neural circuitry that links brainstem respiratory centers with higher-order regions involved in emotion processing. Specifically, the brainstem, limbic system (including the amygdala and hippocampus), and cortical areas form an integrated network that governs both emotional arousal and respiratory modulation (Homma & Masaoka, 2008b).

Within the brainstem, the lateral parabrachial nucleus (LPB) plays a pivotal role in coordinating respiratory patterns with affective pain and emotional states. The LPB interacts with structures like the central amygdala, facilitating the integration of nociceptive (pain-related) inputs and emotional cues with breathing rhythms (Liu et al., 2021; Bass & Gardner, 1985). This underscores the multifunctional nature of the respiratory system—not just as a homeostatic regulator but as an affective barometer.

Boiten et. al. (1994) further conceptualized respiratory patterns as reflective of broad affective dimensions, including calm versus excitement, relaxation versus tenseness, and active versus passive coping. Such categorizations help decode the nuanced interplay between physiology and psychology, highlighting how respiration acts as both a consequence and a contributor to emotional states. Significantly, experimental manipulation of breathing—such as slowing the breath or deepening inhalations—can elicit corresponding emotional changes, supporting the notion of a bidirectional relationship between respiration and affect (Philippot et al., 2002).

These findings carry profound implications for emotion theories, particularly those emphasizing peripheral feedback mechanisms like the James-Lange theory of emotion, which posits that bodily states can inform emotional experience (Critchley & Harrison, 2013). Moreover, they offer practical applications for emotion regulation strategies, many of which integrate conscious respiratory control. Techniques such as paced breathing, diaphragmatic breathing, and mindfulness-based breath awareness leverage these physiological pathways to modulate emotional reactivity and enhance psychological resilience (Porges, 2007).

Understanding breath as the body's first language of emotion not only enriches our comprehension of mind-body interactions but also provides actionable tools for therapeutic intervention. By engaging with breath intentionally, individuals can navigate the currents of emotion with greater awareness and agency, transforming an automatic process into a mindful practice of self-regulation.

Respiratory Sinus Arrhythmia: A Marker of Emotional Flexibility and Regulation

A critical physiological indicator of the interplay between respiration and emotional regulation is respiratory sinus arrhythmia (RSA)—the naturally occurring variation in heart rate that synchronizes with the breathing cycle. Specifically, heart rate accelerates during inhalation and decelerates during exhalation, a pattern reflecting parasympathetic (vagal) influence on cardiac function (Porges, 2007; Shaffer et al., 2014). RSA is widely recognized as a non-invasive biomarker of vagal tone and emotional adaptability; higher RSA levels are associated with superior emotion regulation, psychological flexibility, and greater resilience in the face of stress (Beauchaine & Thayer, 2015; Porges, 2007). Conversely, diminished RSA is linked to heightened vulnerability to anxiety, depression, and other affective disorders, reflecting compromised parasympathetic function and reduced capacity for autonomic regulation (Thayer & Lane, 2000).

Interventions that promote coherent breathing—a practice characterized by slow, rhythmic, and evenly paced inhalations and exhalations—have been shown to enhance RSA. Typically, breathing at a frequency of around 5 to 6 breaths per minute optimizes heart rate variability (HRV) and fosters a state of autonomic balance (Lehrer & Gevirtz, 2014). This breathing rate aligns with the body's baroreflex resonance frequency, which maximizes the synchronization between cardiac and respiratory rhythms, thereby bolstering parasympathetic activation and emotional stability.

Therapeutically, the recognition of breath as both a mirror and modulator of emotional states has informed a variety of clinical interventions. By observing clients' breathing patterns, clinicians can gain valuable insights into their emotional arousal and regulatory capacity. Techniques such as biofeedback capitalize on this principle by teaching individuals to monitor and adjust their physiological responses, including breathing, heart rate, and muscle tension, to mitigate anxiety, panic, and mood dysregulation (Goessl et al., 2017). Through real-time feedback mechanisms, clients learn to foster breath control, thereby enhancing RSA and facilitating greater autonomic flexibility.

Additionally, breathwork therapies, encompassing practices such as pranayama (yogic breath control), integrative breath retraining, and coherent breathing, systematically utilize breathing techniques to restore nervous system balance and improve psychological well-being (Zaccaro et al., 2018). Pranayama, for example, includes structured breathing exercises that range from energizing techniques like *Kapalabhati* to calming practices such as *Nadi Shodhana*, each designed to influence physiological states and mental clarity (Sengupta, 2012). These practices not only enhance vagal tone and RSA but also cultivate interoceptive awareness—the conscious perception of internal bodily states—thereby deepening an individual's capacity for self-regulation and emotional insight (Farb et al., 2015).

In sum, the therapeutic potential of breath-based interventions is underpinned by their capacity to engage core autonomic mechanisms such as RSA. By training clients to modulate their breathing patterns, clinicians can provide them with accessible and effective tools for enhancing emotional resilience, reducing stress reactivity, and fostering overall mental health.

4. BREATHING DYSFUNCTIONS: THE VICIOUS CYCLE OF EMOTION, TRAUMA, AND RESPIRATORY DYSFUNCTION

While breath serves as a powerful regulator of physiological and emotional states, it remains particularly vulnerable to disruption under conditions of psychological distress. Conversely, breathing disturbance is known to aggravate clinical conditions, particularly the ones where anxiety is a chief symptom. Dysfunctional breathing patterns—including chronic hyperventilation, shallow thoracic breathing, and habitual breath-holding—are frequently observed in individuals grappling with anxiety, trauma, and prolonged stress exposure (Gardner, 1996; Meuret et al., 2010). These maladaptive patterns not only reflect the body's attempt to cope with internal turmoil but also contribute to a self-perpetuating cycle where dysregulated breathing amplifies emotional instability, which in turn further distorts respiratory function.

A salient example of this cycle is hyperventilation syndrome (HVS), characterized by excessive and inappropriate expulsion of carbon dioxide (CO_2) through rapid or deep breathing. This reduction in arterial CO_2 levels—termed hypocapnia—can provoke a range of distressing physiological symptoms, including dizziness, paresthesia (tingling sensations), chest tightness, and palpitations, many of which mimic or exacerbate panic attacks (Gardner, 1996; Meuret et al., 2010). The physiological sensations induced by hypocapnia often elicit heightened fear and catastrophic interpretations, reinforcing both anxiety and dysfunctional breathing in a feedback loop (Meuret et al., 2017).

Trauma-related disorders, particularly post-traumatic stress disorder (PTSD), are also marked by irregular and maladaptive breathing patterns. Individuals with PTSD may unconsciously engage in shallow, erratic, or inhibited breathing, reflective of the body's fight, flight, or freeze responses (Wilkinson et al., 2019). In these cases, the breath, rather than serving as a grounding anchor, becomes a somatic trigger that reactivates traumatic memories and physiological hyperarousal. Research indicates that such dysregulated breathing in PTSD is associated with autonomic imbalance, specifically a diminished parasympathetic (vagal) tone and heightened sympathetic dominance, which together sustain the cycle of hypervigilance and emotional dysregulation (Zaccaro et al., 2018; Porges, 2007).

From a psychological standpoint, dysfunctional breathing is intricately connected to emotional suppression and somatic holding patterns. The breath may become constrained as a defensive mechanism to avoid fully experiencing overwhelming emotions or body-based memories, especially those associated with trauma or unresolved grief (Levine, 2010; van der Kolk, 2014).

In particular pathologies like Obsessive-Compulsive Disorder (OCD), peculiarities of breathing such as habitual breath-holding may become a compulsion, though some researches argue for its therapeutic implications instead (Datillo, 2006). On the contrary, breath holding along with excessive sighing, or uneven respiratory rhythms often signal internal conflicts, unprocessed affect, and chronic tension held within the body (Wilkinson et al., 2019).

Recognizing these breathing dysfunctions is paramount in therapeutic contexts that aim for holistic healing. Breath retraining interventions, employed across modalities such as cognitive-behavioral therapy (CBT), somatic experiencing, and specialized breathwork therapies, seek to restore a fluid, diaphragmatic, and balanced breathing pattern (Meuret et al., 2010; Levine, 2010). For instance, capnometry-assisted respiratory training (CART) in CBT frameworks directly targets hyperventilation by teaching clients to normalize CO_2 levels, thereby reducing anxiety symptoms (Meuret et al., 2017). Similarly, somatic therapies focus on increasing clients' awareness of their breath and body, helping them release patterns of muscular and respiratory constriction linked to emotional trauma (Payne, et. al., 2015).

By re-establishing healthier breathing patterns, clients can not only enhance autonomic regulation but also reforge a mindful connection between body and emotion, fostering resilience and psychological well-being. As breath becomes less of a battleground and more of a resource, individuals gain access to an embodied sense of safety and emotional coherence.

5. BIOPSYCHOSOCIAL PERSPECTIVES ON BREATH

The biopsychosocial perspective on breathing and emotions offers a comprehensive framework that captures the intricate interplay of physiological, psychological, and social dimensions in the regulation of respiratory patterns. Rather than viewing breathing solely as a reflexive physiological function, this perspective recognizes it as a dynamic process shaped by an individual's emotional states, cognitive appraisals, personality traits, and social environments (Gilbert, 2003; Homma & Masaoka, 2008b).

At the biological level, respiratory regulation is orchestrated through the interplay between brainstem mechanisms, particularly the pre-Bötzinger complex, and higher brain centers such as the limbic system, cortical structures as previously discussed. These interconnected neural circuits modulate respiratory output in response to emotional arousal, ensuring that breathing patterns adapt to the organism's internal and external demands.

Psychologically, individual differences in personality traits—such as trait anxiety, neuroticism, and emotional reactivity—can predispose individuals to specific breathing patterns. This phenomenon has been discussed previously as 'Behavioural Breathing' (Litchfeild & Reamer, 2019) For instance, people high in anxiety sensitivity are more likely to engage in shallow or rapid breathing, exacerbating physiological arousal and perpetuating cycles of emotional dysregulation (Gilbert, 2003; Ley, 1999). Cognitive processes, including attentional biases and maladaptive beliefs about bodily sensations, further influence how individuals perceive and modulate their breathing, particularly under stress or anxiety-provoking conditions (Ley, 1999). In studies, breathing has been differentiated from respiration on the basis of chemical-metabolic changes and some, even on the learnt (behavioural) basis (Litchfeild & Reamer, 2019). Some researches highlight the importance of respiratory variability that, referring to the natural fluctuations in breathing patterns, has emerged as a valuable but often underexplored indicator of emotional regulation capacity. Greater respiratory variability is typically associated with flexible emotional responding and adaptive autonomic control, whereas rigid or monotonous breathing patterns may reflect psychological distress or autonomic dysfunction (Vlemincx et al., 2013). Within this context, sighing serves a critical homeostatic function. More than a mere respiratory event, sighing is hypothesized to act as a reset mechanism, restoring variability in breathing and facilitating emotional recalibration after stress or emotional perturbation (Vlemincx et al., 2013). Frequent sighing, however, when coupled with anxiety or depression, may also signal underlying emotional distress, necessitating nuanced interpretation in both research and clinical practice.

Importantly, Litchfeild & Reamer (2019) reinforce that breathing behavior is not fixed but can be conditioned and modified through Pavlovian and operant mechanisms

(Ley, 1999). Classical conditioning paradigms demonstrate how neutral stimuli can become associated with specific breathing responses, contributing to maladaptive patterns in anxiety disorders. For example, individuals with panic disorder may develop conditioned hyperventilation responses to cues associated with prior panic attacks. Operant conditioning, conversely, enables the reinforcement of adaptive breathing behaviors through positive feedback and behavioral interventions. This plasticity in breathing underscores the potential for therapeutic interventions aimed at retraining dysfunctional respiratory patterns, which can have cascading benefits for emotional well-being and cognitive functioning (Meuret et al., 2017). While significant, this observation challenges the erstwhile assumption that breathing and respiration are bio-physiological in nature. Dysfuntional breathing as a learned phenomenon, rather than a reflex, draws attention to the psychosocial influences on breathing. Modelling is therefore an important factor while understanding how breathing is observed and learned as a corollary of associations.

The social context further shapes breathing and emotional expression. Interpersonal interactions, cultural norms regarding emotional display, and social stressors all influence respiratory patterns, either exacerbating or alleviating dysregulated breathing. Socially mediated practices such as group breathwork, yoga, and mindfulness-based stress reduction (MBSR) capitalize on the social dimension of breathing to foster collective emotional regulation and resilience (Zaccaro et al., 2018). Further, breathing has been identified as a social and political act that extends far beyond a mere biological function as it connects individuals through a complex relational and systemic interactions. Certain interdisciplinary studies provide robust evidence for this claim. For instance, Niclas Kaiser & Butler, (2021) proposed a "Social Breathing" model illustrating how breath involves automatic, implicit, and embodied exchanges between social partners. This exchange, in a way, connects them across space. Mar Pérezts et al. (2025), argue that breathing shapes questions of life and death while rooting these in collective intra-actions.

The social dimensions of respiration have been demonstrated across diverse contexts, illustrating that breathing is embedded within sociocultural practices rather than existing solely as an involuntary physiological act. For instance, in clinical and healthcare settings, breathing is closely monitored, regulated, and interpreted through biomedical, caregiving, and institutional frameworks, positioning it as a marker of bodily distress, vulnerability, and intervention (Harris Solomon, 2021). Similarly, breathing functions as a subtle but essential communicative resource in everyday conversational interaction, contributing to turn-taking, interpersonal alignment, and embodied coordination (Amélie Rochet-Capellan & Fuchs, 2014). Beyond interpersonal and clinical domains, breathing also emerges as a politically charged modality, mobilized within collective action, public protest, and socio-ecological activism to articulate forms of resistance, solidarity, and shared emotional states

(Tsaknaki, 2021). Taken together, these scholarly contributions underscore that breathing constitutes a complex socio-material phenomenon, linking embodied experience to broader political, environmental, and relational networks.

This integrated biopsychosocial model emphasizes the need for multidimensional approaches in both research and clinical settings when examining the nexus of breathing and emotion. Understanding how biological, psychological, and social factors converge to influence respiratory patterns can inform more effective interventions for anxiety, mood disorders, and stress-related conditions.

The Physiology of Breath and Emotion

Breathing is is deeply intertwined with emotional states, serving both as a mirror of affect and a mechanism for emotional regulation. The respiratory system responds dynamically to fluctuations in mood, stress, and cognitive states, reflecting the bi-directional relationship between breath and emotion mediated by complex neurophysiological pathways (Homma & Masaoka, 2008b).

How Emotions Shape Breathing Patterns

Different emotional states manifest through distinct breathing patterns, which can serve as both diagnostic signals and therapeutic entry points. For instance:

- **Anxiety** is typically characterized by rapid, shallow breathing, predominantly thoracic rather than diaphragmatic. This hyperventilatory pattern contributes to hypocapnia (reduced carbon dioxide levels), which can intensify symptoms like dizziness, palpitations, and heightened anxiety—a feedback loop that sustains distress (Meuret et al., 2010).
- **Grief** is often accompanied by sighing, a pattern of deeper and prolonged exhalation that may reflect both a physiological reset and an emotional release mechanism (Vlemincx et al., 2013).
- **Calm and relaxation** are associated with deep, slow breathing, enhancing parasympathetic activity, particularly via vagal tone, which promotes a state of physiological homeostasis and psychological ease (Porges, 2007).

Moreover, negative and high-arousal emotions, such as fear and anger, are known to increase respiratory variability and sigh frequency, and can alter end-tidal carbon dioxide levels and expiratory time (Vlemincx et al., 2015). These physiological markers underscore how emotions modulate respiratory physiology in both subtle and pronounced ways.

Respiratory Patterns as Diagnostic Signals

In psychotherapy and biofeedback, breathing patterns can serve as diagnostic indicators of emotional dysregulation or underlying psychopathology. For example, clients with anxiety disorders, PTSD, or depression often exhibit restricted, shallow, or erratic breathing, which can signal autonomic dysregulation (Wilkinson et al., 2019). Biofeedback therapies utilize real-time data on respiratory patterns and other autonomic markers to help clients become aware of and adjust their breathing, thus improving emotional regulation (Goessl, et. al, 2017). Despite its effectiveness, biofeedback has gathered little evidence in rectifying dysfunctional breathing, owing to its multifactorial etiology. As biofeedback techniques are incorporated to enhance an understanding of one's breathing pattern, it allows for an integration of other psychological factors influencing breathing. The psychological impact manifests through multiple domains: affective (emotional disturbances), behavioral (maladaptive breathing patterns), and cognitive (perceptual processing of breathing) (Yii & Koh, 2013). While promising, the research suggests more comprehensive studies are needed to fully map these complex interactions.

Breath Regulation Techniques: Coherent Breathing and Emotional Balance

Controlled breathing techniques, such as coherent breathing and box breathing, have been shown to positively influence RSA and heart rate variability (HRV), contributing to improved emotional balance and stress reduction (Lehrer & Gevirtz, 2014). Coherent breathing involves slow, rhythmic breaths typically at a pace of 5–6 breaths per minute, optimizing the synchronization between respiratory and cardiovascular rhythms. Similarly, box breathing—where inhalation, breath-hold, exhalation, and subsequent hold are all timed equally—can stabilize the autonomic nervous system, reducing stress and enhancing focus (Zaccaro et al., 2018).

Additionally, experimental research demonstrates that slow-paced breathing can improve motor performance and HRV under emotionally stressful conditions, suggesting its utility not only in emotional regulation but also in enhancing performance in high-pressure environments (Buchanan & Janelle, 2022).

At the neural level, the lateral parabrachial nucleus—particularly the subset of neurons expressing μ-opioid receptors—has been identified as a critical integrative hub that links respiratory regulation with affective pain and emotional processing in animal models (Bass & Gardner, 1985; Liu et al., 2021). This line of work substantially enriches our understanding of the neurobiological substrates through which breathing is intertwined with emotional experience. Collectively, these findings underscore the therapeutic relevance of breath-based interventions, suggesting that the modulation of respiratory rhythms serves not only as a strategy for alleviating distress but also as a foundational mechanism for cultivating emotional resilience, promoting psychological well-being, and stabilizing autonomic function.

Although breathing is rooted in biophysiological processes, research exploring its psychosocial dimensions has increasingly highlighted the extent to which respiration is embedded within, and shaped by, social environments, relational dynamics, and cultural practices.

6. BREATH IN PHILOSOPHICAL AND CULTURAL TRADITIONS

Breath has long occupied a central place in philosophical inquiry, spiritual practices, and cultural traditions, symbolizing life, consciousness, and the delicate threshold between existence and transcendence. Across civilizations, breath is not merely a physiological necessity but a metaphysical bridge that connects the body, mind, and spirit, while offering insight into the human condition, impermanence, and interconnection.

Breath as Life-Force Across Traditions

The conceptualization of breath as a life-force is widespread, evident in diverse linguistic and philosophical traditions. In Indian philosophy and yogic traditions, *prana* refers to the vital energy that permeates all living beings, carried and cultivated through the breath. Similarly, in Traditional Chinese Medicine (TCM), *qi* (or *chi*) represents the vital energy circulating within the body, intricately linked to respiratory function and overall health (Draeger-Muenke & Muenke, 2012). The ancient Greek notion of *pneuma* encompasses both breath and spirit, signifying the animating principle of life. In the Hebrew tradition, *ruach* embodies the dual meanings of "breath" and "spirit," emphasizing the divine source of life and the essence of human existence (Nair, 2007). These parallel traditions reflect a shared understanding that breath is more than air—it is the substrate of vitality, consciousness, and spiritual presence.

Breath in Spiritual and Contemplative Traditions

Breath also occupies a central role in spiritual and contemplative practices across world religions. In Sufism, breath (*nafas*) is an instrument of remembrance (*dhikr*), a means of attuning the heart to divine presence and cultivating spiritual awareness. Zen Buddhism utilizes breath-focused meditation (*zazen*) to anchor the practitioner in the present moment, dissolving ego-boundaries and deepening awareness of impermanence. In Christian mysticism, controlled breathing accompanies contemplative prayer and the pursuit of union with the divine, as seen in the Hesychast tradition, where breath synchronizes with the Jesus Prayer to quiet the mind and open the heart.

These practices illustrate that breath is a medium of transcendence, fostering a state of inner silence, receptivity, and communion with forces greater than the self. In many indigenous cultures, ritual breath practices and intentional silence serve to connect individuals with ancestors, nature, and the cosmos, reinforcing communal bonds and ecological stewardship.

Breath, Silence, and Cultural Rituals

The significance of breath is also evident in cultural rituals that intertwine breathing with silence and mindfulness. Among indigenous communities, breath is incorporated in ceremonial practices to evoke altered states of consciousness, healing, and spiritual connection. Similarly, breath awareness in meditative disciplines, such as mindfulness meditation, emphasizes the quiet observation of each inhalation and exhalation, cultivating presence and a deepened sense of self-in-world.

The Turkish Alevi community exemplifies the cultural centrality of breath through their ritual practice of *nefes*, where spiritual songs guided by breath are vehicles for cultivating listening, empathy, and tolerance. Such practices underscore the potential of breath not only as a personal spiritual tool but also as a medium for interpersonal and intercultural dialogue, nurturing coexistence in diverse societies.

Breath as Existential Metaphor

Philosophically, breath serves as an existential metaphor for presence, impermanence, and rebirth. The simple yet profound act of breathing mirrors the ephemeral nature of life, where each breath taken is both an affirmation of living and a reminder of life's transient quality (Nair, 2007).

The idea of an "Age of Breath", proposed by Škof and Holmes (2013), envisions a cultural and spiritual reawakening rooted in breath awareness—encouraging sensitivity to others, to nature, and to cultural plurality. Feminist philosopher Luce Irigaray extends this by advocating for a "culture of breath", emphasizing breathing as an ethical and existential practice that fosters interpersonal relationships, respect for difference, and embodied presence (Irigaray, 2002).

In this light, breath becomes a symbol of renewal, adaptability, and relational being—a continuous cycle of taking in and letting go, reflecting not only physiological but also existential truths.

7. EMOTIONAL CURRENTS: THE FLOWING SELF

Emotion as Fluid, Not Fixed: Insights from Affect Theory, Somatic Psychology, and Phenomenology

Contemporary understandings of emotion challenge traditional notions of fixed, discrete emotional states, favoring instead a fluid and dynamic model of affective experience. Drawing from affect theory, somatic psychology, and phenomenology, emotions are increasingly conceptualized as embodied flows—processes that arise, shift, and dissipate within the body's internal milieu in response to both internal rhythms, such as breath, and external emotional triggers (Denzin, 1985; Knoblauch, 2017, 2019).

Somatic Psychology: Emotions as Moving Bodily States

In somatic psychology, emotions are seen not as static categories but as bodily sensations and physiological states in motion. This view emphasizes that emotional experiences are deeply rooted in the body's autonomic responses, muscular tension, posture, and most pertinently, breathing patterns. Breath, as a constantly shifting rhythm within the body, mirrors and modulates these emotional flows. Practices that engage the breath—such as somatic therapies, breathwork, and mindful movement—can thus reshape emotional experience by re-patterning the body's habitual responses (Payne et. al., 2015).

Interplay Between Breath Rhythms and Emotional Triggers

The interplay between internal breath rhythms and external emotional stimuli reveals a continuous, bidirectional exchange between physiological states and environmental contexts. For example, an unexpected threat can trigger rapid, shallow breathing, while intentionally slowing the breath can modulate the emotional response to that threat (Homma & Masaoka, 2008a). The concept of "affect navigation," introduced by Knoblauch (2017, 2019), describes this adaptive process whereby individuals navigate complex emotional landscapes through subtle shifts in bodily states, particularly breathing and posture.

This rhythmic patterning of emotions, where the body's internal states sync or clash with external affective cues, underscores the field-like quality of emotions—a notion adapted from psychoanalytic and phenomenological traditions to describe emotions as transient yet structured phenomena that occupy and move through the body's space (Knoblauch, 2017; Kauffman, 2015).

Phenomenology and the Lived Experience of Emotions

Phenomenology offers valuable insights into the lived experience of emotional states as felt flows. Denzin (1985) identifies four layers of lived emotion, including bodily feelings, interpretive frameworks, emotional expressions, and reflective self-awareness, emphasizing that emotions are not simply reactions but multi-layered experiences shaped by consciousness and social interactions.

For example, the experience of anxiety is often described phenomenologically as a tightening or constriction of breath and chest, a bodily sense of impending collapse or suffocation. Grief, on the other hand, manifests as deep sighs, heaviness in the chest, and a sense of emptiness, while joy is felt as expansive breathing, lightness, and openness in the body. These phenomenological descriptions of emotion align with research on the psychophysiology of breathing, which demonstrates how different affective states produce distinct breathing patterns (Philippot et al., 2002; Homma & Masaoka, 2008a).

Kauffman (2015) extends this understanding through a biophysical and phenomenological lens, proposing a new dualism that integrates classical notions of the embodied mind with the possibility of quantum consciousness, further emphasizing the non-linear, dynamic nature of emotional processes.

Building on these foundations, phenomenology stresses that emotions are not isolated episodes but are woven into the fabric of everyday existence. Emotions, in this view, are not simply internal states but intentional acts directed towards the world—they disclose meanings, values, and relationships that are significant to the subject. For example, fear is not just a physiological arousal but a mode of being-towards something threatening. Similarly, love is not just a feeling but a way of inhabiting the world that renders certain beings and experiences precious and irreplaceable.

Merleau-Ponty's concept of the lived body (*corps vivant*) deepens this perspective by highlighting how the body is not an object in the world but the very medium through which the world is encountered and felt. Through the body, emotions unfold as gestures, postures, and breathing rhythms that both express and constitute our engagement with the world. For instance, an anxious person does not merely feel anxious inside; their posture may close in on itself, their movements may become hesitant, and their breathing shallow—a full-body expression of their existential state.

Additionally, phenomenological accounts emphasize temporality in emotional experience. Emotions are not static but unfold over time, having their own internal rhythms and durations. Grief, for example, is not a momentary sadness but a prolonged reconfiguration of one's temporal horizon—a pervasive sense that time itself has slowed, become heavy, or even broken. In contrast, moments of elation or joy may be experienced as an acceleration of time, where one feels lifted into a heightened present.

The intersubjective dimension of emotions is also central to phenomenology. Emotions are often co-constituted through interactions with others. The smile of a friend, the scorn of a stranger, or the touch of a loved one can all elicit profound emotional responses, revealing how our emotional lives are entangled with social contexts and relations. This intersubjectivity extends to collective emotions, where shared affective experiences, such as mourning in public rituals or collective joy in celebrations, create a communal atmosphere that transcends individual subjectivity.

Moreover, the language of the body in emotion is not universal but culturally mediated. Different cultures cultivate specific emotional repertoires, including distinct ways of expressing and experiencing emotions. The social shaping of the body, including posture, gesture, and breath, aligns with cultural norms about what emotions are acceptable or desirable to express. Thus, while the body grounds emotional experience, it is also inscribed with social meanings and expectations.

Phenomenological inquiry also attends to the ways in which emotions are reflective and self-revealing. Emotional experiences often prompt introspection and existential questioning. For example, feelings of melancholy or ennui can lead individuals to reflect on the meaning of their lives, their relationships, and their sense of purpose. In this sense, emotions serve not only as responses to the world but as windows into the self, shaping one's self-understanding and personal narratives.

Finally, contemporary extensions of phenomenology, particularly in the fields of affect theory and embodied cognition, continue to explore the complex interplay between bodily states, consciousness, and environmental contexts. These perspectives suggest that emotional life is best understood not through reductionist frameworks that isolate neural or biochemical factors but through a holistic appreciation of the lived body as dynamically situated within a social and material world.

Phenomenology, therefore, provides a rich, nuanced account of emotions as dynamic, embodied, temporal, and socially embedded phenomena. It challenges simplistic dichotomies between mind and body, feeling and thinking, interiority and exteriority, offering instead a vision of emotional life as deeply integrated with the ways we inhabit and make sense of our worlds.

Breath, Dyspnea, and Affective Dimensions

The link between breath and emotional fluidity is also evident in the experience of dyspnea, or breathlessness. Dyspnea is not a uniform sensation but a multidimensional experience, involving both sensory and affective components. The affective dimension, in particular, is highly susceptible to emotional influences such as anxiety, fear, and frustration, which intensify the subjective unpleasantness of breathing discomfort (von Leupoldt et al., 2006; Stevens et al., 2019). In clinical observations, air hunger emerges as the dominant sensation during acute dyspnea episodes, frequently accompanied by panic, anxiety, and helplessness (Basara et al., 2018; Stevens et al., 2019).

Moreover, psychological factors, including psychiatric comorbidities, significantly modulate the intensity and periodicity of dyspnea, often independent of the underlying pulmonary pathology (Janson-Bjerklie et al., 1986). Gender differences also surface, with females reporting higher intensity of dyspnea compared to males, suggesting complex biopsychosocial interplays in the perception of breathlessness (Janson-Bjerklie et al., 1986).

These findings affirm that the perception of breath and its associated discomfort cannot be disentangled from the emotional and psychological contexts in which they arise, further validating affect theory's emphasis on the fluid, embodied, and context-dependent nature of emotional experience.

8. PRACTICES OF AWARENESS: LISTENING TO THE BREATH

The simple yet profound act of listening to the breath forms the cornerstone of many contemplative, therapeutic, and self-regulatory practices across cultures. Breath-focused techniques are increasingly recognized not just for their capacity to calm the mind and body, but for their potential to reshape psychological functioning, foster resilience, and promote deeper self-awareness. These practices harness the intentional observation and modulation of breath, turning an automatic physiological process into a gateway for grounding, emotional regulation, and neuroplastic change.

Breath-Focused Practices

1. Mindfulness Meditation

Mindfulness meditation often begins with the instruction to "focus on the breath," using it as an anchor to stabilize attention. This non-judgmental observation of the breath's natural rhythm cultivates present-moment awareness and facilitates a decentering from ruminative or anxious thought patterns (Kabat-Zinn, 2003). Neuroscientific studies reveal that breath-based mindfulness enhances interoception—the brain's ability to sense internal bodily states—thereby improving emotional regulation and fostering functional connectivity in brain regions associated with attention and self-regulation, such as the prefrontal cortex and insula (Farb et al., 2013).

2. Somatic Experiencing

Developed by Peter Levine, Somatic Experiencing uses gentle breath awareness in tandem with body tracking to help clients discharge trauma-related arousal trapped in the nervous system (Payne, et. al., 2015). By observing subtle changes in breathing alongside somatic sensations, individuals learn to renegotiate traumatic memories, restoring autonomic balance. Breath, in this context, becomes both a regulator and informant of embodied states, enabling the safe processing of distressing experiences.

3. Holotropic and Rebirthing Breathwork

Holotropic breathwork, developed by Stanislav Grof, and Rebirthing Breathwork, popularized by Leonard Orr, employ intensified breathing patterns to facilitate access to non-ordinary states of consciousness. Through accelerated and continuous breathing, practitioners may evoke vivid emotional catharsis, biographical insights, and transcendent experiences often associated with feelings of wholeness or spiritual awakening (Armand & Braud, 2008). Although research on these methods remains emergent, anecdotal evidence suggests their potential for processing unresolved psychological material and inducing profound states of integration.

4. Yogic Pranayama

Pranayama, the yogic science of breath control, comprises a variety of techniques designed to regulate the pranic energy through deliberate breathing patterns. Techniques such as *Kapalabhati (forceful exhalation), Nadi Shodhana (alternate nostril breathing)*, and *Bhramari (humming breath)* influence autonomic balance, enhance cognitive focus, and modulate mood (Joshi & Telles, 2009). Studies have shown that practices like Kapalabhati can increase P300 peak amplitude, a neural marker associated with attentional engagement and cognitive processing (Joshi & Telles, 2009).

Psychological and Neurophysiological Mechanisms

Breath-focused practices engage critical psychological and neurophysiological mechanisms, particularly interoception, grounding, and neuroplasticity. Interoceptive awareness facilitated by breath monitoring strengthens the capacity to detect and interpret internal cues, which is essential for effective emotion regulation (Farb et al., 2013). Grounding through breath offers a stabilizing counterbalance to dissociative states, common in trauma, by re-establishing a safe connection with the body.

Furthermore, repeated engagement with breath awareness practices induces neuroplasticity, reinforcing pathways in the brain that support calm, focused attention and emotional resilience (Tang, Holzel, & Posner, 2015). Such practices are increasingly being integrated into clinical interventions for anxiety, depression, and PTSD.

Breath as Method and Metaphor in Therapeutic Journeys

Beyond its physiological functions, breath serves simultaneously as a method of intervention and a metaphorical lens through which therapeutic change can be understood. The cyclical movement of inhalation and exhalation parallels psychological processes of engagement and withdrawal, tension and release, resistance and surrender, as well as fragmentation and reintegration. This rhythmic oscillation offers a somatic template for understanding how individuals navigate affective states, relational patterns, and internal conflicts over time.

Within psychotherapeutic practice, breath becomes a site where embodied experience and psychological meaning converge. Many therapeutic modalities—from psychodynamic to humanistic, mindfulness-based, and somatic approaches—use breath as a way to foster awareness of internal states, regulate affect, and create a grounding anchor during emotionally charged exploration. Attending to the breath can mark a shift from reactive patterns toward reflective presence, enabling clients to "make space" for complex emotions without being overwhelmed by them. This process reflects a core aim of psychotherapy: cultivating a stance of curiosity and compassion toward one's inner life.

Breath also functions metaphorically as a symbol of psychological openness. Deepening or expanding the breath during therapy can represent a willingness to encounter previously unarticulated thoughts, sensations, or memories. Conversely, constricted breathing patterns often mirror states of fear, suppression, or unresolved conflict. By gently tracking the breath, therapists help clients notice how bodily rhythms embody longstanding narratives of protection or vulnerability, thereby integrating somatic insight with cognitive and emotional understanding.

In this sense, breath is not simply an adjunct to therapeutic technique but a foundational pathway through which individuals learn to regulate arousal, process emotion, and cultivate resilience. It supports the development of interoceptive awareness—an essential component of self-regulation and mental health—and reinforces the therapeutic process of moving toward greater coherence, integration, and psychological flexibility.

Emerging Technologies and Future Directions

Modern technologies are increasingly being integrated into breath-based therapeutic practices, extending and refining techniques that have long been cultivated in contemplative and clinical traditions. Biofeedback systems and breath-aware wearable devices now offer continuous, real-time information about respiratory rhythms, heart rate variability, and physiological markers of stress and arousal, thereby transforming subjective awareness into observable, trackable data (Prpa et al., 2020). Within psychotherapeutic settings, such tools are not merely adjuncts but function as mediators that help bridge the gap between bodily experience and psychological insight.

By visualizing subtle fluctuations in breathing patterns, clients gain a clearer understanding of how emotional states manifest somatically and how intentional breath modulation can shift nervous system activation. This aligns with core principles in cognitive-behavioral, somatic, and mindfulness-based therapies, which emphasize the regulation of autonomic arousal as a foundational component of emotional stability. Wearable technologies further support individualized intervention by allowing therapists and clients to collaboratively identify stress triggers, recognize maladaptive breathing habits, and develop personalized strategies for cultivating calmer, more coherent respiratory patterns.

Modern technologies such as AI-driven applications and wearable devices are increasingly being recognized as significant adjuncts to breath-training interventions, offering new pathways for enhancing mental and emotional well-being. Building on long-standing therapeutic insights into the role of respiration in self-regulation, these digital tools introduce levels of precision, accessibility, and personalization that were previously difficult to achieve in traditional clinical practice.

A growing body of empirical work highlights the effectiveness of such innovations (Eleni Mitsea et al., 2024). For example, mobile applications like *Breeze* utilize smartphone microphones and signal-processing algorithms to detect inhalation and exhalation phases with an accuracy of 75.5% (C. Shih et al., 2019). This capacity for real-time respiratory monitoring allows users to engage in structured breathwork exercises with immediate feedback, supporting core therapeutic aims such as increased interoceptive awareness and improved self-regulation. Parallel developments in wearable breath sensors further expand these possibilities. These devices can continuously track respiratory rate, tidal patterns, and even biochemical markers relevant to stress and well-being, underscoring their potential utility for both preventative mental health care and ongoing therapeutic support (Dohyung Kim et al., 2024).

Emerging evidence indicates that these technologies positively influence several psychological domains, including attentional control, emotional regulation, and stress management (Eleni Mitsea et al., 2024). From a psychotherapeutic perspective, such benefits resonate with established models that emphasize the role of breath in down-regulating sympathetic arousal, supporting cognitive flexibility, and fostering reflective capacity. Importantly, researchers have noted that integrating multiple technological modalities—such as pairing wearable sensors with app-guided training—may produce synergistic effects, enhancing learning and facilitating more sustained behavioral change. These digital interventions appear promising across varied populations, including employees in high-demand work environments, students navigating academic stress, and individuals with disabilities who may require adaptive, accessible forms of self-regulation practice.

Collectively, these advances illustrate how AI and wearable technologies are reshaping the landscape of breath-based interventions. By merging long-standing therapeutic principles with contemporary digital capabilities, they point toward a future in which breath training becomes increasingly personalized, data-informed, and integrative within broader mental health care.

The integration of these technological innovations with long-standing breathing practices reflects a broader convergence between tradition and contemporary science. While ancient systems such as yogic pranayama and meditative breathwork emphasized awareness, discipline, and introspective attunement, modern devices enhance these practices by providing immediate feedback loops that strengthen learning and self-regulation. The result is a more nuanced, data-informed approach to mental health in which breath becomes a measurable, modifiable, and deeply experiential pathway toward psychological resilience and emotional well-being.

9. POETICS OF BREATH AND EMOTION

Breath, as both a physiological rhythm and a symbolic motif, permeates the arts, shaping the rhythm, pacing, and emotive resonance of creative expression. In poetry, theater, dance, and other movement arts, breath operates as an invisible thread—weaving together words, gestures, and silences into a textured language of emotional depth. It provides a non-verbal lexicon, where meaning is not only spoken or written but felt through the body's inherent cadences. Breath is thus not merely a biological necessity but a foundational component of artistic articulation, deeply embedded within the phenomenology of human experience (Cave, 2021).

Poetry: Line Breaks, Pauses, and the Breath of Language

In poetry, the structure of lines and pauses is intimately tied to the rhythm of breath. Line breaks, enjambment, and caesuras create spaces for inhalation and exhalation, turning the act of reading into a somatic experience. This organization of text mirrors the body's rhythms, with breath guiding the tempo of comprehension and affective response (Heine, 2018). Ancient rhetorical traditions emphasized breath control as essential to effective oration, a lineage that persists in poetry where the voice's pacing animates the text.

The ancient Greeks, for instance, developed intricate systems of prosody that accounted for breath patterns within poetic delivery, ensuring that oral recitations resonated not only intellectually but viscerally (Kennedy, 2013). Similarly, in Indian classical poetics, the Sanskrit concept of 'Alap' in musical renditions of poetry involves elongated breath-driven phrases that build emotional intensity over time (Patel, 2017).

In modernist literature, particularly in the works of writers like H.D. (Hilda Doolittle) and Ezra Pound, the "musicality of breath" became a stylistic device, enabling the written word to capture the organic flow of thought and feeling. Heine (2017) notes that modernist prose often structures rhythm not solely through syntactic order but via "breathing pauses," creating intervals within the text that allow emotions to surface between phrases. These intentional gaps produce an emotive atmosphere, inviting readers to dwell in the unsaid and the unspoken.

In Japanese literature, breath plays a unique role in evoking corporeal presence. Mewhinney (2023) describes how breath-oriented writing in Japanese fiction creates "organic rhythms" that immerse readers, enabling them to conspire with the text—breathing alongside its pace, its silences, and its sudden gasps of emotion. The haiku tradition, with its brevity and reliance on seasonal and transient imagery, also exemplifies the use of breath to encapsulate fleeting emotional states (Shirane, 2012).

Moreover, poets such as Adrienne Rich and Denise Levertov have explicitly discussed the significance of breath in crafting poetic cadence. Levertov (1992) spoke of the "line as breath unit," suggesting that the integrity of a poem's line structure derives from the physiological experience of breathing, thereby intertwining the reader's body with the text.

Theater: Voice, Pacing, and Emotional Delivery

In the theater, breath is fundamental to voice production, emotional delivery, and the pacing of dialogue. Actors are trained to harness breath to modulate tone, volume, and timing, crafting performances that convey subtle shifts in affect. An actor's breath control can evoke tension, intimacy, or power, enabling the audience to physically feel the weight of a character's internal states.

For example, a whispered line, shaped by minimal breath, can convey vulnerability, while a shouted phrase, bolstered by deep inhalation, embodies authority or anger. Breath, in this sense, becomes an instrument of presence, drawing audiences into a shared somatic space where emotion is transmitted through the resonances of the voice.

Practitioners of method acting, derived from Konstantin Stanislavski's system, emphasize breath as a pathway to emotional authenticity. Stanislavski posited that breath could summon genuine emotions from an actor's psyche, thereby bridging the gap between performer and character (Carnicke, 2009). Similarly, contemporary vocal coaches like Kristin Linklater focus on freeing the natural voice through breath work, facilitating a more resonant and emotionally honest performance (Linklater, 2006).

Breath also serves as a temporal marker in theater, dictating the rhythm of exchanges between characters and the unfolding of dramatic tension. Playwrights such as Harold Pinter famously utilized pauses—infused with breath—to create an atmosphere of ambiguity and psychological intensity (Esslin, 2001). These "Pinter pauses" demonstrate how the absence of speech, sustained by the actor's breath, can speak volumes, intensifying the audience's emotional engagement.

Dance and Movement Arts

In dance and movement arts, breath orchestrates movement, ensuring that gestures are not mechanical but infused with life and emotion. Breath dictates the ebb and flow of motion, enhancing the expressiveness of the body. Choreographers like Martha Graham emphasized the synergy between breath and movement, teaching that "movement begins in the breath," thereby rooting dance in the body's visceral rhythms.

Graham's technique is predicated on the concept of 'contraction and release,' which directly corresponds to patterns of exhalation and inhalation, allowing dancers to embody emotional narratives physically (Franko, 2012). This approach underscores the idea that breath is not just an internal mechanism but an externalized form of storytelling through the body.

Contemporary somatic practices, such as Contact Improvisation, further explore this connection, where dancers remain attuned to their own breath and that of their partners, creating an interactive, breathing dialogue of bodies. The resulting movements are improvisational, fluid, and deeply responsive to emotional undercurrents. Practices like the Feldenkrais Method and Alexander Technique also integrate breath awareness to enhance bodily alignment, movement efficiency, and emotional expression (Batson & Schwartz, 2007).

Moreover, in non-Western traditions such as the Indian classical dance form Bharatanatyam, breath control is integral to the execution of intricate rhythmic patterns and expressive gestures known as 'Abhinaya,' which convey emotional states (Meduri, 2005). Similarly, Tai Chi and Qigong, rooted in Chinese martial arts and healing practices, incorporate breath regulation to harmonize body movements, cultivate internal energy (Qi), and express serenity and strength (Wayne & Kaptchuk, 2008).

Breath as Non-Verbal Language of Emotional Expression

Across these art forms, breath emerges as a non-verbal language of emotional expression—one that communicates beyond words. Whether shaping the line breaks of a poem, pacing an actor's monologue, or initiating the arc of a dancer's gesture, breath carries the invisible pulse of feeling. Yoo (2019) captures this beautifully, describing breath as a "life-giving force in writing," animating words with vitality and transforming the writer's body into an expressive instrument.

Additionally, breath's connection to emotion is deeply rooted in the physiological interplay between respiration and the autonomic nervous system. Research in psychophysiology indicates that specific breathing patterns can modulate emotional states, with slow, deep breathing activating the parasympathetic system, promoting calmness and emotional regulation (Jerath et al., 2015). This intersection of physiology and poetics suggests that breath, whether consciously manipulated by artists or naturally synchronized with creative acts, serves as a bridge between the inner affective world and external expression.

Moreover, the poetics of breath reflects the fragility and impermanence of human experience. Each breath, transient and necessary, parallels the fleeting nature of emotion—rising, peaking, and dissolving. In this way, breath in the arts does not merely accompany emotion; it materializes it, rendering the ephemeral visible and palpable.

This notion is echoed in phenomenological philosophies, such as those of Maurice Merleau-Ponty, who emphasized the embodied nature of perception and expression, where breath situates the self within a dynamic world of lived experience (Merleau-Ponty, 1962). Artistic practices that foreground breath thus invite a deeper attunement to the present moment, cultivating what Thich Nhat Hanh (2013) describes as "mindful breathing," a practice of returning to presence and experiencing life fully.

In conclusion, breath operates as a crucial axis in the poetics of emotion across artistic disciplines. It serves as both a physiological necessity and a profound medium of expression, translating the ineffable into sensory and emotional resonance. Whether in the cadence of poetry, the timbre of theatrical delivery, or the fluidity of dance, breath shapes the contours of human expression, offering a silent yet potent voice to the emotional landscapes we traverse.

10. CONCLUSION – RETURNING TO THE WAVE

Throughout this chapter, we have traced the delicate yet powerful intertwining of breath and emotion, observing how they do not simply run parallel to each other like separate streams but move in tandem, more akin to entwined waves—each shaping, influencing, and echoing the other. Breathing is not merely a background physiological process, nor is emotion solely a mental state. Instead, they constitute a dynamic system of reciprocal influence, where the rhythms of inhalation and exhalation carry emotional tones, and affective shifts ripple back to alter the breath.

Understanding this entanglement reveals that the breath is far more than a passive reflection of our inner life. It is a medium of modulation, a tool for navigating psychological states, a diagnostic signal in therapy, and an expressive force in the arts. Emotions ride the currents of the breath, just as waves rise and fall on the surface of the ocean, each movement unique yet patterned by deeper, often unconscious forces.

To return to the wave as an image is to acknowledge that breath and emotion are not static elements to be 'managed' or 'controlled' in isolation. They are processes of ongoing movement, oscillating between tension and release, contraction and expansion, agitation and calm.

The breath is the tide of the body, always in flux yet always returning, a gentle rhythm that calls us back to presence no matter how turbulent the emotional sea becomes.

This insight bears significant implications across several domains—emotional health, psychotherapy, education, and even cultural understanding. Breath literacy, or the capacity to become aware of, interpret, and skillfully engage one's breathing, is an underappreciated yet essential competence in our time. Just as we teach reading and writing to navigate the external world, so too must we cultivate the literacy of breath to navigate our internal landscapes.

In the context of emotional health, breath literacy enables individuals to recognize early signs of distress encoded in their respiratory patterns—whether it is the shallow panting of anxiety, the constricted holding of anger, or the sighs of resignation and grief. Knowing how to gently adjust the breath offers a form of immediate intervention, providing regulation from within rather than reliance on external solutions alone. Practices such as coherent breathing, mindfulness, or pranayama are not merely techniques; they are invitations to dialogue with oneself, to become attuned to the body's whispers before they escalate into cries for help.

In psychotherapy, breath serves as both a mirror and a tool. A therapist attentive to a client's breath gains a portal into the unspoken—the suppressed emotions, the body memories, the unprocessed traumas that manifest as irregular or dysfunctional breathing patterns. Interventions that include breath retraining, somatic experiencing, or body-oriented therapies leverage this knowledge to foster healing. By teaching clients to 'ride the breath wave', therapy becomes not just an intellectual exercise but an embodied journey of restoring rhythm and balance.

In education, integrating breath awareness into curricula, especially for children and adolescents, holds promise for cultivating emotional intelligence and resilience. Simple practices of pausing to breathe can equip young people with lifelong tools for managing stress, enhancing concentration, and fostering empathy. In a world increasingly driven by speed and stimulation, breath-centered education could offer a counter-rhythm of reflection, patience, and connection—qualities essential for navigating the complexities of the human condition.

On a broader cultural and philosophical level, re-centering breath reawakens a sense of interconnectedness between self, others, and the environment.

Many indigenous and spiritual traditions have long recognized that the breath is shared—between people, between species, between the animate and inanimate. The air we inhale has traveled across continents, oceans, and forests; it carries the trace of other lives, other histories, a collective wave moving through time and space. In this way, to attend to one's breath is also to participate in a shared planetary rhythm, reminding us that well-being is not merely personal but relational and ecological.

Returning to the image of the wave, the breath reminds us that life itself is cyclical. We rise with the inhalation, we fall with the exhalation, and in that ongoing ebb and flow, we are constantly being offered the chance to return—to ourselves, to presence, to the immediacy of now. The wave does not resist the pull of gravity nor the push of the wind; it moves with them, embodying a wisdom that we, too, can learn through breath. To breathe consciously is to ride the wave of being, embracing its crests and troughs with curiosity rather than fear.

In closing, the cultivation of breath literacy is not merely a health practice or therapeutic technique. It is a philosophical orientation, a way of living with attentiveness to the rhythms that define us, seen and unseen. It teaches us that just as waves return to shore, so too can we return—again and again—to presence, to balance, to the simple, profound act of breathing. In the end, the breath is both the journey and the homecoming, the pulse of life that continues, with or without our attention, inviting us to listen, to feel, and to be.

REFERENCES

Ashhad, S., Kam, K., Negro, C. A. D., & Feldman, J. L. (2022). Breathing Rhythm and Pattern and Their Influence on Emotion. *Annual Review of Neuroscience*, *45*(1), 223–247. Advance online publication. DOI: 10.1146/annurev-neuro-090121-014424 PMID: 35259917

Basara, L., Jokic Begic, N., Popovic Grle, S., Jakopovic, M., & Samarzija, M. (2018). DYSPNEA FROM NEUROPSYCHYATRIC PERSPECTIVE: A NARRATIVE REVIEW. *Psychiatria Danubina*, *30*(1), 11–20. DOI: 10.24869/psyd.2018.11 PMID: 29546853

Bass, C., & Gardner, W. (1985). Emotional influences on breathing and breathlessness. *Journal of Psychosomatic Research*, *29*(6), 599–609. DOI: 10.1016/0022-3999(85)90069-8 PMID: 3910805

Batson, G., & Schwartz, R. E. (2007). Revisiting the value of somatic education in dance training through an inquiry into practice schedules. *Journal of Distance Education*, *7*(2), 47–56.

Beauchaine, T. P., & Thayer, J. F. (2015). Heart rate variability as a transdiagnostic biomarker of psychopathology. *International Journal of Psychophysiology : Official Journal of the International Organization of Psychophysiology*, *98*(2), 338–350.

Berger, A. J. (1990). Recent advances in respiratory neurobiology using in vitro methods. *American Journal of Physiology. Lung Cellular and Molecular Physiology*, *259*(2), L24–L29. DOI: 10.1152/ajplung.1990.259.2.L24 PMID: 2200281

Boiten, F. A., Frijda, N. H., & Wientjes, C. J. (1994). Emotions and respiratory patterns: Review and critical analysis. *International Journal of Psychophysiology*, *17*(2), 103–128. DOI: 10.1016/0167-8760(94)90027-2 PMID: 7995774

Buchanan, T. L., & Janelle, C. M. (2022). Emotions and ensuing motor performance are altered by regulating breathing frequency: Implications for emotion regulation and sport performance. *Frontiers in Psychology*, *13*, 963711.

Carnicke, S. M. (2009). Stanislavsky and Female Actors: Women in Stanislavsky's Life and Art. By Maria Ignatieva. Lanham, Md.: University Press of America, 2008. xx, 140 pp. Notes. Bibliography. Index. $23.00, paper. *Slavic Review*, *68*(4), 985–986.

Critchley, H. D., & Harrison, N. A. (2013). Visceral influences on brain and behavior. *Neuron*, *77*(4), 624–638. DOI: 10.1016/j.neuron.2013.02.008 PMID: 23439117

Denzin, N. K. (1985). Emotion as Lived Experience. *Symbolic Interaction*, *8*(2), 223–240. DOI: 10.1525/si.1985.8.2.223

Dick, T. E., Dutschmann, M., Feldman, J. L., Fong, A. Y., Hülsmann, S., Morris, K. M., Ramirez, J. M., & Smith, J. C. (2018). Facts and challenges in respiratory neurobiology. *Respiratory Physiology & Neurobiology*, *258*, 104–107. DOI: 10.1016/j.resp.2015.01.014 PMID: 25644207

Draeger-Muenke, R., & Muenke, M. (2012). The healing energy of breath in traditional Chinese Medicine and other eastern traditions. In *Functional Respiratory Disorders: When Respiratory Symptoms Do Not Respond to Pulmonary Treatment* (pp. 301–323). Humana Press.

Esslin, M. (2001). Beckett and the Quest for Meaning. *Samuel Beckett Today/Aujourd'hui, 11*, 27-30.

Farb, N. A. S., Segal, Z. V., & Anderson, A. K. (2013). Mindfulness meditation training alters cortical representations of interoceptive attention. *Social Cognitive and Affective Neuroscience*, *8*(1), 15–26. DOI: 10.1093/scan/nss066 PMID: 22689216

Farb, N., Daubenmier, J., Price, C. J., Gard, T., Kerr, C., Dunn, B. D., & Mehling, W. E. (2015). Interoception, contemplative practice, and health. *Frontiers in Psychology*, *6*, 763.

Feldman, J. L., & Del Negro, C. A. (2006). Looking for inspiration: New perspectives on respiratory rhythm. *Nature Reviews. Neuroscience*, *7*(3), 232–241.

Franko, M. (2012). *Martha Graham in Love and War: the life in the work*. OUP USA.

Gardner, W. N. (1996). The pathophysiology of hyperventilation disorders. *Chest*, *109*(2), 516–534.

Gilbert, C. (2003). Book Review. *Behavior Modification*, *27*(5), 755–760. DOI: 10.1177/0145445503256326 PMID: 14531162

Haddad, G. G., & Farber, J. P. (1991). *Developmental neurobiology of breathing*.

Hanh, T. N. (2013). *Peace of mind: Becoming fully present*. Parallax Press.

Heine, S. (2017). animi Velut Respirant. *Comparative Literature*, *69*(4), 355–369. DOI: 10.1215/00104124-4260409

Heine, S. (2018). Ebb and Flow: Breath-Writing from Ancient Rhetoric to Jack Kerouac and Allen Ginsberg. *Palgrave Studies in Literature. Science & Medicine*, •••, 91–112. DOI: 10.1007/978-3-319-99948-7_5

Homma, I., & Masaoka, Y. (2008a). Breathing rhythms and emotions. *Experimental Physiology*, *93*(9), 1011–1021. DOI: 10.1113/expphysiol.2008.042424 PMID: 18487316

Homma, I., & Masaoka, Y. (2008b). Breathing rhythms and emotions. *Experimental Physiology*, *93*(9), 1011–1021. DOI: 10.1113/expphysiol.2008.042424 PMID: 18487316

Irigaray, L. (2002). *Between east and west: From singularity to community*. Columbia University Press.

Janson-Bjerklie, S., Carrieri, V. K., & Hudes, M. (1986). The sensations of pulmonary dyspnea. *Nursing Research*, *35*(3), 154–161.

Jerath, R., Crawford, M. W., Barnes, V. A., & Harden, K. (2015). Self-regulation of breathing as a primary treatment for anxiety. *Applied Psychophysiology and Biofeedback*, *40*(2), 107–115.

Joshi, M., & Telles, S. (2009). A Nonrandomized Non-Naive Comparative Study of the Effects of Kapalabhati and Breath Awareness on Event-Related Potentials in Trained Yoga Practitioners. *Journal of Alternative and Complementary Medicine (New York, N.Y.)*, *15*(3), 281–285. DOI: 10.1089/acm.2008.0250 PMID: 19243275

Kabat-Zinn, J. (2003). Mindfulness-based interventions in context: past, present, and future.

Kaiser, N., & Butler, E. (2021). Introducing social breathing: A model of engaging in relational systems. *Frontiers in Psychology*, *12*, 571298.

Kauffman, K. P. (2015). Emotional sentience and the nature of phenomenal experience. *Progress in Biophysics and Molecular Biology*, *119*(3), 545–562. DOI: 10.1016/j.pbiomolbio.2015.08.003 PMID: 26272799

Kim, D., Lee, J., Park, M. K., & Ko, S. H. (2024). Recent developments in wearable breath sensors for healthcare monitoring. *Communications Materials*, *5*(1), 1–14. DOI: 10.1038/s43246-024-00480-w

Knoblauch, S. H. (2017). The Fluidity of Emotions and Clinical Vulnerability: A Field of Rhythmic Tensions. *Psychoanalytic Perspectives*, *14*(3), 283–308. DOI: 10.1080/1551806X.2017.1342421

Knoblauch, S. H. (2019). Fluidity of emotions and vulnerability in the therapeutic situation: A field of rhythmic tensions. *Psyche*, *73*(4), 235–263.

Lehrer, P. M., & Gevirtz, R. (2014). Heart rate variability biofeedback: How and why does it work? *Frontiers in Psychology*, *5*, 756.

Levertov, D. (1992). *New & selected essays* (Vol. 749). New Directions Publishing.

Levine, P. A. (2010). *In an unspoken voice: How the body releases trauma and restores goodness*. North Atlantic Books.

Ley, R. (1999). The modification of breathing behavior: Pavlovian and operant control in emotion and cognition. *Behavior Modification, 23*(3), 441–479.

Linklater, K. (2006). Freeing the natural voice: Imagery and art in the practice of voice and language (Revised & expanded ed.). Drama Publishers / Quite Specific Media Group.

Liu, S., Ye, M., Pao, G. M., Song, S. M., Jhang, J., Jiang, H., Kim, J.-H., Kang, S. J., Kim, D.-I., & Han, S. (2021). Divergent brainstem opioidergic pathways that coordinate breathing with pain and emotions. *Neuron, 110*(5), 857–873.e9. Advance online publication. DOI: 10.1016/j.neuron.2021.11.029 PMID: 34921781

McCrimmon, D. R., Mitchell, G. S., & Alheid, G. F. (2008). Overview: The neurochemistry of respiratory control. *Respiratory Physiology & Neurobiology, 164*(1-2), 1–2. DOI: 10.1016/j.resp.2008.07.021 PMID: 18721910

Meduri, A. (Ed.). (2005). *Rukmini Devi Arundale, 1904-1986: A visionary architect of Indian culture and the performing arts*. Motilal Banarsidass Publishing House.

Merleau-Ponty, M. (1962). An unpublished work by Maurice Merleau-Ponty. *Revue de Metaphysique et de Morale, 67*(4), 401–409.

Meuret, A. E., Rosenfield, D., Seidel, A., Bhaskara, L., & Hofmann, S. G. (2010). Respiratory and cognitive mediators of treatment change in panic disorder: Evidence for intervention specificity. *Journal of Consulting and Clinical Psychology, 78*(5), 691.

Meuret, A. E., Kroll, J., & Ritz, T. (2017). Panic disorder comorbidity with medical conditions and treatment implications. *Annual Review of Clinical Psychology, 13*, 209–240.

Mewhinney, M. (2023). The Rhythm of Breath in Natsume Sōseki's Recollecting and Such. *Literature, 3*(1), 94–111. DOI: 10.3390/literature3010008

Mitsea, E., Drigas, A., & Skianis, C. (2024). Artificial Intelligence, Immersive Technologies, and Neurotechnologies in Breathing Interventions for Mental and Emotional Health: A Systematic Review. *Electronics (Basel), 13*(12), 2253. DOI: 10.3390/electronics13122253

Nair, S. (2007). *Restoration of Breath*. https://doi.org/DOI: 10.1163/9789401205177

Payne, P., Levine, P. A., & Crane-Godreau, M. A. (2015). Somatic experiencing: Using interoception and proprioception as core elements of trauma therapy. *Frontiers in Psychology*, *6*, 93. DOI: 10.3389/fpsyg.2015.00093 PMID: 25699005

Pérezts, M., Fotaki, M., Shymko, Y., & Islam, G. (2025). Breathe and let breathe: Breathing as a political model of organizing. *Organization*, *32*(1), 136–153.

Philippot, P., Chapelle, G., & Blairy, S. (2002). Respiratory feedback in the generation of emotion. *Cognition and Emotion*, *16*(5), 605–627. DOI: 10.1080/02699930143000392

Porges, S. W. (2007). The polyvagal perspective. *Biological Psychology*, *74*(2), 116–143. DOI: 10.1016/j.biopsycho.2006.06.009 PMID: 17049418

Prpa, M., Stepanova, E. R., Schiphorst, T., Riecke, B. E., & Pasquier, P. (2020). Inhaling and Exhaling: How Technologies Can Perceptually Extend our Breath Awareness. *Proceedings of the 2020 CHI Conference on Human Factors in Computing Systems*. DOI: 10.1145/3313831.3376183

Rochet-Capellan, A., & Fuchs, S. (2014). Take a breath and take the turn: How breathing meets turns in spontaneous dialogue. *Philosophical Transactions of the Royal Society of London. Series B, Biological Sciences*, *369*(1658).

Sengupta, P. (2012). Health impacts of yoga and pranayama: A state-of-the-art review. *International Journal of Preventive Medicine*, *3*(7), 444.

Shaffer, F., McCraty, R., & Zerr, C. L. (2014). A healthy heart is not a metronome: An integrative review of the heart's anatomy and heart rate variability. *Frontiers in Psychology*, *5*, 1040.

Shih, C. H., Tomita, N., Lukic, Y. X., Reguera, Á. H., Fleisch, E., & Kowatsch, T. (2019). Breeze: Smartphone-based acoustic real-time detection of breathing phases for a gamified biofeedback breathing training. *Proceedings of the ACM on Interactive, Mobile, Wearable and Ubiquitous Technologies*, *3*(4), 1–30.

Shirane, H. (2012). *Traditional Japanese literature: An anthology, beginnings to 1600*. Columbia University Press.

Škof, L., & Holmes, E. A. (Eds.). (2013). *Breathing with Luce Irigaray*. Bloomsbury Publishing Plc., DOI: 10.5040/9781472547965

Solomon, H. (2021). Living on borrowed breath: Respiratory distress, social breathing, and the vital movement of ventilators. *Medical Anthropology Quarterly*, *35*(1), 102–119.

Stevens, J. P., Sheridan, A. R., Bernstein, H. B., Baker, K., Lansing, R. W., Schwartzstein, R. M., & Banzett, R. B. (2019). A Multidimensional Profile of Dyspnea in Hospitalized Patients. *Chest, 156*(3), 507–517. DOI: 10.1016/j.chest.2019.04.128 PMID: 31128117

Tang, Y. Y., Hölzel, B. K., & Posner, M. I. (2015). The neuroscience of mindfulness meditation. *Nature Reviews. Neuroscience, 16*(4), 213–225.

Thayer, J. F., & Lane, R. D. (2000). A model of neurovisceral integration in emotion regulation and dysregulation. *Journal of Affective Disorders, 61*(3), 201–216.

Tsaknaki, V. (2021, June). The breathing wings: An autobiographical soma design exploration of touch qualities through shape-change materials. In *Proceedings of the 2021 ACM Designing Interactive Systems Conference* (pp. 1266-1279).

Van der Kolk, B. (2014). The body keeps the score: Brain, mind, and body in the healing of trauma. *New York, 3*, 14-211.

Vlemincx, E., Abelson, J. L., Lehrer, P. M., Davenport, P. W., Van Diest, I., & Van den Bergh, O. (2013). Respiratory variability and sighing: A psychophysiological reset model. *Biological Psychology, 93*(1), 24–32. DOI: 10.1016/j.biopsycho.2012.12.001 PMID: 23261937

von Leupoldt, A., Mertz, C., Kegat, S., Burmester, S., & Dahme, B. (2006). The impact of emotions on the sensory and affective dimension of perceived dyspnea. *Psychophysiology, 43*(4), 382–386. DOI: 10.1111/j.1469-8986.2006.00415.x PMID: 16916434

Wayne, P. M., & Kaptchuk, T. J. (2008). Challenges inherent to t'ai chi research: Part I—t'ai chi as a complex multicomponent intervention. *The Journal of Alternative and Complementary Medicine: Paradigm, Practice, and Policy Advancing Integrative Health, 14*(1), 95–102.

Yii, A. C., & Koh, M. S. (2013). A review of psychological dysfunction in asthma: Affective, behavioral and cognitive factors. *The Journal of Asthma : Official Journal of the Association for the Care of Asthma, 50*(9), 915–921.

Yoo, J. (2019). Learning to Write Through an Awareness of Breath. *Qualitative Inquiry, 107780041984653*. Advance online publication. DOI: 10.1177/1077800419846533

Zaccaro, A., Piarulli, A., Laurino, M., Garbella, E., Menicucci, D., Neri, B., & Gemignani, A. (2018). How breath-control can change your life: A systematic review on psycho-physiological correlates of slow breathing. *Frontiers in Human Neuroscience, 12*, 353. Advance online publication. DOI: 10.3389/fnhum.2018.00353 PMID: 30245619

Chapter 11

Yoga and the Mind–Body Connection: Integrative Perspectives on Neurophysiology, Mental Health, and Embodied Awareness

Dilshith Azeezul Kabeer
http://orcid.org/0000-0003-3317-1167
Pondicherry University, India

W. Vinu
http://orcid.org/0000-0001-6745-9893
Pondicherry University, India

K. K. Shareef
Pondicherry University, India

M. K. Aravind
Pondicherry University, India

N. K. Ashif Ali
Pondicherry University, India

ABSTRACT

The chapter presents a unified examination of yoga and its body-mind approach by exploring neural mechanisms, psychological and philosophical aspects. It examines how yoga facilitates the body-mind connection through yogic texts and scientific study, such as breath regulation (pranayama), postural awareness (asana) and meditative focus (dhyana). This study applies polyvagal theory, interoceptive awareness,

DOI: 10.4018/979-8-3373-4187-3.ch011

neuroplasticity and the biopsychosocial framework. Research in neuroscience and mental health shows yoga's efficacy in addressing anxiety, depression, trauma and stress. The chapter highlights yoga as an evidence-based non-drug intervention combining traditional Eastern knowledge with Western science to benefit mental health holistically. This part outlines present-day yoga research restrictions, including cultural knowledge appropriateness, methodological challenges, and future directions. This research supports yoga as an effective practice for developing unified mind-body relationships, emotional resilience and psychological health in both individuals and collective contexts.

1 INTRODUCTION

In the modern world, individuals face anxiety and depression, trauma-related and stress-related illnesses. In orderly, mental and physical health, highlighting the problems separately. They have different views on the connection between mind and body. In Western belief, there is a solid entity between the mind and body influenced by Cartesian dualism. This systematic view, ensuing physical laws, while the mind is observed as the source of consciousness, is set apart and superior. The mind-body connection in the Eastern tradition of yoga and Advaita Vedanta emphasise deep and strong. Consciousness (chitta), life energy (prana), and physical body (shirira) are the yoga sutras of Patanjali. These concepts of human reality are explained in the Upanishads. In this Eastern tradition, physical states are interconnected to thoughts and emotions. These concepts explain that mental problems can affect physical health, and also that physical exercise enhances mental stability. The following characteristics convey that yoga is not only a physical exercise, but it is a total well-being through the integration of yoga.

1.1 Integration in the Modern Health System

Modern medicine has made huge advancements in treating diseases, but it still often separates physical health and mental health. It considers them as different areas with special kinds of treatment. Conversely, the increasing figure of psychosomatic disorders, where emotional stress indications up as physical symptoms, shows the need for a more joined approach to healthcare. In modern years, experts have known the requirement for models that consider biological, psychological, and social elements in health and illness. Yoga is an excellent illustration of how these elements can work together. It includes using the body postures, breath control, and focused attention (Maity et al., 2024). Studies have shown that yoga balances the autonomic nervous system for the body and controls stress hormones to enhance emotional strength in the mind. Integrating mind-body practices such as yoga into modern healthcare can support more holistic care and better reflect contemporary understanding of health as a whole-person experience (Chinnusamy et al., 2025).

1.2 Psychosomatic and Psychospiritual Aspects in Yoga

The main parts of yoga are the Asana (posture), Pranayama (breathing techniques), and Dhyana (meditation). These components work together to develop body awareness and regulate physical functions, then automatically relax the mind. In the same way, this technique helps people recognise themselves better and supports overall well-being. Yoga meets individuals as having several connected stages, termed Koshas. Modern research studies help this idea by showing that yoga affects brain zones that assist in managing emotions, develop heart functions, and support changes in the brain that make it stronger. Yoga involves a psychospiritual feature that emphasises self-exploration, living morally, and recognising our relationship to all around us. The approach helps people change after their personal conjunction and get a feeling more attached to society. Yoga supports sympathy, mindfulness, and awareness in creating a peaceful world.

This chapter discusses the mind-body connection in yoga. Proposing both a philosophical experience and research helps in its capability to integrate these characteristics. The chapter begins by examining yoga's historical and philosophical foundations, including concepts such as non-dualism, the five koshas, and the gunas. It then explores how yoga influences physiological and psychological functioning, how it controls the autonomic nervous system, stabilises hormones, and alters brain connections. The chapter converges on the three key practices, such as asana (posture), pranayama (breathing), and dhyana (meditation), and how to cultivate awareness of our bodies and inner feelings. Conclusively, the chapter examines the justifications and limitations of current methodologies. Also, recommend future research practice areas and highlight the need for culturally sensitive and interdisciplinary techniques. This translational progression of yoga, from its philosophical foundations to evidence-based applications in contemporary societal contexts, is schematically represented in Figure 4.1, illustrating its expanding role in promoting global well-being.

Figure 1. Flowchart showing how traditional yoga has evolved from ancient wisdom to scientific validation, leading to therapeutic applications and promoting global well-being.

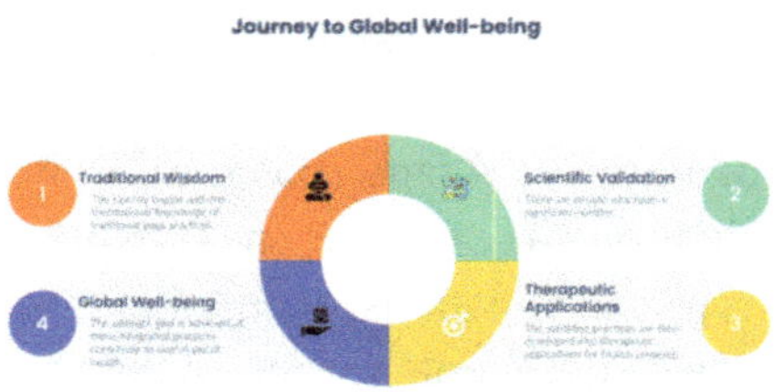

2 PHILOSOPHICAL FOUNDATIONS OF MIND-BODY IN YOGA

2.1 Understanding Non-Dualism in Yoga

At the core of yogic philosophy lies the standard of non-dualism (advaita), which asserts the fundamental unity of awareness and material existence. Contrasting dualistic systems that isolate mind and matter, Advaita posits that both are manifestations of a singular underlying reality, Brahman, or pure consciousness. In this perspective, the separation between body and mind is an illusion (maya). Yoga deals with a simple way to bring together the mind and body, helping people understand their natural completeness. Through regular practice, the constant changes in the mind (chitta vritti) can calm down, allowing a clear association between inner awareness and the external world. Contemporary cognitive science supports this view, showing that mental processes connect closely with physical states. Therefore, yoga's non-dual method contributes a solid, practical way to unite the mind and body, assisting in overcoming the separation that frequently leads to human suffering.

2.2 Five Sheaths of Pancha Kosha

The pancha kosha model, explained in the Taittiriya Upanishad, deals with an understanding support of human presence that integrates physical, energetic, mental, intellectual, and bliss dimensions. The five sheaths of human experience are:

1. Annamaya kosha: The physical body, constant by food.

2. Pranayama kosha: The vital energy layer, leading physiological functions through prana.
3. Manomaya kosha: The mental-emotional sheath, covering feelings and emotions.
4. Vijnanamaya kosha: The intellect and discernment layer.
5. Anandamaya kosha: This is the state of true pleasure and association with something better.

2.3 Gunas in Yoga

Yogic philosophy states that everything, involving the mind and body, is made up of three qualities called gunas:

1. Clarity, harmony, balance (Sattva)
2. Activity, passion, restlessness (Rajas)
3. Inertia, darkness, ignorance (Tamas)

These three gunas cooperate and shape a person's mental and physical state. Excessive Rajas lead to anxiety or hyperactivity, and too much Tamas causes lethargy or depression. Sattva is the ideal state in yoga and also represents balance, lightness, and clear thinking, promoting well-being and spiritual progress. Yoga practices are obviously proposed to reduce Tamas and Rajas while increasing Sattva. Body balance and energy are kept through Asanas. Meditation sharpens awareness, and the pranayama supports the flow of life energy (prana). Yoga practitioners can better control their inner state by learn about gunas, and it helps them accomplish harmony between mind and body (M. Pascoe & Bauer, 2015).

2.4 Key Yoga Concepts of Chitta, Prana, and Sharira

A clear explanation is provided by yoga, how the mind and body work together. Chitta means the whole mind, which involves retention, thinking and feelings. Prana indicates the life force that stimulates the body and keeps it functioning. Sharira denotes the body itself, perceived as an existing, intentional entity rather than just an unconscious object. Highlighting the holistic view in yoga, consider how thoughts, emotions, and physical states are associated. The thoughts and emotions (chitta) always disturb the flow of life energy (prana). From the disturbance of chitta, create physical tension or illness. Conversely, it causes stress in the mind if prana is disrupted. The target of yoga is to relax the chitta by adjusting prana and improving the physical body (sharira).

2.5 Classical Insights Sources

The connection of mind and body is associated with the yoga sutras of Patanjali and the Bhagavat Gita, which are the fundamental texts. In the yoga sutras, Patanjali's sutras state that yoga is the ending of mental variations, which means relaxing the mind. The mind relaxation technique is achieved by ethical behaviour, postures, breath mechanism, extracting the senses, concentrating, and meditating. For the fundamental consciousness, these phases connect the body and mind. Bhagavat Gita emphasises bhakti yoga, which signifies devotion, and karma yoga means taking action without being involved in the outcome. It expresses how it focuses on internal harmony, emotional state, and good actions (Pandurangi et al., 2017). Having reviewed yoga's philosophical foundations, the following section explores the corresponding neurophysiological mechanisms.

3 NEUROPHYSIOLOGICAL MECHANISMS OF THE MIND-BODY INTERFACE

The mind-body interface, from the neurophysiological perspective, is the two-way, dynamic interaction between the body and brain, including the integration of cognitive, emotional, and physiological processes. This is supported by neural networks and signalling pathways connecting major central brain regions, including the prefrontal cortex, amygdala, insula, and anterior cingulate cortex, to the autonomic nervous system, which regulates heart rate, respiration, and stress responses. Recent studies indicate heightened activation in the insular cortex and anterior cingulate cortex among long-term yoga practitioners, thereby endorsing enhanced interoceptive awareness and emotional regulation (Campelo et al., 2025). Yoga, as a mind-body intervention, modulates central and autonomic nervous system pathways. It promotes the activity of localities concerned with interoception, the processing of emotions, and attentional controls and balances the parasympathetic system and reduces sympathetic activation. This chapter outlines the neuromodulator mechanisms and neuroanatomical substrates involved in the mind-body interaction and reviews evidence related to the long-term neuroplastic changes induced by yoga practice that underlie its benefits to mental health, emotional regulation, and physiological functioning. Overall, yoga has effects on both top-down and bottom-up processes due to the control of autonomic, hormonal, and neural networks. These changes in the vagal tone, cortisol patterns, and insular activity prove that yoga enhances self-regulation.

3.1 Brain Regions Involved in Yoga Practice

Yoga and meditation activities involve a circuit of brain areas that are part of the neurophysiological foundation of the mind-body interface. The most prominent of them is the prefrontal cortex (PFC) (front part of the brain responsible for planning, decision-making, self-control, and higher thinking) with its subdivisions and the dorsolateral, ventrolateral, and orbitofrontal regions that are always in use during practice. The PFC contributes to executive operation, attentional management and emotional management. It has been found that long-term yogic practitioners exhibit greater volume of gray matter and oxygenation of the brain in them, indicating greater structural neuroplasticity and neural efficiency. Both the anterior cingulate cortex (ACC) (a brain region that helps regulate emotions, focus attention, make decisions, and detect errors) and the insular cortex (a brain region involved in bodily awareness) play significant roles as well. The ACC is implicated in conflict monitoring and controlled cognition, and the insula in interoceptive awareness, conscious awareness of internal body conditions. Due to increased white matter connections between the ACC, insula, and amygdala in meditators, there is an indication of improved integration of emotion and attention (Perez-Diaz et al., 2024).

Hippocampus and amygdala, which are key in memory and emotion processing, also show structural modifications with the prolonged practice of yoga. The diminished volume of the amygdala, especially in the right hemisphere, has been related to the attenuated emotional reactivity and stress responsiveness. Striatum and caudate, which are part of the basal ganglia, also happen to have functional connectivity which enables improvements in behaviour regulation and attention flexibility. The Functional neuroimaging (fMRI, EEG) displays more connectivity in attention and control networks, and less default mode network activity. Electrophysiological experiments also depict that there is an increase in theta, alpha, and beta in the brains of skilled practitioners, and such a process is reflected in the increase in self-awareness, emotional stability, and cognitive clarity. In combination, these modifications constitute a well-grounded neural basis of the psychological advantages of yoga.

3.2 The Vagus Nerve and the Autonomic Nervous System

The main afferent pathway of the parasympathetic nervous system (PNS), which stimulates a state of relaxation, healing and physiologic homeostasis, is the vagus nerve. The words vagal tone denote the functional action of the vagus nerve. The higher the vagal tone, the more important a parasympathetic response and better management of stress, emotional stability, and faster restoration to baseline in response to arousal. A common measure in this respect is the heart rate variability

(HRV), which measures the variability in time between successive heartbeats and is considered to be a biomarker of vagal tone. Greater HRV is indicative of good vagal functioning and resiliency in responding to stress. Yoga, specifically via the means of pranayama (breath training), mindfulness and deep relaxation, activates vagal afferents, thus enhancing parasympathetic state and decreasing sympathetic arousal. Autonomic rebalancing helps reduce the allostatic load, which is the physiologic burden of chronic stress and aids systemic regulation and psychological resilience. Several studies carried out empirically in clinical trials and physiological studies have proven the good performance of yoga in the enhancement of vagal tone and HRV (Udupa & Sathyaprabha, 2018).

3.3 Hormonal and Neurochemical Mediators

This part explores how yoga controls the neurophysiological mechanisms that border the mind and the body, especially through the processes of hormonal and neurochemical mechanisms. Yoga activities have been revealed to cause a decrease in cortisol, which is a major stress hormone, and an increase in oxytocin, which favours emotional attachment and social interactions, and promotes melatonin that aids sleep regulation. The hormonal effects also carry a worth of enhanced stress coping and emotional well-being. The neurochemical brain mechanism of yoga has been attributed to significant levels of increased levels of gamma-aminobutyric acid (GABA) neurotransmitters, serotonin and dopamine neurotransmitters, which influence mood regulation, emotional stability and cognitive capacity. Yoga further seems to increase brain-derived neurotrophic factor (BDNF). BDNF is a neurotropic growth factor which plays a pivotal role in neuroplasticity, neuron learning, and the level of resilience (Brems, 2020). The physiological effects are partly assisted by the effect of yoga on the hypothalamic-pituitary-adrenal (HPA) axis (the body's central stress-response system), which facilitates the recovery of the stress response and thus a shift towards parasympathetic nervous system preponderance. Such a transition helps one to relax, recover and restore autonomic balance. At the clinical level, these alterations are associated with decreases in anxiety and symptoms of depression, enhanced emotional control, and cognitive functioning. Key neurochemical mechanisms of yoga are summarized in Table 4.1 and illustrated in Figure 4.2.

Table 1. Summary of Key Neurochemicals Influenced by Yoga Practices.

Neurochemical	Function	Yoga Influence
GABA	Calming, reduces anxiety	↑ with asana and meditation (Streeter et al., 2010).
Serotonin	Mood regulation	↑ with meditation and breathwork (Lee et al., 2014)
Cortisol	Stress hormone	↓ with yoga, especially breathwork and meditation (Thirthalli et al., 2013).
Dopamine	Motivation, reward	↑ with regular yoga practice (Kjaer et al., 2002)
Norepinephrine	Alertness, arousal	↓ with yoga, balancing stress response
Endorphins	Pain relief, well-being	↑ with yoga and meditation (Saleem et al., 2025).

Figure 2. Yoga-Induced Modulation of Neurotransmitters and Brain Systems Relevant to Mental Health.

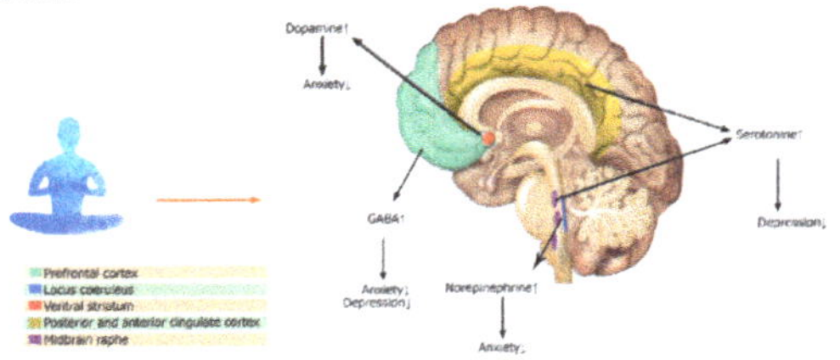

Adapted from (Nourollahimoghadam et al., 2021).

3.4 Polyvagal Theory: Safety, Regulations, and Social Engagement

Polyvagal Theory is a theory by Stephen Porges which offers a neurobiological understanding of the autonomous nervous system (ANS) underpins emotional regulation, safety, and social engagement. The most important of the tenets of the theory is the notion of neuroception (the nervous system's unconscious detection of safety or threat), the unconscious assessment of the environment as either safe or threatening, and the mediating effects of the ventral vagal complex in helping foster calm, good relationships and emotional regulation. Activation of the ventral vagus leads to an increase in the social connections and psychological resilience of people (M. B. Sullivan et al., 2018). The features of Yoga, such as mindful movement, controlled breathing, and rhythmical engagement, can activate the ventral vagal pathway and evoke internal feelings of safety. Such activation is beneficial as it promotes the social engagement system at the same time that it calms sympathetic arousal and dorsal vagal shutdown, conditions related to immobilisation, dissociation, and emotional numbing that are commonly seen in people who are trauma-affected. Under trauma-informed practices, a combination of the Polyvagal Theory and yoga can present an effective concept of regaining the balance of our autonomous system and promoting embodied self-directive activities. It places yoga not only as a physical or relaxation practice or as a means of relaxation but as a therapeutic approach that involves fundamental neurophysiological pathways involved with safety, connectedness, and healing. In post-traumatic recovery, yoga, which is based on the polyvagal principles, may play a great role in attaining a shift in defensive states towards greater regulatory, resilient and prosocial functioning.

3.5 Neuroplasticity and Long-Term Psychophysiological Change

Yoga has gained wider acceptance in its possible neuroplastic impacts with reported growth in the volume of the gray matter and thickening of the cortex in the brain regions involving the hippocampus, prefrontal cortex (PFC), and insular cortex, which are critical areas involved in memory, executive function, and interoceptive awareness. Regular yoga practice seems to promote the integration processes of both the top-down (cognitive control) and bottom-up (sensory and emotional processing), achieving long-term adaptation in the psychophysiological aspect. The existing neuroimaging evidence indicates that yoga leads to an increase in the functional interconnectedness of fundamental brain networks, such as the default mode one (DMN), and can potentially curtail age-related or disease-related neural decline. Molecularly, yoga boosts the activity of neuroplasticity markers such as brain-derived neurotrophic factor (BDNF) as well as telomerase activities, whereas decreasing the stressful hormones like cortisol and inflammatory markers like interleukin-6 (IL-6). These results indicate that yoga could play a role in gene expression and epigenetic pathways implicated in inflammation and stress regulation, and cellular health. The neurobiological outcome is associated with positive mood state, less anxiety and depressive symptoms, and increased resilience, which may underlie the potential of yoga as a comprehensive intervention towards mental and cognitive health (Tolahunase et al., 2018).

The above-described neurophysiological mechanisms are put into practice through the triad of asana, pranayama, and dhyana. The next section looks at how those practices operationalise neural, autonomic, and somatic regulation.

4 THE TRIAD OF PRACTISING

Embodied yoga practice is grounded in the triad of asana (physical postures), pra ayama (breath regulation), and dhyana (meditation), which presents a holistic framework of psychophysiological regulation and overall well-being. While distinct in method, these components are complementary as they work in synergy to balance body, breath, and mind. Asana develops physical strength, flexibility, and somatic awareness and promotes emotional balance. The process of Pranayama regulates the autonomic nervous system, reduces stress and enhances the activation of the parasympathetic system with the help of breathing techniques. Dhyana leads to mindfulness, emotional resilience and cognitive stability by fostering non-reactive present-centred awareness (Liu et al., 2025). collectively, the practices allow managing both physical and psychological stressors, reinforcing one another's effects, and strengthening their influences on emotional regulation, cognitive function, and overall health. This section of the chapter looks at the role of individual practices and how the combination makes a whole system of self-regulation, mental clarity and transformation.

4.1 Asana and Proprioceptive Feedback

Asana, or the physical postures of the yoga practice, is responsible for enhancing proprioceptive awareness, the internal ability of the body to perceive its position, movement, and balance. By the practice of conscious and aware movement, asana activates proprioceptive pathways like the sensorimotor cortex, cerebellum, and spinal reflex arcs and thus improves neuromuscular coordination and posture control (Nayan Rishi, 2024). This is done through sensory neurons that carry signals from muscles and joints through the medial lemniscus pathway to the somatosensory cortex, where conscious proprioceptive experience is integrated and processed. Regular repetition of asana strengthens these neural pathways and leads to improved balance, motor flexibility, and physical stability. In addition to the neuromuscular benefits, asana enables one to perform bottom-up regulation of the nervous system. The exclusive attention to the bodily sensations during practice conditions the mindfulness in the present moment, decreasing anxiety and promoting emotional stability. Therefore, the somatic dimension of asana renders it a gateway and key to physical, emotional regulation and takes part in a collective mind-body wellbeing through proprioception system clarification. A simple posture, such as Balasana (Child's Pose), encourages parasympathetic activation and is commonly used in therapeutic settings.

4.2 Pranayama and Breath-Driven Autonomic Regulation

Pranayama, the breath regulation, is the yogic science that includes techniques like Nadi Shodhana (alternate nostrils breathing), Ujjayi and Bhramari. These techniques show different modulatory influences on the autonomic nervous system (ANS) (Nivethitha et al., 2016). These practices have proven to slow the heart rate, increase heart rate variability (HRV), and ensure an active equilibrium exists between the sympathetic and the parasympathetic action. For example, slow diaphragmatic breathing stimulates vagal pathways, which can immediately reduce heart rate and feelings of anxiety. Specifically, the slow performance of pranayama promotes the dominance of the parasympathetic system over sympathetic arousal and helps to maintain the autonomic homeostasis and lower stress (Pal et al., 2004). The fundamental processes include the excitation of various cerebral areas, including the brainstem, involved in autonomic and respiratory rhythm control and the insular cortex, which is used to integrate interoceptive awareness, and the prefrontal cortex, linked to higher-order cognitive regulation and emotion modulation. Through these neural pathways, conscious breath control enhances vagal tone and influences cardiovascular function and emotional regulation (Betka et al., 2022). Through these neural pathways which conscious breathing can increase vagal tone and affect the cardiovascular system and emotional regulation. The effectiveness of pranayama in the decrease of blood pressure in hypertensive individuals, and in the improvement of the symptoms of anxiety and panic conditions and reduction of stress-related consequences, was confirmed with clinical research. As a non-invasive, accessible intervention, pranayama provides a breath-based solution to autonomic self-regulation, strengthening psychophysiological resilience and psychological well-being. It has been incorporated in the therapeutic and preventive health model, thus the evidence of its application as a holistic mind-body practice.

4.3 Dyana: Attentional Training and Neural Coherence

Dhyana attentional meditation was acknowledged as powerful in enhancing executive functioning and the capacity of emotional regulation through the optimal tuning of cognitive control and adaptive stress response functioning. Neuroimaging and electrophysiological neuroscience studies indicate that during dhyana, fronto-parietal networks engaged in sustained attention, the salience network is modulated to improve attentional saliency, and the default mode network (DMN), which usually correlates with mind-wandering and self-referential processing, is deactivated. In numerous EEG studies, it was frequently repeated that when meditating, a person has more alpha waves and theta waves. These waves indicate some form of relaxed alertness and concentrated internal conscious awareness.

Dhyana has also been linked with the positive effects on short-term memory, mood, and cognitive functioning, and some early evidence indicates epigenetic changes that facilitate long-term neural plasticity (Pragya et al., 2021). Collectively, these results bring dhyana into the conceptual framework of a powerful method of inducing neural coherence, attentional flexibility, and emotional resiliency, supporting integrated psychophysiological health.

4.4 Synergic Effects: Beyond Single-Component Models

An integrated model of yoga conceptualises the triad of asana (postures), pranayama (breath regulation), and dhyana (meditation) as a dynamic psychophysiological loop, wherein each element reinforces and amplifies the effects of the others through continuous interaction between body, breath, and mind. This cooperation has synergistic effects, positively reinforcing interoceptive awareness, emotion resilience and cognitive regulation with a resulting effect that is greater as compared to the impacts of isolated practices. Inter-disciplinary empirical studies and meta-analyses confirm that the technical effect of multi-component yoga interventions on psychological well-being, physiological health, and cognitive processing variables is more integrative in terms of improvement as compared to single-component interventions. Holistic practice is important since Integrated protocols have proven effective in improving mental health, academic performance, and social well-being. This model theoretically embraces top-down and bottom-up mechanisms of self-regulation, which enhance autonomic balance and long-term psychophysiological flexibility. These effects are also congruent with the classical yogic idea of sadhana, that is, the unity of the body, breath and the mind as the foundation of self-realisation and holistic transformation. Modern research supports this holistic view more, and yoga is validated as a multidimensional tool to promote optimal well-being. (Voss et al., 2023).

4.5 Classical and Contemporary Interpretations of Integration

Classical interpretations of yoga as described in Patanjali's A tanga Yoga and the Hatha Yoga Pradipika present a unified path where ethical precepts (yama and niyama), physical postures (asana), breath management (pranayama) and meditation (dhyana) are combined in order to achieve mental stillness (citta-v tti-nirodha) and spiritual recognition. In these contexts, asana and pranayama serve as preparatory stages for meditative absorption and mind-body-spirit and soul unification. By contrast, contemporary readings tend to separate out yoga into distinct modalities such as exercise-oriented asana, mindfulness-oriented meditation, or autonomous breathwork, witnessing both worldwide dissemination and accommodation to modern lifestyles. This evolution has also challenged how the balance between accessibility and authenticity is maintained, and has created worries that such fragmentation will disrupt the unifying ethos that pervades classical yoga. To connect this gap, it is important to respect the philosophical origin of yoga and, at the same time, justify integrated practices through empirical research. Notably, both the traditional and modern yoga varieties produce similar positive results according to systematic reviews. The balanced model proposed by scholars allows embracing both classical ideals and scientific research in the practice of yoga, where yoga can be explained as an evidence-informed, whole approach to practice that holds a compatible view of yoga with classical traditions and modern health paradigms.

5 NEUROPHYSIOLOGY OF EMBODIED AWARENESS AND INTEROCEPTION

5.1 The Essence of Embodied Awareness

Embodied awareness refers to the active engagement with one's body as the primary ground for perception, emotion and identity fundamentally rooted in the lived experience of the body. It moves beyond traditional dualistic views of mind and body by highlighting how individuals live through their bodies. Rather than viewing the body as a mere vessel or object, embodied awareness recognises the body as the locus of lived experience, where perception and meaning are generated through direct interaction with the world around them. In addition, individuals cultivate embodied awareness and muscle tone through asana (postures), pranayama (breath control, and Dhyana (meditation). Asanas build strength and flexibility, while pranayama promotes mindful breathing, reducing stress and enhancing emotional regulatio. Through Dhyana they foster mental clarity and presence. Together these practices improve physical fitness and psychological well-being and fostering a harmonious connection between body and mind. A randomised trial (Eusebio et al., 2022) showed that after 10 weeks, there was a significant improvement in proprioceptive accuracy and interoceptive sensitivity. And also, yoga helps a person transition from automatic and scattered thinking to a more unified awareness of their body and mind. It opens better emotional stability and stress management while reinforcing a stable sense of himself. This embodied awareness improves mental resilience and overall well-being by integrating sensory and cognitive and emotional aspects of experience.

5.2 Inner and Outer Awareness: Exploration of Interception, proprioception, and Mindfulness

Individuals use three major systems to understand their body states: proprioception, interoception and mindfulness. Each system plays uniquely to self-awareness and managing emotions.

Proprioception: proprioception is the sensory system that helps us know where our body is and how it moves and muscle tension. It is essential for controlling our movements and spatial orientation but also plays a significant role in emotional regulation and social responsiveness. Proprioception helps us be aware of our bodies, which supports our social and emotional connections. Therapies that focus on improving proprioceptive feedback such as movement exercises and muscle relaxation that can help people control their emotions better. Proprioception also influences emotional responses and interpersonal behaviour. The signals from our joints and muscles tell our brain about body's state and it helps us be aware about our self (Shafir, 2016).

Interoception: Interoception refers to the process by which the nervous system detects and understands what happens inside our bodies. Those includes heart rate, respiration and visceral sensations. The consciousness of our bodily states and the emotional experiences depend on this process. By integrating multi-modal internal bodily signals, the system facilitates homeostasis while enhancing self-awareness. Whereas most interoceptive signals operate beneath conscious awareness, their perception by conscious creatures has a large impact on affect, cognition, and behaviour. The interoceptive system continuously provides information about the organism's state (Solano Durán et al., 2024).

Mindfulness: Mindfulness refers to paying attention to the present moment experience without judgment including our bodily sensations. It enhances self-awareness of our feelings and bodily signals. These practices of mindfulness also positively improve control and understanding of the body's position. Additionally, mindfulness supports emotional regulation by fostering greater awareness and acceptance of emotional states. These mindfulness programs can decrease mental illness issues by enhancing body awareness and emotional parameters. While the link between mindfulness and measurable body awareness is mindset, therefore it supports recognizing bodily signals in our conscious experience.

5.3 Insular Cortex Functionality in Interoception: A Neural Interface Between Body and Mind

The insular cortex is crucial for processing internal body signals and help us become aware of them. It receives information from the body's organs and sends it through the thalamus. The posterior insula maps basic sensation such as temperature and pain. Damage to the insula, especially on the right side can hider awareness of internal signals and affect our sense of self. Its connections are vital for balancing our body and emotions. These changes help them better understanding manage their emotions, maintain a balanced nervous system and their feeling. Paying attention to interoceptive sensations such as through breath awareness and moving mindfully those helps the insula in our brain work better and improves self-perception. Therefore, the insula acts not just as a hub for sensory integration, but also as a pathway for improving our feelings and strength our emotions. This practice can boost our mental stability and mental health also through mindful activities.

5.4 Yoga-Based Interventions for Trauma Recovery: Reconnecting Body and self in Dissociative State

Trauma often makes one's ability to inhabit the body safely and consciously. Survivors often disconnect from their sensations, emotions and sense of identity due to changes in certain brain areas that increase stress response. Here yoga helps us to re-embodiment through movement, breathing and stillness. Trauma-sensitive yoga (TSY) emphasizes safety, awareness of internal sensations, and individual limits. Instructors avoid physical adjustment and encourage participants to move at their own pace and allowing individuals to regain control over their experience. These regular practices calm the body and restore balance. By focusing on internal cues, participants learn to manage sensations and emotions better. Clinicians often use guided breath awareness with trauma survivors because it helps patients safely reconnect with bodily sensations without becoming overwhelmed (English et al., 2022). Some studies explored that trauma-informed yoga can reduce PTSD symptoms, improve variability of heart rate, and enhance mental and emotional clarity. Desperate talking therapies, yoga addresses memories stored in the body. By developing a safe connection with themselves, yoga empowers individuals and serves as a powerful tool for healing and self-awareness.

5.5 Embodied Cognition and Mind-Body Interface

Embodied cognition offers the role of the body in influencing our thoughts, feelings and actions by showing that mental processes emerge from interactions between the body brain and environment. This idea challenges the separation of mind and body and emphasizes can influence our facial expressions and mental state and how posture breathing movement. Empirical studies show that standing up straight can improve self-esteem and mood. Yoga puts this into practice by using specific postures, breath control, and stillness to influence our feelings. Backwards bends can enhance the energy of the body, and forward bends help relax. By aligning body-based interventions with neural and psychological mechanisms, yoga offers a bottom-up pathway to cognitive enhancement and emotional regulation. Therefore, connecting body-centred practices with mental processes yoga offers a way to manage emotions and improve thinking while complementing traditional therapies and enhancing mental well-being.

6 IMPACT OF YOGA ON MENTAL HEALTH: EMPIRICAL AND CLINICAL INSIGHTS

6.1 Mind-Body Disconnection and Mental Health Disorder

Mental Health Disorder: A mental health disorder is a clinically significant disturbance in an individual's integration of cognition, emotional regulation or behavior that reflects a dysfunction in psychological, biological, or developmental processes. A phenomenon commonly referred to as mind-body disconnection. In such a state, individuals may feel emotionally detached from their physical sensations or experience their bodies as unfamiliar or unsafe. These disorders affect how people think, feel, and act, and they often impair social, academic, or occupational functioning.

Mind-Body Disconnection: Mind-body disconnection happens when the link between our mental processes is disrupted. Such as thoughts, emotions and physical sensations break down (e.g., heartbeat, muscle tension). This disconnection can affect overall well-being and mental health. To regain this connection, people can try practices like yoga and somatic therapies. These activities can help restore awareness and create a more integrated sense of self. Under, Table 4.2 outlines key neurobiological correlates of mind–body disconnection in mental health disorders.

Table 2. Neurobiological Correlates of Mind-Body Disconnection in Mental Health Disorders.

Mental Health Disorder	Manifestations of Mind-Body Disconnection	Neurobiological Correlates	Reference
Depression	→ Emotional numbness → Sense of disembodiment → Fatigue and lower energy → Diminishing interoceptive awareness	→ Reduce activity in the insula → Altered hypothalamic-pituitary-adrenal (HPA) axis functions → Decrease vagal tone	(Ruggiero et al., 2025)
Anxiety	→ Persistent hyperarousal → Misinterpretation of internal bodily sensations → Somatic symptoms like panic and restlessness	→ Heightened amygdala reactivity → Dysregulated activity in the anterior cingulate cortex (ACC) and insula	(Roberts & Mulvihill, 2024)
Post-Traumatic Stress Disorder (PTSD)	→ Dissociation and detachment from bodily experiences → Avoidance of somatic cues → Feeling of bodily alienation	→ Trauma-induced dysregulation in the insula, prefrontal cortex (PFC) and hippocampus	(Henigsberg et al., 2019)
Chronic Stress	→ Reduced parasympathetic response → Chronic muscle tension → Sleep disturbance and insomnia	→ Lowered heart rate variability (HRV) → Elevated cortisol level → Autonomic nervous system	(Philippi et al., 2024) [REMOVED HYPERLINK FIELD]

6.2 Treatment for Anxiety, Depression, PTSD, Chronic Stress with the help of Yoga

Yoga is a useful addition to treatment for various mental health disorders like, anxiety, depression, PTSD, and chronic Stress. Rooted in integrative mind-body practices, yoga modulates the autonomic nervous system, enhances interoceptive awareness, and helps mental stability through a combination of movements. It combines movement (asana), (pranayama) breath control, and (Dhyana) meditative focus. Empirical studies show that practicing yoga regularly can lower cortisol levels and therefore increase heart rate variability, and encourage a calm state in the body. These factors change and reduce stress and emotional regulation. Yoga can help with anxiety and depression by enhancing thinking and feelings. Through breathwork, movements and meditation. It supports fostering mindfulness, self-compassion, and body awareness. There are so many findings that structured yoga can significantly reduce symptoms, and often matches traditional therapies. For PTSD, trauma-informed yoga can lessen symptoms like hyper-alertness, disconnection, and upsetting memories. This approach calms the nervous system, therefore builds emotional tolerance and aids trauma recovery (Yang et al., 2023). Yoga supports managing chronic stress by enhancing brain adaptability, stress-related systems like the HPA axis. This leads to better resilience and mental clarity.

6.3 Biomarker-Based Evaluation of Mental Health Interventions: (HRV, EEG, Cortisol)

Heart rate variability: Serves as a reliable indicator of whether the autonomic nervous system (ANS) is working, especially the vagal nerve. A higher HRV means more activity from the parasympathetic system, which plays a crucial role in emotional regulation. Yoga practices, mainly those that emphasize breath control and mindfulness techniques has been shown to significantly improve heart rate variability. This improvement in heart rate variability indicates a less sympathetic nervous system activity and better ability to handle stress (Kuppusamy et al., 2020).

Electroencephalography (EEG): Findings from various studies have shown that yoga benefits contribute to elevated levels of alpha and theta brainwaves in those who participate. Yoga reduces feelings of stress, depression, and PTSD by supporting relaxation while also enhancing focus. Combining yoga with other treatments may increase results by addressing both mental and physical health needs. This makes yoga a useful addition to mental health care for those managing with depression, stress and PTSD. It is a valuable option for managing the conditions (Zhu et al., 2022).

Cortisol: Cortisol is the main stress hormone in the human body. This is produced by the hypothalamic-pituitary-adrenal (HPA) axis. It mainly increases when a person experiences chronic stress. Regular yoga practices can lower both baseline and reactive cortisol levels in the body. It means that yoga can support our lower body respond to stress and system (Erkin & Kocaçal, 2024). Below, Neurophysiological and biomarker responses to yoga are summarized in Table 4.3 and schematically illustrated in Fig. 4.3.

Table 3. Neurophysiological and Biomarker Responses to Yoga.

Biomarker	Effect of Yoga	Implications for Mental Health	Reference
Heart Rate Variability	Increase HRV indicating enhanced parasympathetic (vagal) activity and autonomic regulation.	Suggests improved emotional regulation, resilience to stress, and lowered anxiety symptoms.	(Woodyard, 2011)
Cortisol (stress Hormone)	Reduces basal and reactive cortisol levels, especially under chronic stress.	Reflects downregulation of the hypothalamic-pituitary-adrenal (HPA) axis, leading to reduced perceived stress.	(M. C. Pascoe et al., 2021)
Alpha Wave Activity (EEG)	Increase alpha and theta EEG patterns during and after yoga sessions.	Associated with calm states, improved focus, and reduced symptoms of anxiety and depression.	(Gaur et al., 2020)
Brain Gray Matter Volume (Hippocampus, PFC)	Increase in gray matter density in the hippocampus, prefrontal cortex and insula after consistent yoga practice.	Supports improved memory, emotion regulation and reduction in PTS symptoms.	(Kishore et al., 2022)

Figure 3. Schematic Illustration of Potential Effects of Yoga on Mind and Body Connection.

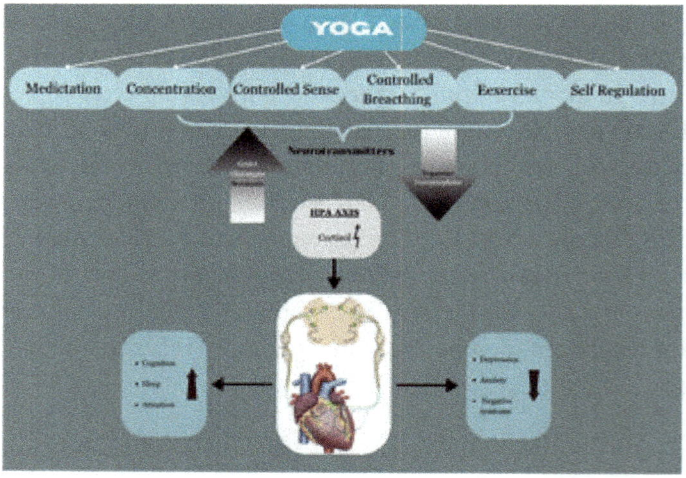

Adapted from (Balasubramaniam et al., 2013).

7 APPLIED CONTEXTS FOR HEALING: THERAPY, TRAUMA AND EDUCATION

7.1 Yoga for Trauma Recovery: Principles and Practices

Trauma-informed yoga is a specific practice for individuals who've been through trauma. It's focused on safety and empowerment, not hard and fast routines or movements that will bring on uncomfortable emotions. Practice aims at creating a safe space and, at the same time, preserving the autonomy of the participants. It also creates body awareness through light movements, grounding, and breathing exercises using careful language not to elicit the memory of trauma in participants. Trauma-informed yoga has been shown to help people deal with themselves, practice self-knowledge, distress coping and emotional regulation. Especially among vulnerable populations, including those who have overcome substance use disorders, childhood trauma survivors, or veterans of military sexual trauma. Benefits have been reported by many participants, including decreased anxiety, increased self-knowledge and regulation, and greater feelings of empowerment and acceptance. The neurobiological rationale for trauma-informed yoga connects to ideas like polyvagal theory and somatic psychology. These suggest that mindful, slow movement helps regulate the autonomic nervous system and reduce hyperarousal. Existing research justifies trauma-informed yoga as a useful resource in recovery therapy (Klukan & Lunsford, 2024).

7.2 Yoga in Educational Institutions: Improving Student Well-being and Overall Performance

The yoga inclusion in schools is an effective non-pharmacological intervention that helps maintain the mental health, mood regulation, and academic activity of students. Yoga programmes in schools that include mindful breathing, meditation and developmentally appropriate physical postures have been found to reduce stress, anxiety, and emotional reactivity in parallel with increasing self-awareness, emotional regulation, and self-confidence. These psychophysiological advantages translate to increased focus, concentration and classroom behaviour, which are essential to academic achievement. Teachers have indicated that they often observe reduced aggression, better self-regulation and an increase in motivation in those students who are habitually practising yoga. Particularly, yoga activities are flexible and can be used at different levels of education and, therefore, many people can participate in yoga, whether in curricula or as extracurricular activities. In addition to the personal results, group Yoga allows fostering an empathetic, collaborative and positive peer relationship which leads to a more nurturing and disciplined academic setting. Overall, Yoga in educational settings offers a wide range of benefits to students, including their holistic health and the creation of a healthier and more conscious learning environment.

7.3 Yoga in Clinical and Community Mental Health Settings

Yoga is being recognised as a helpful addition to mental treatments for various conditions like depression, anxiety and PTSD. Numerous research explanations demonstrate that yoga improves well-being, mental and emotional concerns and tends to result in alleviated tension and anxiety. Yoga is used together with Cognitive Behavioural Therapy (CBT) and Dialectical Behaviour Therapy (DBT), and used in clinical setups to balance emotions and stress levels safely (Chourse, 2025). Especially for trauma survivors.

The practice of yoga exercise within a community, including various groups, such as schools, shelters, and correction centres, has been shown to be beneficial towards the mood and mental health of individuals. Especially in older and younger adults. Yoga enhances self-compassion and attention while relating to physical health by regulating the autonomic nervous system. Although the current research on the subject of yoga in a diverse population is restricted, yoga remains a promising approach to enhancing mental health (Chobe et al., 2020).

7.4 Designing Inclusive, Safe and Culturally Sensitive Programs

When establishing yoga programs that are truly inclusive and culturally sensitive, one should plan in a considerate and practical way to address the various needs of the participants. There have been successful programs in which the community organisations and individuals have co-created the program, as has been experienced in programs on Latina women with cancer and programs on indigenous girls. It makes everyone feel included by suggesting modifications, requesting body alterations and utilising inclusive language, creating a feeling of belonging to make members feel appreciated, being respectful of cultural rituals and working with leaders without engaging in cultural appropriation. In schools, a secular model can improve accessibility and meet the legal threshold. Training facilitators in trauma-informed care, anti-oppression and intercultural competencies enhances physiological safety, trust and higher engagement, improving yoga as a more accessible and empowering experience for all participants (Kachroo & Deguire, 2024).

7.5 Case Studies or Program Models

The application of yoga in the realms of mental health is confirmed by many successful case studies and models. Especially, trauma-informed yoga interventions applied in correlational and inpatient psychiatric settings have been proven to be effective and well-liked, since participants have reported better skills in managing their emotions, feeling less anxious, and enhanced feelings of belonging and overall well-being. In an educational context, dynamic mindfulness and yoga interventions in schools have established reductions in student stress and behavioral problems, playing a role in protective mental health care. Clinical model, including designed yoga interventions for medical students. In addition, treatment through yoga has been related with better emotional steadiness and relapse prevention, aligning with conclusions that yoga can reduce stress and improve psychological well-being in both clinical and non-clinical populations. These examples support its role as a restorative and preventative tool in mental health and wellness and underscore yoga's flexibility to meet educational, clinical and cultural needs (M. C. Pascoe et al., 2021).

Although the empirical and clinical findings reviewed above show important benefits, for the translation of these results into robust practice and policy, it is relevant to confront methodological, cultural, and scalability challenges, which are outlined in this section with their directions for future research.

8 CHALLENGES AND FUTURE DIRECTIONS

8.1 Scientific Limitations

Aggregate numbers of research display yoga's benefits. Conversely, some studies have serious problems. Yoga certainly has the practical effects, which are small groups of participants, a lack of appropriate the real causes. Changes in yoga types, session length, and teacher experience add to the challenge of attaining consistent results. Additionally, much of the research predominantly depends on self-reported psychological assessments, which are susceptible to expectation bias and social desirability effects. While more randomised controlled trials (RCTs) are being conducted, they frequently do not have the constant strict controls and blinding methods found in medication studies. Standardised instruments for assessing constructs like interoception, mindfulness, or embodied awareness remain insufficient, resulting in diversity in outcome measures. This creates challenges in assigning any advantages that come specifically from yoga, social support, and people's expectations, which are not additional factors. Yoga is typically seen as one thing, even though it includes movement, breathwork, meditation, and philosophical ideas. This makes it hard to figure out which parts provide certain outcomes. Obviously, required a well-designed, significant, multi-site study to perfectly validate. Most of the evidence comes from Western clinical settings, which limits its cultural generalisability and shows how important it is to have study methods that are more diverse and sensitive to many cultures (Chourse, 2025).

8.2 Misunderstanding and Cultural Concerns

Yoga is progressively prevalent across the world. On the other hand, many people reduce yoga to just a physical practice or a method to mitigate stress. This approach of people ignores ethical, spiritual, and philosophical heritages. The simplified approach to yoga can underestimate its actual purpose and turn away communities that see yoga as a sacred tradition. It often happens with cultural insensitivity when yoga is brought to Western countries. Sometimes, old yoga practices are repeated without mentioning where they came from or what they mean. To keep yoga real, you need to have respectful conversations with people from other cultures and honour the traditions of yoga. In other words, help practices that recognise yoga's rich tradition while adapting it thoughtfully for modern audiences (Bartholomew, 2020).

8.3 Cultural and Methodological Considerations

Most yoga programs applied in Western clinical practice focus on physical postures, excluding critical philosophical and ethical elements of the original practice. Such an adaptation risks the erosion of cultural meaning and diminishes holistic philosophy. Methodologically, underrepresented groups, such as rural populations, low-income communities, and indigenous groups, are very seldom included in research regarding yoga, limiting generalisability. Besides, due to different research designs, inconsistent outcome measures, and multiple possible meanings associated with the concept of yoga, studies are hardly comparable. Therefore, such studies will have a lack of cultural sensitivity and methodological consistency that needs addressing to ensure authenticity and validate scientific interpretation.

8.4 Scientific Balancing with Tradition in Yoga Practice

In research and clinical settings, yoga is used more frequently. It is significant to balance science with traditional practices. The systematic techniques are important for confirming reproducibility and comparability through studies. However, yoga's adaptability, experience, and spiritual value are enhanced by strict rules. To maintain the holistic nature of yoga, while meeting the requirements of evidence-based practice, researchers, clinicians, and traditional yoga instructors need to work together.

The combination of different fields like neuroscience, psychology, education, and yoga philosophy indicates both the difficulty of yoga and the different experiences of its experts. These frameworks that are systematically solid, aesthetically aware, and respectful of philosophy, the field can support the responsible and ethical use of yoga in healthcare and social wellness (Vollbehr et al., 2023).

8.5 Recommendations and Future Directions

In the health and education system, future research should emphasise how specific practices on yoga, like breathing exercises (pranayama), physical posture (asana), and meditation, connection of our mind and body. For the numerous advantages, extensive and ingenious studies involving diverse groups of people have been conducted to prove that yoga works and to gain a deeper understanding of it. Future research should involve clusters that are often ignored, such as children, aged people, downgraded communities, and individuals with traumatic pasts, to design relevant models for everyone. In the framework of public health, health organisations need to consider the inclusion of yoga in preventive and rehabilitation care, mainly in mental health plans, care for aged people, and school wellness programs. These frameworks are also significant in guarding from commercial manipulation and cultural misrepresentation. The yoga programs designed in schools and clinics should be understanding to trauma and traditionally suitable, adapting to the requirements of all participants. Conclusively, training education for yoga instructors should deliver a comprehensive education covering not just yoga poses but also yogic philosophy, ethics, anatomy, mental support and mind-body connection. Creating a mutual guarantee standard will assist in building a group of yoga instructors who are experienced and respect the spiritual quality of yoga.

9 CONCLUSION

In this chapter, the concept of yoga has been discussed as a unified psycho-physiological system which bridges the dual realms of body and mind. Based on the ancient Indian philosophy and today increasingly proven useful by the latest neuroscience, yoga has turned out to be a multidimensional tool that helps reinstate the integrity of both physical, emotional, and cognitive domains.

The discussion began by challenging the historical separation of the mind and body, contrasting Western dualism with holistic principles existing in the tradition of yoga. Yoga presents a complex philosophy of embodied awareness through its philosophical corpus, including the Pancha Koshas, Gunas, and synthesis of Chitta, Pra a and Sharira. Building on this, the chapter analysed the neurophysiological foundation of the mind-body interface. Brain images, autonomic markers such as vagal tone, and hormonal mediators demonstrate the effect of yoga on top-down (cognitive) and bottom-up (somatic) processes. The triad of practice, asana, pranayama, and dhyana, emerged as central to regulating stress, enhancing neuroplasticity, and fostering emotional resilience. Furthermore, the emerging empirical evidence is showing a role of yoga as an adjunct to the treatment of anxiety, depression, trauma, and chronic stress, both through subjective experience and measurable biomarkers like HRV and cortisol.

Yoga is not just a system of physical training, nor is it a spiritual philosophy; it is an active psychophysiological system that unifies both voluntary and involuntary functions. Yoga integrates the autonomic and the central nervous system through energising attentional networks, engaging the vagus nerve and regulating neuroendocrine pathways. This dual engagement of the top-down (e.g., focused awareness, intention) and bottom-up (e.g., breath, movement, interoception) processes identifies yoga as the connection between consciousness and physiology. It enables a condition of inner coherence, adaptive regulation, and embodied awareness that are all intrinsic features of psychological well-being and health. The mind-body interaction is being verified by multimodal approaches such as functional magnetic resonance imaging (fMRI), heart rate variability (HRV), electroencephalography (EEG), and psychometric tests, thus unequivocally demonstrating the interfacing of traditional practices and modern scientific standards . Such integrative ability can be particularly useful during a time in which mental health issues are multi-factorial and demand holistic responses. The focus of yoga on self-regulation, presence and inner transformation aligns with modern theories of resilience and salutogenesis, which drives its usefulness in practice, in clinical practice, educational, and community settings.

The yoga practice and research of the future will be interdisciplinary. In order to actually live up to its potential, there will have to be ongoing collaboration between clinicians, philosophers, neuroscientists, and traditional yoga scholars. It will have to be done with scientific accuracy as well as sensitivity to culture, so yoga will not sacrifice its spiritual essence in translation. Possibilities of the future involve incorporating yoga into international mental health policies, trauma treatment, and prevention models of psychosocial health, especially during low-resource or diverse cultural situations. Yoga can thus be understood as a globally shared but locally embedded practice, a living tradition that cultivates mental clarity, emotional balance, and somatic healing across communities and cultures.

REFERENCES

Balasubramaniam, M., Telles, S., & Doraiswamy, P. M. (2013). Yoga on Our Minds: A Systematic Review of Yoga for Neuropsychiatric Disorders. *Frontiers in Psychiatry, 3*. Advance online publication. DOI: 10.3389/fpsyt.2012.00117 PMID: 23355825

Bartholomew, O. (2020). *Investigation of the "Cultural Appropriation" of Yoga*. International ResearchScape Journal., DOI: 10.25035/irj.07.01.02

Betka, S., Adler, D., Similowski, T., & Blanke, O. (2022). Breathing control, brain, and bodily self-consciousness: Toward immersive digiceuticals to alleviate respiratory suffering. *Biological Psychology, 171*, 108329. DOI: 10.1016/j.biopsycho.2022.108329 PMID: 35452780

Brems, C. (2020). Yoga as a Mind-Body Practice. In *Nutrition, Fitness, and Mindfulness* (pp. 137–155). Springer International Publishing. DOI: 10.1007/978-3-030-30892-6_10

Campelo, G., de Araújo, J. R., Aristizabal, J. P., de Souza, W., & de Castilho, G. M. (2025). Long-term effects of yoga-based practices on neural, cognitive, psychological, and physiological outcomes in adults: A scoping review and evidence map. *BMC Complementary Medicine and Therapies, 25*(1), 92. DOI: 10.1186/s12906-025-04825-x PMID: 40050913

Chinnusamy, M., Sukumar, A., & Nanduri, V. (2025). Role of yoga prana vidya in healing psychosomatic disorders: a multiple case study in a family setting. *International Journal of Advances in Medicine*. DOI: 10.18203/2349-3933.ijam20251083

Chobe, S., Chobe, M., Metri, K., Patra, S. K., & Nagaratna, R. (2020). Impact of Yoga on cognition and mental health among elderly: A systematic review. *Complementary Therapies in Medicine, 52*, 102421. DOI: 10.1016/j.ctim.2020.102421 PMID: 32951703

Chourse, S. (2025). THE IMPACT OF YOGA ON MENTAL HEALTH: A SYSTEMATIC REVIEW. *International Ayurvedic Medical Journal, 13*(02), 433–438. DOI: 10.46607/iamj2013022025

English, A., McKibben, E., Sivaramakrishnan, D., Hart, N., Richards, J., & Kelly, P. (2022). A Rapid Review Exploring the Role of Yoga in Healing Psychological Trauma. *International Journal of Environmental Research and Public Health, 19*(23), 16180. DOI: 10.3390/ijerph192316180 PMID: 36498254

Erkin, Ö., & Kocaçal, E. (2024). The impact of laughter yoga as a NIC on health parameters in nurses and nursing students: A systematic review. *BMC Complementary Medicine and Therapies*, *24*(1), 378. DOI: 10.1186/s12906-024-04663-3 PMID: 39472871

Eusebio, J., Forbes, B., Sahyoun, C., Vago, D. R., Lazar, S. W., & Farb, N. (2022). Contemplating movement: A randomized control trial of yoga training for mental health. *Mental Health and Physical Activity*, *23*, 100483. DOI: 10.1016/j.mhpa.2022.100483

Gaur, S., Panjwani, U., & Kumar, B. (2020). EEG Brain Wave Dynamics: A Systematic Review and Meta Analysis on Effect of Yoga on Mind Relaxation. *Journal of Biomedical Research & Environmental Sciences*, *1*(7), 353–362. DOI: 10.37871/jbres1166

Henigsberg, N., Kalember, P., Petrović, Z. K., & Šečić, A. (2019). Neuroimaging research in posttraumatic stress disorder – Focus on amygdala, hippocampus and prefrontal cortex. *Progress in Neuro-Psychopharmacology & Biological Psychiatry*, *90*, 37–42. DOI: 10.1016/j.pnpbp.2018.11.003 PMID: 30419321

Kachroo, M. J., & Deguire, D. (2024). Braiding Indigenous Yoga. *Indigenous Religious Traditions*, *2*(1), 27–46. DOI: 10.1558/irt.27583

Kishore, D. M., Bindu, S., & Manjunath, N. K. (2022). Estimation of Yoga Postures Using Machine Learning Techniques. *International Journal of Yoga*, *15*(2), 137–143. DOI: 10.4103/ijoy.ijoy_97_22 PMID: 36329766

Kjaer, T. W., Bertelsen, C., Piccini, P., Brooks, D., Alving, J., & Lou, H. C. (2002). Increased dopamine tone during meditation-induced change of consciousness. *Brain Research. Cognitive Brain Research*, *13*(2), 255–259. DOI: 10.1016/S0926-6410(01)00106-9 PMID: 11958969

Klukan, K., & Lunsford, D. (2024). Trauma-Informed Yoga: A Scoping Review. *Occupational Therapy in Mental Health*, *40*(4), 430–454. DOI: 10.1080/0164212X.2023.2276148

Kuppusamy, M., Kamaldeen, D., Pitani, R., Amaldas, J., Ramasamy, P., Shanmugam, P., & Vijayakumar, V. (2020). Effects of yoga breathing practice on heart rate variability in healthy adolescents: A randomized controlled trial. *Integrative Medicine Research*, *9*(1), 28–32. DOI: 10.1016/j.imr.2020.01.006 PMID: 32025489

Lee, M., Moon, W., & Kim, J. (2014). Effect of Yoga on Pain, Brain-Derived Neurotrophic Factor, and Serotonin in Premenopausal Women with Chronic Low Back Pain. *Evidence-Based Complementary and Alternative Medicine, 2014*(1). DOI: 10.1155/2014/203173

Liu, L., Liu, C., Tang, L., Wang, X., & Feng, Q. (2025). From contemplation to serenity: How yoga meditation improves the mental health of female college students? *Frontiers in Psychology*, *16*, 1545943. Advance online publication. DOI: 10.3389/fpsyg.2025.1545943 PMID: 40129498

Maity, S., Abbaspour, R., Bandelow, S., Pahwa, S., Alahdadi, T., Shah, S., Chhetri, P., Jha, A., Nauhria, S., Nath, R., Nayak, N., & Nauhria, S. (2024). The psychosomatic impact of Yoga in medical education: A systematic review and meta-analysis. *Medical Education Online*, *29*(1), 2364486. Advance online publication. DOI: 10.1080/10872981.2024.2364486 PMID: 38861675

Nivethitha, L., Mooventhan, A., & Manjunath, N. (2016). Effects of various Prā āyāma on cardiovascular and autonomic variables. *Ancient Science of Life*, *36*(2), 72. DOI: 10.4103/asl.ASL_178_16 PMID: 28446827

Nourollahimoghadam, E., Gorji, S., Gorji, A., & Khaleghi Ghadiri, M. (2021). Therapeutic role of yoga in neuropsychological disorders. *World Journal of Psychiatry*, *11*(10), 754–773. DOI: 10.5498/wjp.v11.i10.754 PMID: 34733640

Pal, G. K., & Velkumary, S., & Madanmohan. (2004). Effect of short-term practice of breathing exercises on autonomic functions in normal human volunteers. *The Indian Journal of Medical Research*, *120*(2), 115–121. PMID: 15347862

Pandurangi, A., Keshavan, M., Ganapathy, V., & Gangadhar, B. (2017). Yoga: Past and Present. *The American Journal of Psychiatry*, *174*(1), 16–17. DOI: 10.1176/appi.ajp.2016.16080853 PMID: 28040996

Pascoe, M., & Bauer, I. (2015). A systematic review of randomised control trials on the effects of yoga on stress measures and mood. *Journal of Psychiatric Research*, *68*, 270–282. DOI: 10.1016/j.jpsychires.2015.07.013 PMID: 26228429

Pascoe, M. C. J., de Manincor, M., Hallgren, M., Baldwin, P. A., Tseberja, J., & Parker, A. G. (2021). Psychobiological Mechanisms Underlying the Mental Health Benefits of Yoga-Based Interventions: A Narrative Review. *Mindfulness*, *12*(12), 2877–2889. DOI: 10.1007/s12671-021-01736-z

Perez-Diaz, O., Góngora, D., González-Mora, J. L., Rubia, K., Barrós-Loscertales, A., & Hernández, S. E. (2024). Enhanced amygdala–anterior cingulate white matter structural connectivity in Sahaja Yoga Meditators. *PLoS One*, *19*(3), e0301283. DOI: 10.1371/journal.pone.0301283 PMID: 38547155

Philippi, C. L., Weible, E., Ehlers, A., Walsh, E. C., Hoks, R. M., Birn, R. M., & Abercrombie, H. C. (2024). Effects of cortisol administration on heart rate variability and functional connectivity across women with different depression histories. *Behavioural Brain Research*, *463*, 114923. DOI: 10.1016/j.bbr.2024.114923 PMID: 38408523

Pragya, S. U., Mehta, N. D., Abomoelak, B., Uddin, P., Veeramachaneni, P., Mehta, N., Moore, S., Jean-Francois, M., Garcia, S., Pragya, S. C., & Mehta, D. I. (2021). Effects of Combining Meditation Techniques on Short-Term Memory, Attention, and Affect in Healthy College Students. *Frontiers in Psychology*, *12*, 607573. Advance online publication. DOI: 10.3389/fpsyg.2021.607573 PMID: 33746830

Nayan Rishi, N. (2024). Bridging the Science Between Yogic Postures (Asanas) and Neurophysiology: A Narrative Review. *Journal of Cancer Research and Cellular Therapeutics, 8*(4), 01–04. DOI: 10.31579/2640-1053/198

Roberts, A. C., & Mulvihill, K. G. (2024). Multiple faces of anxiety: A frontal lobe perspective. *Trends in Neurosciences*, *47*(9), 708–721. DOI: 10.1016/j.tins.2024.07.001 PMID: 39127569

Ruggiero, V., Dell'Acqua, C., Cremonese, E., Giraldo, M., & Patron, E. (2025). Under the surface: Low cardiac vagal tone and poor interoception in young adults with subclinical depressive symptoms. *Journal of Affective Disorders*, *375*, 1–9. DOI: 10.1016/j.jad.2025.01.057 PMID: 39826615

Saleem, Y., Noushad, S., Ahmed, S., & Ansari, B. (2025). Psychophysiological Biomarkers for the Effects of Yoga as an Alternative Therapy among Healthcare Professionals with Chronic Low Back Pain: A Randomized Controlled Trial. *Journal of Nature and Science of Medicine*, *8*(1), 74–80. DOI: 10.4103/jnsm.jnsm_39_24

Shafir, T. (2016). Using Movement to Regulate Emotion: Neurophysiological Findings and Their Application in Psychotherapy. *Frontiers in Psychology*, *7*. Advance online publication. DOI: 10.3389/fpsyg.2016.01451 PMID: 27721801

Solano Durán, P., Morales, J.-P., & Huepe, D. (2024). Interoceptive awareness in a clinical setting: The need to bring interoceptive perspectives into clinical evaluation. *Frontiers in Psychology*, *15*, 1244701. Advance online publication. DOI: 10.3389/fpsyg.2024.1244701 PMID: 38933585

Streeter, C. C., Whitfield, T. H., Owen, L., Rein, T., Karri, S. K., Yakhkind, A., Perlmutter, R., Prescot, A., Renshaw, P. F., Ciraulo, D. A., & Jensen, J. E. (2010). Effects of Yoga Versus Walking on Mood, Anxiety, and Brain GABA Levels: A Randomized Controlled MRS Study. *Journal of Alternative and Complementary Medicine (New York, N.Y.)*, *16*(11), 1145–1152. DOI: 10.1089/acm.2010.0007 PMID: 20722471

Sullivan, M. B., Erb, M., Schmalzl, L., Moonaz, S., Noggle Taylor, J., & Porges, S. W. (2018). Yoga Therapy and Polyvagal Theory: The Convergence of Traditional Wisdom and Contemporary Neuroscience for Self-Regulation and Resilience. *Frontiers in Human Neuroscience*, *12*, 67. Advance online publication. DOI: 10.3389/fnhum.2018.00067 PMID: 29535617

Thirthalli, J., Naveen, G., Rao, M., Varambally, S., Christopher, R., & Gangadhar, B. (2013). Cortisol and antidepressant effects of yoga. *Indian Journal of Psychiatry*, *55*(7), 405. DOI: 10.4103/0019-5545.116315 PMID: 24049209

Tolahunase, M. R., Sagar, R., Faiq, M., & Dada, R. (2018). Yoga- and meditation-based lifestyle intervention increases neuroplasticity and reduces severity of major depressive disorder: A randomized controlled trial. *Restorative Neurology and Neuroscience*, *36*(3), 423–442. DOI: 10.3233/RNN-170810 PMID: 29614706

Udupa, K., & Sathyaprabha, T. N. (2018). *Influence of Yoga on the Autonomic Nervous System.*, DOI: 10.4018/978-1-5225-2788-6.ch005

Vollbehr, N., Schmidt, A., Bartels-Velthuis, A., Ostafin, B., & Hoenders, H. (2023). The ethics of yoga in (mental) healthcare: Beyond the traditional Eightfold path. *Complementary Therapies in Medicine*, *102979*, 102979. Advance online publication. DOI: 10.1016/j.ctim.2023.102979 PMID: 37640167

Voss, S., Cerna, J., & Gothe, N. P. (2023). Yoga Impacts Cognitive Health: Neurophysiological Changes and Stress Regulation Mechanisms. *Exercise and Sport Sciences Reviews*, *51*(2), 73–81. DOI: 10.1249/JES.0000000000000311 PMID: 36342265

Woodyard, C. (2011). Exploring the therapeutic effects of yoga and its ability to increase quality of life. *International Journal of Yoga*, *4*(2), 49. DOI: 10.4103/0973-6131.85485 PMID: 22022122

Yang, Y., Cao, D., Lyu, T., & Gao, W. (2023). Meta-analysis of a mindfulness yoga exercise intervention on depression – based on intervention studies in China. *Frontiers in Psychology*, *14*, 1283172. Advance online publication. DOI: 10.3389/fpsyg.2023.1283172 PMID: 38148781

Zhu, L., Li, L., Li, X., & Wang, L. (2022). Mind–Body Exercises for PTSD Symptoms, Depression, and Anxiety in Patients With PTSD: A Systematic Review and Meta-Analysis. *Frontiers in Psychology*, *12*, 738211. Advance online publication. DOI: 10.3389/fpsyg.2021.738211 PMID: 35153889

Compilation of References

Agorastos, A., Kellner, M., Baker, D. G., & Stiedl, O. (2015). Comprehensive Guide to Post-Traumatic Stress Disorder. *Comprehensive Guide to Post-Traumatic Stress Disorder*, 1–15. 10.1007/978-3-319-08613-2_30-1

Akobeng, A. K. (2016). Understanding type i and type II errors, statistical power and sample size. *Acta Paediatrica. International Journal of Pediatrics*, *105*(6), 605–609. DOI: 10.1111/apa.13384 PMID: 26935977

Aleksić Veljković, A., Katanić, B., & Masanovic, B. (2021). Effects of a 12-Weeks Yoga Intervention on Motor and Cognitive Abilities of Preschool Children. *Frontiers in Pediatrics*, *9*, 799226. Advance online publication. DOI: 10.3389/fped.2021.799226 PMID: 34926359

Alpert, J. L. (2012). Loss of humanness: The ultimate trauma. *American Journal of Psychoanalysis*, *72*(2), 118–138. Advance online publication. DOI: 10.1057/ajp.2012.8 PMID: 22617097

Álvarez-Pérez, Y., Rivero-Santana, A., Perestelo-Pérez, L., Duarte-Díaz, A., Ramos-García, V., Toledo-Chávarri, A., Torres-Castaño, A., León-Salas, B., Infante-Ventura, D., González-Hernández, N., Rodríguez-Rodríguez, L., & Serrano-Aguilar, P. (2022). Effectiveness of mantra-based meditation on mental health: A systematic review and meta-analysis. *International Journal of Environmental Research and Public Health*, *19*(6), 3380. DOI: 10.3390/ijerph19063380 PMID: 35329068

Anālayo. (2003). *Satipa hāna: The Direct Path to Realization*. Windhorse Publications.

Anderson, K., & Li, M. (2023). Digital detox mindfulness interventions for technology-related anxiety: A randomized controlled trial. *Journal of Behavioral Addictions*, *17*(2), 245–258.

Ankad, R., Herur, A., Patil, S., Shashikala, G., & Chinagudi, S. (2011). Effect of short-term pranayama and meditation on cardiovascular functions in healthy individuals. *Heart Views : the Official Journal of the Gulf Heart Association, 12*(2), 58. DOI: 10.4103/1995-705X.86016 PMID: 22121462

Arnsten, A. F. T. (2009). Stress signalling pathways that impair prefrontal cortex structure and function. *Nature Reviews. Neuroscience, 10*(6), 410–422. DOI: 10.1038/nrn2648 PMID: 19455173

Arora, S., & Bhattacharjee, J. (2008). Modulation of immune responses in stress by Yoga. *International Journal of Yoga, 1*(2), 45. DOI: 10.4103/0973-6131.43541 PMID: 21829284

Ashhad, S., Kam, K., Negro, C. A. D., & Feldman, J. L. (2022). Breathing Rhythm and Pattern and Their Influence on Emotion. *Annual Review of Neuroscience, 45*(1), 223–247. Advance online publication. DOI: 10.1146/annurev-neuro-090121-014424 PMID: 35259917

Austin, J. H. (1998). *Zen and the brain: Toward an understanding of meditation and consciousness* (pp. xxiv, 844). The MIT Press.

Babiy, Z., Frey, B. N., Bieling, P. J., McCabe, R. E., & Green, S. M. (2025). Mindfulness-Based Interventions and Neuroplasticity: A Review of Network Connectivity in Healthy and Clinical Samples. *Mindfulness, 16*(4), 783–796. DOI: 10.1007/s12671-025-02549-0

Badoni, P., Kumar, N., Singh, R., Gupta, K., Kalra, P., & Arora, V. (2025). Exploring the synergy of yoga and ayurveda in metaverse. In *Exploring the Metaverse* (pp. 165–187). Elsevier., https://www.sciencedirect.com/science/article/pii/B9780443241321000119 DOI: 10.1016/B978-0-443-24132-1.00011-9

Badve, R., Varadharajan, E., Govindasamy, K., Dongre, S., Velusamy, S., Kambitta Valappil, I. N., Karmakar, D., Çitozi, R., & Geantă, V. A. (2025). Considering the Impact of Yoga on Psychological Well-being and Quality of Life in Perimenopausal Women: A Randomized Controlled Trial. *Physical Education Theory and Methodology, 25*(2), 331–339. DOI: 10.17309/tmfv.2025.2.14

Baer, R. A., Smith, G. T., Hopkins, J., Krietemeyer, J., & Toney, L. (2006). Using self-report assessment methods to explore facets of mindfulness. *Assessment, 13*(1), 27–45. DOI: 10.1177/1073191105283504 PMID: 16443717

Baer, R. A., Smith, G. T., Lykins, E., Button, D., Krietemeyer, J., Sauer, S., Walsh, E., Duggan, D., & Williams, J. M. G. (2008). Construct validity of the five-facet mindfulness questionnaire in meditating and nonmeditating samples. *Assessment, 15*(3), 329–342. DOI: 10.1177/1073191107313003 PMID: 18310597

Bahi, C., Irrmischer, M., Franken, K., Fejer, G., Schlenker, A., Deijen, J. B., & Engelbregt, H. (2024). Effects of conscious connected breathing on cortical brain activity, mood and state of consciousness in healthy adults. *Current Psychology (New Brunswick, N.J.), 43*(12), 10578–10589. DOI: 10.1007/s12144-023-05119-6

Bai, Z., Luo, S., Zhang, L., Wu, S., & Chi, I. (2020). Acceptance and Commitment Therapy (ACT) to reduce depression: A systematic review and meta-analysis. *Journal of Affective Disorders, 260*(September 2019), 728–737. DOI: 10.1016/j.jad.2019.09.040

Baicker, K., Cutler, D., & Song, Z. (2010). Workplace wellness programs can generate savings. *Health Affairs (Project Hope), 29*(2), 304–311. DOI: 10.1377/hlthaff.2009.0626 PMID: 20075081

Baier, K. (2019). Swami Vivekananda. Reform Hinduism, nationalism and scientistic yoga. *Interdisciplinary Journal for Religion and Transformation in Contemporary Society, 5*(1), 230–257. DOI: 10.30965/23642807-00501012

Baka, E., Tan, Y., Wong, B. L. H., Xing, Z., & Yap, P. (2025). A scoping review of digital interventions for the promotion of mental health and prevention of mental health conditions for young people. *Oxford Open Digital Health, 3*, oqaf005. Advance online publication. DOI: 10.1093/oodh/oqaf005 PMID: 40230873

Balaji, P. A., Varne, S. R., & Ali, S. S. (2012). Physiological effects of yogic practices and transcendental meditation in health and disease. *North American Journal of Medical Sciences, 4*(10), 442. https://www.ncbi.nlm.nih.gov/pmc/articles/PMC3482773/. DOI: 10.4103/1947-2714.101980 PMID: 23112963

Balasubramaniam, M., Telles, S., & Doraiswamy, P. M. (2013). Yoga on Our Minds: A Systematic Review of Yoga for Neuropsychiatric Disorders. *Frontiers in Psychiatry, 3*. Advance online publication. DOI: 10.3389/fpsyt.2012.00117 PMID: 23355825

Balcombe, L., & De Leo, D. (2020). Digital mental health challenges and the horizon ahead for solutions (Preprint). *JMIR Mental Health*. https://doi.org/DOI: 10.2196/preprints.26811

Banzett, R. B., Mulnier, H. E., Murphy, K., Rosen, S. D., Wise, R. J. S., & Adams, L. (2000). Breathlessness in humans activates insular cortex. *Neuroreport, 11*(10), 2117–2120. DOI: 10.1097/00001756-200007140-00012 PMID: 10923655

Barbezat, D. P., & Bush, M. (2014). *Contemplative practices in higher education: Powerful methods to transform teaching and learning* (pp. xxiii, 231). Jossey-Bass/ Wiley.

Barik, S., & Nayak, T. (2024). Workplace spirituality: Exploring past, present and future through bibliometric analysis. *Benchmarking*, *31*(9), 3216–3241. DOI: 10.1108/BIJ-04-2022-0251

Barrett, L. F. (2017). *How emotions are made: The secret life of the brain* (pp. xv, 425). Houghton Mifflin Harcourt.

Bartholomew, O. (2020). *Investigation of the "Cultural Appropriation" of Yoga*. International ResearchScape Journal., DOI: 10.25035/irj.07.01.02

Barua, R. (2025). Harmonizing Body and Mind: Investigating the Combined Impact of Yoga and Mindfulness Meditation on Depression, Anxiety, Stress. In *Global Innovations in Physical Education and Health* (pp. 203–232). IGI Global Scientific Publishing. https://www.igi-global.com/chapter/harmonizing-body-and-mind/361163

Basara, L., Jokic Begic, N., Popovic Grle, S., Jakopovic, M., & Samarzija, M. (2018). DYSPNEA FROM NEUROPSYCHYATRIC PERSPECTIVE: A NARRATIVE REVIEW. *Psychiatria Danubina*, *30*(1), 11–20. DOI: 10.24869/psyd.2018.11 PMID: 29546853

Bass, C., & Gardner, W. (1985). Emotional influences on breathing and breathlessness. *Journal of Psychosomatic Research*, *29*(6), 599–609. DOI: 10.1016/0022-3999(85)90069-8 PMID: 3910805

Basu-Ray, I. (2021). A Mechanistic Model for Yoga as a Preventive and Therapeutic Modality. *International Journal of Yoga*, *14*(2), 152–157. DOI: 10.4103/ijoy.IJOY_136_20 PMID: 34188388

Batson, G., & Schwartz, R. E. (2007). Revisiting the value of somatic education in dance training through an inquiry into practice schedules. *Journal of Distance Education*, *7*(2), 47–56.

Baumeister, R. F., Vohs, K. D., Aaker, J. L., & Garbinsky, E. N. (2013). Some key differences between a happy life and a meaningful life. *The Journal of Positive Psychology*, *8*(6), 505–516. DOI: 10.1080/17439760.2013.830764

Beauchaine, T. P., & Thayer, J. F. (2015). Heart rate variability as a transdiagnostic biomarker of psychopathology. *International Journal of Psychophysiology : Official Journal of the International Organization of Psychophysiology*, *98*(2), 338–350.

Beer, J. M., Smith, K. N., Kennedy, T., Mois, G., Acena, D., Gallerani, D. G., McDonnell, K. K., & Owens, O. L. (2020). A Focus Group Evaluation of Breathe Easier: A Mindfulness-Based mHealth App for Survivors of Lung Cancer and Their Family Members. *American Journal of Health Promotion, 34*(7), 770–778. DOI: 10.1177/0890117120924176 PMID: 32406241

Berardi, C., Antonini, M., Jordan, Z., Wechtler, H., Paolucci, F., & Hinwood, M. (2024). Barriers and facilitators to the implementation of digital technologies in mental health systems: A qualitative systematic review to inform a policy framework. *BMC Health Services Research, 24*(1), 243. DOI: 10.1186/s12913-023-10536-1 PMID: 38408938

Berger, A. J. (1990). Recent advances in respiratory neurobiology using in vitro methods. *American Journal of Physiology. Lung Cellular and Molecular Physiology, 259*(2), L24–L29. DOI: 10.1152/ajplung.1990.259.2.L24 PMID: 2200281

Berkovich-Ohana, A. (2017). A case study of a meditation-induced altered state: Increased overall gamma synchronization. *Phenomenology and the Cognitive Sciences, 16*(1), 91–106. DOI: 10.1007/s11097-015-9435-x

Berne, E. (2013). *Transactional analysis in psychotherapy: A systematic individual and social psychiatry.* (Original work published 1961)

Bertelli, R. (2019). Does the cognitive-behavioural model of learning share features of Buddha's and Krishnamurti's teachings? Using the concept of automatic maladaptive thoughts as an example. *Advances in Social Sciences Research Journal, 6*(2). Advance online publication. DOI: 10.14738/assrj.62.6222

Berthon, P. R., & Pitt, L. F. (2019). Types of mindfulness in an age of digital distraction. *Business Horizons, 62*(2), 131–137. DOI: 10.1016/j.bushor.2018.10.003

Beshai, S. (2024). Mindfulness and CBT: A conceptual integration bridging ancient wisdom and modern cognitive theories of psychopathology. *Frontiers in Psychology, 15*, 1489798. Advance online publication. DOI: 10.3389/fpsyg.2024.1489798 PMID: 39723397

Betka, S., Adler, D., Similowski, T., & Blanke, O. (2022). Breathing control, brain, and bodily self-consciousness: Toward immersive digiceuticals to alleviate respiratory suffering. *Biological Psychology, 171*(July 2021), 108329. DOI: 10.1016/j.biopsycho.2022.108329

Bhagabati, D., & Kumar, A. (2016). Evolving society and mental health. *Open Journal of Psychiatry & Allied Sciences, 7*(2), 117. Advance online publication. DOI: 10.5958/2394-2061.2016.00018.5

Bhagat, O. L., Kharya, C., Jaryal, A., & Deepak, K. K. (2017). Acute effects on cardiovascular oscillations during controlled slow yogic breathing. *The Indian Journal of Medical Research, 145*(4), 503–512. DOI: 10.4103/ijmr.IJMR_830_15 PMID: 28862183

Bhar, G. C. (2020). *Why things go wrong in life: Spiritual viewpoints*. Indian Science Cruiser., DOI: 10.24906/isc/2020/v34/i3/203784

Bhati, R., Mandal, M., & Singh, T. (2025). Ancient Indian perspectives and practices of mental well-being. *Frontiers in Psychology, 16*, 1616802. DOI: 10.3389/fpsyg.2025.1616802 PMID: 40528855

Bhavanani, A. B. (2014). Diverse dimensions of Yoga. *Yoga Mimamsa, 46*(1–2), 3–8. DOI: 10.4103/0044-0507.137846

Bianco, S., Barilaro, P., & Palmieri, A. (2016). Traditional meditation, mindfulness and psychodynamic approach: An integrative perspective. *Frontiers in Psychology, 7*. Advance online publication. DOI: 10.3389/fpsyg.2016.00552 PMID: 27148153

Bijlenga, D., Kulcu, S., Van Gellecum, T., Eryigit, Z., & Kooij, J. S. (2017). Persistence and adherence to psychostimulants, and psychological well-being up to 3 years after specialized treatment of adult attention-deficit/hyperactivity disorder: A naturalistic follow-up study. *Journal of Clinical Psychopharmacology, 37*(6), 689–696. DOI: 10.1097/JCP.0000000000000787 PMID: 29049077

Bing-Canar, H., Pizzuto, J., & Compton, R. J. (2016). Mindfulness-of-breathing exercise modulates EEG alpha activity during cognitive performance. *Psychophysiology, 53*(9), 1366–1376. DOI: 10.1111/psyp.12678 PMID: 27245493

Binsale, L. J. (2017). *Self-concept clarity, trauma and psychopathology* (Doctoral dissertation). Lancaster University.

Bishop, S. R., Lau, M., Shapiro, S., Carlson, L., Anderson, N. D., Carmody, J., Segal, Z. V., Abbey, S., Speca, M., Velting, D., & Devins, G. (2004). Mindfulness: A Proposed Operational Definition. *Clinical Psychology : a Publication of the Division of Clinical Psychology of the American Psychological Association, 11*(3), 230–241. DOI: 10.1093/clipsy.bph077

Boiten, F. A., Frijda, N. H., & Wientjes, C. J. (1994). Emotions and respiratory patterns: Review and critical analysis. *International Journal of Psychophysiology, 17*(2), 103–128. DOI: 10.1016/0167-8760(94)90027-2 PMID: 7995774

Bornemann, B., & Singer, T. (2017). Taking time to feel our body: Steady increases in heartbeat perception accuracy and decreases in alexithymia over 9 months of contemplative mental training. *Psychophysiology, 54*(3), 469–482. DOI: 10.1111/psyp.12790 PMID: 27925645

Bowles, N. I., Davies, J. N., & Van Dam, N. T. (2022). Dose–response Relationship of Reported Lifetime Meditation Practice with Mental Health and Wellbeing: A Cross-sectional Study. *Mindfulness, 13*(10), 2529–2546. DOI: 10.1007/s12671-022-01977-6 PMID: 36193220

Boyatzis, R., & McKee, A. (2005). *Resonant Leadership: Renewing Yourself and Connecting with Others Through Mindfulness, Hope and CompassionCompassion*. Harvard Business Press.

Brahmaprana, P. (2001). Vedanta: Death and the art of dying. *CrossCurrents*.

Brahmbhatt, A., & Kumavat, P. P. (2024). Yoga and Mindfulness Practices: Their Role in Modern Mental Health and Wellness Programs. *Research Review Journal of Indian Knowledge Systems, 1*(2), 09–17. DOI: 10.31305/rrjiks.2024.v1.n2.002

Bremer, B., Wu, Q., Mora Álvarez, M. G., Hölzel, B. K., Wilhelm, M., Hell, E., Tavacioglu, E. E., Torske, A., & Koch, K. (2022). Mindfulness meditation increases default mode, salience, and central executive network connectivity. *Scientific Reports, 12*(1), 1–15. DOI: 10.1038/s41598-022-17325-6 PMID: 35918449

Brems, C. (2020). Yoga as a Mind-Body Practice. In *Nutrition, Fitness, and Mindfulness* (pp. 137–155). Springer International Publishing. DOI: 10.1007/978-3-030-30892-6_10

Brewer, J. A., Worhunsky, P. D., Gray, J. R., Tang, Y.-Y., Weber, J., & Kober, H. (2011). Meditation experience is associated with differences in default mode network activity and connectivity. *Proceedings of the National Academy of Sciences of the United States of America, 108*(50), 20254–20259. DOI: 10.1073/pnas.1112029108 PMID: 22114193

Broderick, P. C., & Frank, J. L. (2014). Learning to BREATHE: An intervention to foster mindfulness in adolescence. *New Directions for Youth Development, 2014*(142), 31–44. DOI: 10.1002/yd.20095 PMID: 25100493

Brown, R. P., & Gerbarg, P. L. (2005). Sudarshan Kriya Yogic Breathing in the Treatment of Stress, Anxiety, and Depression: Part II—Clinical Applications and Guidelines. *Journal of Alternative and Complementary Medicine (New York, N.Y.), 11*(4), 711–717. DOI: 10.1089/acm.2005.11.711 PMID: 16131297

Brown, R. P., & Gerbarg, P. L. (2005). Sudarshan Kriya yogic breathing in the treatment of stress, anxiety, and depression: Part I-neurophysiologic model. *Journal of Alternative and Complementary Medicine (New York, N.Y.)*, *11*(1), 189–201. DOI: 10.1089/acm.2005.11.189 PMID: 15750381

Brown, R. P., Gerbarg, P. L., & Muench, F. (2013). Breathing Practices for Treatment of Psychiatric and Stress-Related Medical Conditions. *The Psychiatric Clinics of North America*, *36*(1), 121–140. DOI: 10.1016/j.psc.2013.01.001 PMID: 23538082

Brown, V. A., Olmstead, R., & Creswell, J. D. (2021). The effects of mindfulness and meditation on autonomic nervous system activity and heart rate variability: A meta-analysis. *Psychosomatic Medicine*, *83*(7), 699–713. DOI: 10.1097/PSY.0000000000000900 PMID: 33395216

Bryant, E. F. (2009). *The Yoga Sūtras of Patañjali: A New Edition, Translation, and Commentary*. North Point Press.

Buchanan, T. L., & Janelle, C. M. (2022). Emotions and ensuing motor performance are altered by regulating breathing frequency: Implications for emotion regulation and sport performance. *Frontiers in Psychology*, *13*, 963711.

Buckner, R. L., Andrews-Hanna, J. R., & Schacter, D. L. (2008). The brain's default network: Anatomy, function, and relevance to disease. *Annals of the New York Academy of Sciences*, *1124*(1), 1–38. DOI: 10.1196/annals.1440.011 PMID: 18400922

Buenrostro-Jáuregui, M. H., Muñóz-Sánchez, S., Rojas-Hernández, J., Alonso-Orozco, A. I., Vega-Flores, G., Tapia-de-Jesús, A., & Leal-Galicia, P. (2025). A Comprehensive Overview of Stress, Resilience, and Neuroplasticity Mechanisms. *International Journal of Molecular Sciences*, *26*(7), 3028. DOI: 10.3390/ijms26073028 PMID: 40243691

Buhle, J. T., Silvers, J. A., Wager, T. D., Lopez, R., Onyemekwu, C., Kober, H., Weber, J., & Ochsner, K. N. (2014). Cognitive Reappraisal of Emotion: A Meta-Analysis of Human Neuroimaging Studies. *Cerebral Cortex (New York, N.Y.)*, *24*(11), 2981–2990. DOI: 10.1093/cercor/bht154 PMID: 23765157

Button, A. J., & De Pretto, M. (2023). A psalm a day keeps the psychiatrist at bay: Measuring the effects of a three-week micro-course based on *lectio divina*. *Pastoral Psychology*, *72*, 1015–1033. DOI: 10.1007/s11089-022-01040-0

Butzer, B., Day, D., Potts, A., Ryan, C., Coulombe, S., Davies, B., Weidknecht, K., Ebert, M., Flynn, L., & Khalsa, S. B. S. (2015). Effects of a classroom-based yoga intervention on cortisol and behavior in second- and third-grade students: A pilot study. *Journal of Evidence-Based Complementary & Alternative Medicine*, *20*(1), 41–49. DOI: 10.1177/2156587214557695 PMID: 25412616

Butzer, B., Ebert, M., Telles, S., & Khalsa, S. B. S. (2015). School-based Yoga Programs in the United States: A Survey. *Advances in Mind-Body Medicine*, *29*(4), 18–26. PMID: 26535474

Buysse, D. J., Reynolds, C. F.III, Monk, T. H., Berman, S. R., & Kupfer, D. J. (1989). The Pittsburgh Sleep Quality Index: A new instrument for psychiatric practice and research. *Psychiatry Research*, *28*(2), 193–213. DOI: 10.1016/0165-1781(89)90047-4 PMID: 2748771

Cacioppo, J. T., & Cacioppo, S. (2018). The growing problem of loneliness. *Lancet*, *391*(10119), 426. DOI: 10.1016/S0140-6736(18)30142-9 PMID: 29407030

Cahn, B. R., Goodman, M. S., Peterson, C. T., Maturi, R., & Mills, P. J. (2017). Yoga, meditation and mind-body health: Increased BDNF, cortisol awakening response, and altered inflammatory marker expression after a 3-month yoga and meditation retreat. *Frontiers in Human Neuroscience*, *11*(June), 1–13. DOI: 10.3389/fnhum.2017.00315 PMID: 28694775

Calderone, A., Latella, D., Impellizzeri, F., de Pasquale, P., Famà, F., Quartarone, A., & Calabrò, R. S. (2024). Neurobiological changes induced by mindfulness and meditation: A systematic review. *Biomedicines*, *12*(11), 2613. DOI: 10.3390/biomedicines12112613 PMID: 39595177

Campanelli, S., Lopes Tort, A., & Lobão-Soares, B. (2020). Pranayamas and their neurophysiological effects. *International Journal of Yoga*, *13*(3), 183. DOI: 10.4103/ijoy.IJOY_91_19 PMID: 33343147

Campelo, G., de Araújo, J. R., Aristizabal, J. P., de Souza, W., & de Castilho, G. M. (2025). Long-term effects of yoga-based practices on neural, cognitive, psychological, and physiological outcomes in adults: A scoping review and evidence map. *BMC Complementary Medicine and Therapies*, *25*(1), 92. DOI: 10.1186/s12906-025-04825-x PMID: 40050913

Canter, P. H. (2003). The therapeutic effects of meditation. *BMJ (Clinical Research Ed.)*, *326*(7398), 1049–1050. DOI: 10.1136/bmj.326.7398.1049 PMID: 12750183

Carmody, J., & Baer, R. A. (2008). Relationships between mindfulness practice and levels of mindfulness, medical and psychological symptoms and well-being in a mindfulness-based stress reduction program. *Journal of Behavioral Medicine*, *31*(1), 23–33. DOI: 10.1007/s10865-007-9130-7 PMID: 17899351

Carnicke, S. M. (2009). Stanislavsky and Female Actors: Women in Stanislavsky's Life and Art. By Maria Ignatieva. Lanham, Md.: University Press of America, 2008. xx, 140 pp. Notes. Bibliography. Index. $23.00, paper. *Slavic Review*, *68*(4), 985–986.

Carpenter, J. K., Conroy, K., Gomez, A. F., Curren, L. C., & Hofmann, S. G. (2019). The relationship between trait mindfulness and affective symptoms: A meta-analysis of the Five Facet Mindfulness Questionnaire (FFMQ). *Clinical Psychology Review*, *74*, 101785. DOI: 10.1016/j.cpr.2019.101785 PMID: 31751877

Carter, M. J. (2017). How self-perceptions of identity change in person, role, and social identities relate to depression. *Identity*, *17*(4), 242–257. DOI: 10.1080/15283488.2017.1379908

Carver, C. S., & Johnson, S. L. (2018). Impulsive reactivity to emotion and vulnerability to psychopathology. *The American Psychologist*, *73*(9), 1067–1078. DOI: 10.1037/amp0000387 PMID: 30525782

Cásedas, L., Pirruccio, V., Vadillo, M. A., & Lupiáñez, J. (2020). Does Mindfulness Meditation Training Enhance Executive Control? A Systematic Review and Meta-Analysis of Randomized Controlled Trials in Adults. *Mindfulness*, *11*(2), 411–424. DOI: 10.1007/s12671-019-01279-4

Caspi, A., Hariri, A. R., Holmes, A., Uher, R., & Moffitt, T. E. (2010). Genetic Sensitivity to the Environment: The Case of the Serotonin Transporter Gene and Its Implications for Studying Complex Diseases and Traits. *The American Journal of Psychiatry*, *167*(5), 509–527. DOI: 10.1176/appi.ajp.2010.09101452 PMID: 20231323

Chadha, M. (2015). The Self and Its States: A Buddhist Perspective on Consciousness. *Philosophy East & West*, *65*(3), 722–740.

Chapman, A. L. (2006). Acceptance and mindfulness in behavior therapy: A comparison of Dialectical Behavior Therapy and Acceptance and Commitment Therapy. *International Journal of Behavioral and Consultation Therapy*, *2*(3), 308–313. DOI: 10.1037/h0100785

Chattopadhyay, A., Gayen, M. T. K., & Sardar, M. C. (2025). *Yoga education and life skills*. Chyren Publication.

Chauhan, D., & Bansal, S. (2024). Bridging Traditions and Trends: Exploring Indian Knowledge Systems and Yoga in the Modern Era. *Sirjana Journal*, *54*(7), 20–36.

Chauhan, P., & Rai, S. (2024). Conceptualizing work–life integration: A review and research agenda. *Asia Pacific Management Review*, *29*(4), 415–426. DOI: 10.1016/j.apmrv.2024.10.002

Chawla, V., Brems, C., Freeman, H., Ravindran, A., & Noordsy, D. L. (2023). The Future of Yoga for Mental Health Care. *International Journal of Yoga*, *16*(1), 38–41. DOI: 10.4103/ijoy.ijoy_25_23 PMID: 37583539

Chen, A. C., & Etkin, A. (2013). Hippocampal network connectivity and activation differentiates post-traumatic stress disorder from generalized anxiety disorder. *Neuropsychopharmacology : Official Publication of the American College of Neuropsychopharmacology*, *38*(10), 1889–1898. DOI: 10.1038/npp.2013.122 PMID: 23673864

Chen, L., Wang, Y., Niu, C., Zhong, S., Hu, H., Chen, P., & Huang, R. (2021). Common and distinct abnormal frontal-limbic system structural and functional patterns in patients with major depression and bipolar disorder. *NeuroImage. Clinical*, *30*, 102663. PMID: 30069426

Chen, M., Liu, X., Wang, S., Liu, Y., Chen, X., Yuan, L., & Liu, T. (2022). Genetic and environmental influences on the relationship between mindfulness and anxiety: A twin study. *Journal of Anxiety Disorders*, *91*, 102615.

Chessick, C. (2007). The Mindful Brain: Reflection and Attunement in the Cultivation of Well-Being. *The American Journal of Psychiatry*, *164*(10), 1619–1620. DOI: 10.1176/appi.ajp.2007.07081292 PMID: 22688157

Chiappelli, F., Arora, R., Barkhordarian, B., & Ramchandani, M. (2012). Evidence-based clinical research: Toward a new conceptualization of the level and the quality of the evidence. *Annals of Ayurvedic Medicine*, *1*(4), 60–64.

Chinnusamy, M., Sukumar, A., & Nanduri, V. (2025). Role of yoga prana vidya in healing psychosomatic disorders: a multiple case study in a family setting. *International Journal of Advances in Medicine*. DOI: 10.18203/2349-3933.ijam20251083

Chobe, S., Chobe, M., Metri, K., Patra, S. K., & Nagaratna, R. (2020). Impact of Yoga on cognition and mental health among elderly: A systematic review. *Complementary Therapies in Medicine*, *52*, 102421. DOI: 10.1016/j.ctim.2020.102421 PMID: 32951703

Chohan, S. K. (2010). Whispering selves and reflective transformations in the internal dialogue of teachers and students. *Journal of Invitational Theory and Practice*.

Chopra, D., Stern, E., Bushell, W. C., & Castle, R. D. (2023). Yoga and pain: A mind-body complex system. *Frontiers in Pain Research (Lausanne, Switzerland)*, *4*, 1075866. Advance online publication. DOI: 10.3389/fpain.2023.1075866 PMID: 36910253

Chouchou, F., Mauguière, F., Vallayer, O., Catenoix, H., Isnard, J., Montavont, A., Jung, J., Pichot, V., Rheims, S., & Mazzola, L. (2019). How the insula speaks to the heart: Cardiac responses to insular stimulation in humans. *Human Brain Mapping*, *40*(9), 2611–2622. DOI: 10.1002/hbm.24548 PMID: 30815964

Chourse, S. (2025). THE IMPACT OF YOGA ON MENTAL HEALTH: A SYSTEMATIC REVIEW. *International Ayurvedic Medical Journal*, *13*(02), 433–438. DOI: 10.46607/iamj2013022025

Chu, I.-H., Lin, Y.-J., Wu, W.-L., Chang, Y.-K., & Lin, I.-M. (2015). Effects of Yoga on Heart Rate Variability and Mood in Women: A Randomized Controlled Trial. *Journal of Alternative and Complementary Medicine (New York, N.Y.)*, *21*(12), 789–795. DOI: 10.1089/acm.2015.0138 PMID: 26505201

Ciołkosz, M. (2015). The Possible Significance of Sensorimotor Synchronisation in Modern Postural Yoga Practice. *Studia Religiologica. Zeszyty Naukowe Uniwersytetu Jagiellońskiego*, *48*(4), 327–340. https://www.ceeol.com/search/article-detail?id=477117

Clayton, M., Spaeth, P. E., Renna, M. E., Fresco, D. M., & Mennin, D. S. (2021). Optimizing cognitive behavioral therapy to reduce the burden of distress disorders within an emotion regulation framework. In *New directions in rational emotive behaviour therapy* (pp. 79–98). https://doi.org/DOI: 10.4324/9781003081593-6

Clifton, C. L., Killen, L. G., Green, J. M., O'neal, E. K., Swain, J. C., & Frisbie, C. M. (2023). Effects of 3 Weeks Yogic Breathing Techniques on Sub-maximal Running Responses. *International Journal of Exercise Science*, *16*(4), 1066–1076. DOI: 10.70252/OLEG4431 PMID: 38288073

Coelho, J., Pécune, F., Micoulaud-Franchi, J., Bioulac, B., & Philip, P. (2025). Promoting mental health in the age of new digital tools: Balancing challenges and opportunities of social media, chatbots, and wearables. *Frontiers in Digital Health*, *7*, 1560580. DOI: 10.3389/fdgth.2025.1560580 PMID: 40182586

Cohen, S., Kamarck, T., & Mermelstein, R. (1983). A global measure of perceived stress. *Journal of Health and Social Behavior*, *24*(4), 385–396. DOI: 10.2307/2136404 PMID: 6668417

Collette, A. (2015). The Felt Sense of Interconnectedness: A qualitative analysis of perceptions on finding resilience in the aftermath of trauma using the mind-body connections of Yoga. *Theses and Dissertations (Comprehensive)*. https://scholars.wlu.ca/etd/1735

Collins, F. S., & Varmus, H. (2015). A new initiative on precision medicine. *The New England Journal of Medicine, 372*(9), 793–795. DOI: 10.1056/NEJMp1500523 PMID: 25635347

Connors, C., Norvell, M., & Wu, A. (2024). The RISE (Resilience in Stressful Events) Peer Support Program: Creating a Virtuous Cycle of Healthcare Leadership Support for Staff Resilience and Well-Being. *Journal of Healthcare Leadership, 16*, 537–542. DOI: 10.2147/JHL.S487709 PMID: 39679177

Cook-Cottone, C., & Perey, I. (2025). Defining Embodiment, Yoga, and Yoga as Embodied Mindfulness. In Cook-Cottone, C., & Tylka, T. L. (Eds.), *Yoga as Embodied Mindfulness: Integrating Research and Practice* (pp. 11–31). Springer Nature Switzerland., DOI: 10.1007/978-3-031-83418-9_2

Craig, A. D. (2002). How do you feel? Interoception: The sense of the physiological condition of the body. *Nature Reviews. Neuroscience, 3*(8), 655–666. DOI: 10.1038/nrn894 PMID: 12154366

Craig, A. D. B. (2009). How do you feel—Now? The anterior insula and human awareness. *Nature Reviews. Neuroscience, 10*(1), 59–70. DOI: 10.1038/nrn2555 PMID: 19096369

Craigie, M., Osseiran-Moisson, R., Hemsworth, D., Aoun, S., Francis, K., Brown, J., Hegney, D., & Rees, C. (2016). The influence of trait-negative affect and compassion satisfaction on compassion fatigue in Australian nurses. *Psychological Trauma: Theory, Research, Practice, and Policy, 8*(1), 88–97. DOI: 10.1037/tra0000050 PMID: 25961866

Cramer, H., Lauche, R., Anheyer, D., Pilkington, K., de Manincor, M., Dobos, G., & Ward, L. (2023). Yoga for anxiety: A systematic review and meta-analysis of randomized controlled trials. *Depression and Anxiety, 40*(3), 234–248. PMID: 29697885

Cramer, H., Lauche, R., Langhorst, J., & Dobos, G. (2013a). Yoga for depression: A systematic review and meta-analysis. *Depression and Anxiety, 30*(11), 1068–1083. DOI: 10.1002/da.22166 PMID: 23922209

Crane, R. S., Brewer, J., Feldman, C., Kabat-Zinn, J., Santorelli, S., Williams, J. M. G., & Kuyken, W. (2017). What defines mindfulness-based programs? The warp and the weft. *Psychological Medicine, 47*(6), 990–999. DOI: 10.1017/S0033291716003317 PMID: 28031068

Critchley, H. D., & Harrison, N. A. (2013). Visceral influences on brain and behavior. *Neuron, 77*(4), 624–638. DOI: 10.1016/j.neuron.2013.02.008 PMID: 23439117

Cropley, M., Dijk, D. J., & Stanley, N. (2020). Job strain, work rumination, and sleep in school teachers. In *Work and rest: A topic for work and organizational psychology* (pp. 181–196). Psychology Press. DOI: 10.4324/9781003059714-4

Cuijpers, P., Karyotaki, E., Weitz, E., Andersson, G., Hollon, S. D., & van Straten, A. (2014). The effects of psychotherapies for major depression in adults on remission, recovery and improvement: A meta-analysis. *Journal of Affective Disorders, 159*, 118–126. DOI: 10.1016/j.jad.2014.02.026 PMID: 24679399

Curran, G. M., Bauer, M., Mittman, B., Pyne, J. M., & Stetler, C. (2012). Effectiveness–implementation hybrid designs: Combining elements of clinical effectiveness and implementation research to enhance public health impact. *Medical Care, 50*(3), 217–226. DOI: 10.1097/MLR.0b013e3182408812 PMID: 22310560

Curtis, K., Weinrib, A., & Katz, J. (2012). Systematic Review of Yoga for Pregnant Women: Current Status and Future Directions. *Evidence-Based Complementary and Alternative Medicine : eCAM, 2012*(1), 715942. DOI: 10.1155/2012/715942 PMID: 22927881

Daniela, M., Catalina, L., Ilie, O., Paula, M., Daniel-Andrei, I., & Ioana, B. (2022). Effects of Exercise Training on the Autonomic Nervous System with a Focus on Anti-Inflammatory and Antioxidants Effects. *Antioxidants, 11*(2), 350. Advance online publication. DOI: 10.3390/antiox11020350 PMID: 35204231

Davidson, R. J., & Goleman, D. (2017). *Altered Traits: Science Reveals How Meditation Changes Your Mind, Brain, and Body*. Avery.

Davidson, R. J., & Lutz, A. (2008). Buddha's Brain: Neuroplasticity and Meditation. *IEEE Signal Processing Magazine, 25*(1), 176–174. DOI: 10.1109/MSP.2008.4431873 PMID: 20871742

Davidson, R. J., & Roeser, R. W. (2022). Contemplative practices and mental training: Prospects for American education. *Child Development Perspectives, 16*(2), 89–95.

de Diego-Cordero, R., Zurrón-Pérez, M. P., Vargas-Martínez, A. M., Lucchetti, G., & Vega-Escaño, J. (2021). The effectiveness of spiritual interventions in the workplace for work-related health outcomes: A systematic review and meta-analysis. *Journal of Nursing Management*, *29*(6), 1703–1712. DOI: 10.1111/jonm.13315 PMID: 33772925

de Lacey, S., Smith, C., & Paterson, C. (2009). Building resilience: A preliminary exploration of women's perceptions of the use of acupuncture as an adjunct to in vitro fertilisation. *BMC Complementary and Alternative Medicine*, *9*(1), 50. DOI: 10.1186/1472-6882-9-50 PMID: 20003370

de Manincor, M., Bensoussan, A., Smith, C. A., Barr, K., Schweickle, M., Donoghoe, L. L., Bourchier, S., & Fahey, P. (2016). Individualized Yoga for Reducing Depression and Anxiety, and Improving Well-Being: A Randomized Controlled Trial. *Depression and Anxiety*, *33*(9), 816–828. DOI: 10.1002/da.22502 PMID: 27030303

De Morree, H. M., Rutten, G. J., Szabo, B. M., Sitskoorn, M. M., & Kop, W. J. (2016). Effects of Insula Resection on Autonomic Nervous System Activity. *Journal of Neurosurgical Anesthesiology*, *28*(2), 153–158. DOI: 10.1097/ANA.0000000000000207 PMID: 26192246

De Vente, W., Olff, M., Van Amsterdam, J. G. C., Kamphuis, J. H., & Emmelkamp, P. M. G. (2003). Physiological differences between burnout patients and healthy controls: Blood pressure, heart rate, and cortisol responses. *Occupational and Environmental Medicine*, *60*(suppl 1), i54–i61. DOI: 10.1136/oem.60.suppl_1.i54 PMID: 12782748

de Witt Huberts, J. C., Evers, C., & de Ridder, D. T. D. (2014). Because I am worth it: A theoretical framework and empirical review of a justification-based account of self-regulation failure. *Personality and Social Psychology Review*, *18*(2), 119–138. DOI: 10.1177/1088868313507533 PMID: 24214148

Decker, J. T., Brown, J. L. C., Ashley, W., & Lipscomb, A. E. (2019). Mindfulness, meditation, and breathing exercises: Reduced anxiety for clients and self-care for social work interns. *Social Work with Groups*, *42*(4), 308–322. DOI: 10.1080/01609513.2019.1571763

Denzin, N. K. (1985). Emotion as Lived Experience. *Symbolic Interaction*, *8*(2), 223–240. DOI: 10.1525/si.1985.8.2.223

Desbordes, G., Negi, L. T., Pace, T. W. W., Wallace, B. A., Raison, C. L., & Schwartz, E. L. (2012). Effects of mindful-attention and compassion meditation training on amygdala response to emotional stimuli in an ordinary, non-meditative state. *Frontiers in Human Neuroscience*, *6*, 292. DOI: 10.3389/fnhum.2012.00292 PMID: 23125828

Dhanaradja, U., Rajasegaran, R., Aghoram, R., Pal, P., Basu, S., Mukherjee, M. P., & Harichandrakumar, K. T. (2025). Effect of 12-week Practice of Anulom Vilom Pranayama as Adjunctive Therapy on the Cardiac Autonomic Balance, Cognition, Psychological Status, and Quality of Life in Individuals with Mild-to-Moderate Parkinson's Disease: A Randomized Controlled Trial. *International Journal of Yoga*, *18*(2), 189–198. Advance online publication. DOI: 10.4103/ijoy.ijoy_176_24 PMID: 41079240

Dhangar, A., Jaiswal, A., Sahu, P., Saraswat, T., & Gera, A. (2025). Personalized Fitness Recommendation System Integrating Yoga, Physiotherapy Exercises and Tips. *2025 3rd International Conference on Disruptive Technologies (ICDT)*, 255–260. DOI: 10.1109/ICDT63985.2025.10986670

Dhaniwala, N. K. S., Dasari, V., & Dhaniwala, M. N. (2020). Pranayama and Breathing Exercises - Types and Its Role in Disease Prevention & Rehabilitation. *Journal of Evolution of Medical and Dental Sciences*, *9*(44), 3325–3330. DOI: 10.14260/jemds/2020/730

Dhar, D., Shrivastava, A., Jha, S., Saini, P., & Chauhan, S. (2025). Effect of a 6-week combined protocol of Bhastrika Pranayama and Nadishodhana Pranayama on dynamic lung function indices of young adults. *National Journal of Physiology, Pharmacy and Pharmacology*, *15*(0), 1. DOI: 10.5455/NJPPP.2025.v15.i3.2

Di Blasi, M., Cavani, P., Pavia, L., Lo Baido, R., La Grutta, S., & Schimmenti, A. (2015). The relationship between self-image and social anxiety in adolescence. *Child and Adolescent Mental Health*, *20*(2), 74–80. DOI: 10.1111/camh.12071 PMID: 32680392

Dick, T. E., Dutschmann, M., Feldman, J. L., Fong, A. Y., Hülsmann, S., Morris, K. M., Ramirez, J. M., & Smith, J. C. (2018). Facts and challenges in respiratory neurobiology. *Respiratory Physiology & Neurobiology*, *258*, 104–107. DOI: 10.1016/j.resp.2015.01.014 PMID: 25644207

Dita, M., & Bubuioc, L. (2024). Neuroplasticity—The metamorphosis of the human brain. *Vector European*, *1*(1), 188–192. DOI: 10.52507/2345-1106.2024-1.35

Doll, A., Hölzel, B. K., Mulej Bratec, S., Boucard, C. C., Xie, X., Wohlschläger, A. M., & Sorg, C. (2016). Mindful attention to breath regulates emotions via increased amygdala–prefrontal cortex connectivity. *NeuroImage*, *134*, 305–313. DOI: 10.1016/j.neuroimage.2016.03.041 PMID: 27033686

Donahoe-Fillmore, B., & Grant, E. (2019). The effects of yoga practice on balance, strength, coordination and flexibility in healthy children aged 10–12 years. *Journal of Bodywork and Movement Therapies*, *23*(4), 708–712. DOI: 10.1016/j.jbmt.2019.02.007 PMID: 31733751

Draeger-Muenke, R., & Muenke, M. (2012). The healing energy of breath in traditional Chinese Medicine and other eastern traditions. In *Functional Respiratory Disorders: When Respiratory Symptoms Do Not Respond to Pulmonary Treatment* (pp. 301–323). Humana Press.

Draganski, B., & May, A. (2008). Training-induced structural changes in the adult human brain. *Behavioural Brain Research*, *192*(1), 137–142. DOI: 10.1016/j.bbr.2008.02.015 PMID: 18378330

Dreyfus, H. L. (2007). Detachment, involvement, and rationality: Are we essentially rational animals? *Human Affairs*, *17*(2), 101–109. DOI: 10.2478/v10023-007-0010-0

Drysdale, A. T., Grosenick, L., Downar, J., Dunlop, K., Mansouri, F., Meng, Y., Fetcho, R. N., Zebley, B., Oathes, D. J., Etkin, A., Schatzberg, A. F., Sudheimer, K., Keller, J., Mayberg, H. S., Gunning, F. M., Alexopoulos, G. S., Fox, M. D., Pascual-Leone, A., Voss, H. U., & Liston, C. (2017). Resting-state connectivity biomarkers define neurophysiological subtypes of depression. *Nature Medicine*, *23*(1), 28–38. DOI: 10.1038/nm.4246 PMID: 27918562

Dubey, S., & Bedi, S. S. (2024). Workplace spirituality: A systematic review and future research agenda. *Journal of Management, Spirituality & Religion*, *21*(1), 1–22. DOI: 10.51327/CQER6430

Dudeja, J. P. (2017). Scientific analysis of mantra-based meditation and its beneficial effects: An overview. *International Journal of Advanced Science. Technology and Engineering Management*, *3*(6), 49101. Advance online publication. DOI: 10.22413/ijastems/2017/v3/i6/49101

Dutschmann, M., & Dick, T. E. (2012). Pontine Mechanisms of Respiratory Control. *Comprehensive Physiology*, *5*(6), 2443–2469. DOI: 10.1002/j.2040-4603.2012.tb00457.x PMID: 23720253

Dutton, M. A., Bermudez, D., Matas, A., Majid, H., & Myers, N. L. (2013). Mindfulness-Based Stress Reduction for Low-Income, Predominantly African American Women With PTSD and a History of Intimate Partner Violence. *Cognitive and Behavioral Practice*, *20*(1), 23–32. DOI: 10.1016/j.cbpra.2011.08.003 PMID: 24043922

Eisenbeck, N., Luciano, C., & Valdivia-Salas, S. (2018). Effects of a Focused Breathing Mindfulness Exercise on Attention, Memory, and Mood: The Importance of Task Characteristics. *Behaviour Change*, *35*(1), 54–70. DOI: 10.1017/bec.2018.9

Elices, M., Soler, J., Feliu-Soler, A., Carmona, C., Tiana, T., Pascual, J. C., & Álvarez, E. (2017). Combining emotion regulation and mindfulness skills for preventing depression relapse: A randomized controlled study. *Borderline Personality Disorder and Emotion Dysregulation*, *4*(13), 13. Advance online publication. DOI: 10.1186/s40479-017-0064-6 PMID: 28690851

Engel, G. L. (1977). The need for a new medical model: A challenge for biomedicine. *Science*, *196*(4286), 129–136. DOI: 10.1126/science.847460 PMID: 847460

English, A., McKibben, E., Sivaramakrishnan, D., Hart, N., Richards, J., & Kelly, P. (2022). A Rapid Review Exploring the Role of Yoga in Healing Psychological Trauma. *International Journal of Environmental Research and Public Health*, *19*(23), 16180. DOI: 10.3390/ijerph192316180 PMID: 36498254

Erkin, Ö., & Kocaçal, E. (2024). The impact of laughter yoga as a NIC on health parameters in nurses and nursing students: A systematic review. *BMC Complementary Medicine and Therapies*, *24*(1), 378. DOI: 10.1186/s12906-024-04663-3 PMID: 39472871

Espenes, K., Tørmoen, A. J., Rognstad, K., Nilsen, K. H., Waaler, P. M., Wentzel-Larsen, T., & Kjøbli, J. (2024). Effect of psychosocial interventions on children and youth emotion regulation: A meta-analysis. *Administration and Policy in Mental Health*, *52*(5), 833–852. DOI: 10.1007/s10488-024-01373-3 PMID: 38717667

Esslin, M. (2001). Beckett and the Quest for Meaning. *Samuel Beckett Today/Aujourd'hui*, *11*, 27-30.

Eusebio, J., Forbes, B., Sahyoun, C., Vago, D. R., Lazar, S. W., & Farb, N. (2022). Contemplating movement: A randomized control trial of yoga training for mental health. *Mental Health and Physical Activity*, *23*, 100483. DOI: 10.1016/j.mhpa.2022.100483

Faraji, J., & Metz, G. A. S. (2024). *The Neuroexistentialism of Social Connectedness and Loneliness*. *PsyArXiv*. DOI: 10.31234/osf.io/3umvb

Farb, N. A. S., Segal, Z. V., & Anderson, A. K. (2013). Mindfulness meditation training alters cortical representations of interoceptive attention. *Social Cognitive and Affective Neuroscience*, *8*(1), 15–26. DOI: 10.1093/scan/nss066 PMID: 22689216

Farb, N. A. S., Segal, Z. V., Mayberg, H. S., Bean, J., McKeon, D., Fatima, Z., & Anderson, A. K. (2007). Attending to the present: Mindfulness meditation reveals distinct neural modes of self-reference. *Social Cognitive and Affective Neuroscience*, *2*(4), 313–322. DOI: 10.1093/scan/nsm030 PMID: 18985137

Farb, N., Daubenmier, J., Price, C. J., Gard, T., Kerr, C., Dunn, B. D., & Mehling, W. E. (2015). Interoception, contemplative practice, and health. *Frontiers in Psychology*, *6*, 763.

Feldman, J. L., & Del Negro, C. A. (2006). Looking for inspiration: New perspectives on respiratory rhythm. *Nature Reviews. Neuroscience*, *7*(3), 232–241.

Fendt-Newlin, M., Jagannathan, A., & Webber, M. (2020). Cultural adaptation framework of social interventions in mental health: Evidence-based case studies from low- and middle-income countries. *The International Journal of Social Psychiatry*, *66*(1), 41–48. DOI: 10.1177/0020764019879943 PMID: 31580173

Feuerstein, G. (2001). *The Yoga Tradition: Its History, Literature, Philosophy and Practice*. Hohm Press.

Feuerstein, G. (2008). *The Yoga Tradition: Its History, Literature, Philosophy, and Practice*. Hohm Press.

Fincham, G. W., Strauss, C., Montero-Marin, J., & Cavanagh, K. (2023). Effect of breathwork on stress and mental health: A meta-analysis of randomised-controlled trials. *Scientific Reports*, *13*(1), 1–14. DOI: 10.1038/s41598-022-27247-y PMID: 36624160

Fitzgerald, J. M., Phan, K. L., Kennedy, A. E., Shankman, S. A., Langenecker, S. A., & Klumpp, H. (2017). Prefrontal and amygdala engagement during emotional reactivity and regulation in generalized anxiety disorder. *Journal of Affective Disorders*, *218*(262), 398–406. DOI: 10.1016/j.jad.2017.05.013 PMID: 28501740

Flett, J. A. M., Hayne, H., Riordan, B. C., Thompson, L. M., & Conner, T. S. (2019). Mobile Mindfulness Meditation: A Randomised Controlled Trial of the Effect of Two Popular Apps on Mental Health. *Mindfulness*, *10*(5), 863–876. DOI: 10.1007/s12671-018-1050-9

Fox, K. C. R., Dixon, M. L., Nijeboer, S., Girn, M., Floman, J. L., Lifshitz, M., Ellamil, M., Sedlmeier, P., & Christoff, K. (2016). Functional neuroanatomy of meditation: A review and meta-analysis of 78 functional neuroimaging investigations. *Neuroscience and Biobehavioral Reviews*, *65*, 208–228. DOI: 10.1016/j.neubiorev.2016.03.021 PMID: 27032724

Fox, K. C. R., Nijeboer, S., Dixon, M. L., Floman, J. L., Ellamil, M., Rumak, S. P., Sedlmeier, P., & Christoff, K. (2014). Is meditation associated with altered brain structure? A systematic review and meta-analysis of morphometric neuroimaging in meditation practitioners. *Neuroscience and Biobehavioral Reviews, 43*, 48–73. DOI: 10.1016/j.neubiorev.2014.03.016 PMID: 24705269

Frankl, V. E. (1963). *Man's search for meaning: An introduction to logotherapy*. Washington Square Press.

Franko, M. (2012). *Martha Graham in Love and War: the life in the work*. OUP USA.

Fredrickson, B. L. (2001). The role of positive emotions in positive psychology: The broaden-and-build theory of positive emotions. *The American Psychologist, 56*(3), 218–226. DOI: 10.1037/0003-066X.56.3.218 PMID: 11315248

Fredrickson, B. L., Boulton, A. J., Firestine, A. M., Van Cappellen, P., Algoe, S. B., Brantley, M. M., Kim, S. L., Brantley, J., & Salzberg, S. (2017). Positive Emotion Correlates of Meditation Practice: A Comparison of Mindfulness Meditation and Loving-Kindness Meditation. *Mindfulness, 8*(6), 1623–1633. DOI: 10.1007/s12671-017-0735-9 PMID: 29201247

Fresco, D. M., & Mennin, D. S. (2018). All together now: Utilizing common functional change principles to unify cognitive behavioral and mindfulness-based therapies. *Current Opinion in Psychology, 28*, 65–70. DOI: 10.1016/j.copsyc.2018.10.014 PMID: 30502664

Fresco, D. M., Mennin, D. S., Heimberg, R. G., & Ritter, M. (2013). Emotion regulation therapy for generalized anxiety disorder. *Cognitive and Behavioral Practice, 20*(3), 282–300. DOI: 10.1016/j.cbpra.2013.02.001 PMID: 27499606

Froeliger, B. E., Garland, E. L., Modlin, L. A., & McClernon, F. J. (2012). Neurocognitive correlates of the effects of yoga meditation practice on emotion and cognition: A pilot study. *Frontiers in Integrative Neuroscience, 6*, 48. https://www.frontiersin.org/journals/integrative-neuroscience/articles/10.3389/fnint.2012.00048/full. DOI: 10.3389/fnint.2012.00048 PMID: 22855674

Froeliger, B., Garland, E. L., & McClernon, F. J. (2012). Yoga meditation practitioners exhibit greater gray matter volume and fewer reported cognitive failures: Results of a preliminary voxel-based morphometric analysis. *Evidence-Based Complementary and Alternative Medicine : eCAM, 2012*, 1–8. Advance online publication. DOI: 10.1155/2012/821307 PMID: 23304217

Gambhirananda, S. (2006). *Shankara's Commentary on the Brahma-Sutra (Brahma Sutra Bhashya)*. Advaita Ashrama.

Ganesan, S., Van Dam, N., Kamboj, S. K., Tsuchiyagaito, A., Sacchet, M. D., Misaki, M., Moffat, B. A., Lorenzetti, V., & Zalesky, A. (2024). High-precision neurofeedback-guided meditation training optimises real-world self-guided meditation practice for well-being. *Neuroscience*. Advance online publication. DOI: 10.1101/2024.10.25.618656 PMID: 39484554

Ganpat, T. S., Nagendra, H. R., & Selvi, V. (2013). Efficacy of yoga for mental performance in university students. *Indian Journal of Psychiatry*, *55*(4), 349. DOI: 10.4103/0019-5545.120550 PMID: 24459305

Gardner, W. N. (1996). The pathophysiology of hyperventilation disorders. *Chest*, *109*(2), 516–534.

Gard, T., Noggle, J. J., Park, C. L., Vago, D. R., & Wilson, A. (2014). Potential self-regulatory mechanisms of yoga for psychological health. *Frontiers in Human Neuroscience*, *8*, 770. DOI: 10.3389/fnhum.2014.00770 PMID: 25368562

Gaur, S., Panjwani, U., & Kumar, B. (2020). EEG Brain Wave Dynamics: A Systematic Review and Meta Analysis on Effect of Yoga on Mind Relaxation. *Journal of Biomedical Research & Environmental Sciences*, *1*(7), 353–362. DOI: 10.37871/jbres1166

Gaur, V., & Jain, N. (2017). Spiritualizing inter-personal relationships: In view of Vedanta. *International Journal of Business Management & Research*, *7*(1), 33–44.

GBD 2019 Mental Disorders Collaborators. (2022). Global, regional, and national burden of 12 mental disorders in 204 countries and territories, 1990-2019: A systematic analysis for the Global Burden of Disease Study 2019. *The Lancet Psychiatry*, *9*(2), 137-150. DOI: 10.1016/S2215-0366(21)00395-3

Geisler, F. C. M., Kubiak, T., Siewert, K., & Weber, H. (2013). Cardiac vagal tone is associated with social engagement and self-regulation. *Biological Psychology*, *93*(2), 279–286. DOI: 10.1016/j.biopsycho.2013.02.013 PMID: 23466587

Gelles, D. (2015). *Mindful work: How meditation is changing business from the inside out*. Houghton Mifflin Harcourt.

Gerbarg, P. L., Dickson, F., Conte, V. A., & Brown, R. P. (2023). Breath-centered virtual mind-body medicine reduces COVID-related stress in women healthcare workers of the Regional Integrated Support for Education in Northern Ireland: A single group study. *Frontiers in Psychiatry*, *14*(June), 1–14. DOI: 10.3389/fpsyt.2023.1199819 PMID: 37377478

Germer, C. K., & Siegel, R. D. (2012). *Wisdom and Compassion in Psychotherapy: Deepening Mindfulness in Clinical Practice*. Guilford Press.

Gerritsen, R. J. S., & Band, G. P. H. (2018). Breath of Life: The Respiratory Vagal Stimulation Model of Contemplative Activity. *Frontiers in Human Neuroscience*, *12*(February), 1–25. DOI: 10.3389/fnhum.2018.00397 PMID: 30356789

Ghaemi, S. N. (2009). The rise and fall of the biopsychosocial model. *The British Journal of Psychiatry*, *195*(1), 3–4. DOI: 10.1192/bjp.bp.109.063859 PMID: 19567886

Gheranda. (2004). *Gheranda Samhita* (J. Mallinson, Trans.). YogaVidya.com. (Original work published ca. 17th century)

Ghista, D. N., Nandagopal, D., Ramamurthi, B., Das, A., Mukherji, A., & Srinivasan, T. M. (1976). Physiological characterisation of the meditative state during intuitional practice (the Ananda Marga system of meditation) and its therapeutic value. *Medical & Biological Engineering & Computing*, *14*(3), 209–214. DOI: 10.1007/BF02478750 PMID: 781406

Ghosh, T., Duraipandian, C., Joseph, S., Kumasi, B., Salvi, N. M., Elayaraja, M., Astuti, Y., Orhan, B. E., Karmakar, D., & Govindasamy, K. (2024). Effects of Yoga and Combined Yoga with Neuro-Linguistic Programming on Psychological Management in Mothers of Adolescents: A Randomized Controlled Trial. *Sport Mont, 22*(3), 99–105. http://www.sportmont.ucg.ac.me/?sekcija=article&artid=2071

Gilbert, C. (2003). Book Review. *Behavior Modification*, *27*(5), 755–760. DOI: 10.1177/0145445503256326 PMID: 14531162

Gkintoni, E., Vassilopoulos, S. P., & Nikolaou, G. (2025). Mindfulness-Based Cognitive Therapy in clinical practice: A systematic review of neurocognitive outcomes and applications for mental health and well-being. *Journal of Clinical Medicine*, *14*(5), 1703. DOI: 10.3390/jcm14051703 PMID: 40095733

Glasgow, R. E., Harden, S. M., Gaglio, B., Rabin, B., Smith, M. L., Porter, G. C., Ory, M. G., & Estabrooks, P. A. (2019). RE-AIM planning and evaluation framework: Adapting to new science and practice with a 20-year review. *Frontiers in Public Health*, *7*, 64. DOI: 10.3389/fpubh.2019.00064 PMID: 30984733

Goldberg, S. B., Riordan, K. M., Sun, S., & Davidson, R. J. (2021). The empirical status of mindfulness-based interventions: A systematic review of 44 meta-analyses of randomized controlled trials. *Perspectives on Psychological Science*, *17*(1), 108–130. DOI: 10.1177/1745691620968771 PMID: 33593124

Goldberg, S. B., Tucker, R. P., Greene, P. A., Davidson, R. J., Wampold, B. E., Kearney, D. J., & Simpson, T. L. (2021). Mindfulness-based interventions for psychiatric disorders: A systematic review and meta-analysis. *Clinical Psychology Review*, *89*, 102082. PMID: 29126747

Goldstein, J. (2013). *Mindfulness: A Practical Guide to Awakening*. Sounds True.

Gonçalves, J. P. B., Peres, M. F. P., Tolentino, E. J. A., Mendes, A. L., Farina, M., & Vallada, H. (2023). The evaluation of religious and spirituality-based therapy compared to secular therapy on mental health: A meta-analysis of randomized controlled trials. *Psychotherapy Research*, *33*(8), 1037–1052. DOI: 10.1080/10503307.2023.2241626

Gone, J. P., Hartmann, W. E., Pomerville, A., Wendt, D. C., Klem, S. H., & Burrage, R. L. (2019). The impact of historical trauma on health outcomes for indigenous populations in the USA and Canada: A systematic review. *The American Psychologist*, *74*(1), 20–35. DOI: 10.1037/amp0000338 PMID: 30652897

Good, D. J., Lyddy, C. J., Glomb, T. M., Bono, J. E., Brown, K. W., Duffy, M. K., Baer, R. A., Brewer, J. A., & Lazar, S. W. (2016). Contemplating Mindfulness at Work: An Integrative Review. *Journal of Management*, *42*(1), 114–142. DOI: 10.1177/0149206315617003

Gordon, K. (2003). The impermanence of being: Toward a psychology of uncertainty. *Journal of Humanistic Psychology*, *43*(1), 96–117. DOI: 10.1177/0022167802250731

Gothe, N. P., Hayes, J. M., Temali, C., & Damoiseaux, J. S. (2016). Differences in brain structure and function among yoga practitioners and controls. *Frontiers in Integrative Neuroscience*, *10*, 26. DOI: 10.3389/fnint.2016.00026 PMID: 29988397

Gothe, N. P., Khan, I., Hayes, J., Erlenbach, E., & Damoiseaux, J. S. (2019). Yoga Effects on Brain Health: A Systematic Review of the Current Literature. *Brain Plasticity*, *5*(1), 105–122. DOI: 10.3233/BPL-190084 PMID: 31970064

Govindasamy, K., Kaur, D., Elayaraja, M., Sethi, D., Kalidas, S., Karmakar, D., Orhan, B. E., Astuti, Y., & Parpa, K. (2024). Immediate Effect of Uddiyana Bandha on Heart Rate Variability in Patients with Hypertension: A Randomised Controlled Study. *Annals of Neurosciences*, *09727531241299258*, 09727531241299258. Advance online publication. DOI: 10.1177/09727531241299258 PMID: 39678718

Goyal, M., Singh, S., Sibinga, E. M. S., Gould, N. F., Rowland-Seymour, A., Sharma, R., Berger, Z., Sleicher, D., Maron, D. D., Shihab, H. M., Ranasinghe, P. D., Linn, S., Saha, S., Bass, E. B., & Haythornthwaite, J. A. (2014). Meditation programs for psychological stress and well-being: A systematic review and meta-analysis. *JAMA Internal Medicine*, *174*(3), 357–368. DOI: 10.1001/jamainternmed.2013.13018 PMID: 24395196

Grabbe, L., Higgins, M. K., Baird, M., & Pfeiffer, K. M. (2021). Impact of a Resiliency Training to Support the Mental Well-being of Front-line Workers: Brief Report of a Quasi-experimental Study of the Community Resiliency Model. *Medical Care*, *59*(7), 616–621. DOI: 10.1097/MLR.0000000000001535 PMID: 33827106

Grant, J. A., Courtemanche, J., Duerden, E. G., Duncan, G. H., & Rainville, P. (2010). Cortical thickness and pain sensitivity in zen meditators. *Emotion (Washington, D.C.)*, *10*(1), 43–53. DOI: 10.1037/a0018334 PMID: 20141301

Grant, M. J., & Booth, A. (2009). A typology of reviews: An analysis of 14 review types and associated methodologies. *Health Information and Libraries Journal*, *26*(2), 91–108. DOI: 10.1111/j.1471-1842.2009.00848.x PMID: 19490148

Grensman, A., Acharya, B. D., Wändell, P., Nilsson, G. H., Falkenberg, T., Sundin, Ö., & Werner, S. (2018). Effect of traditional yoga, mindfulness-based cognitive therapy, and cognitive behavioral therapy, on health related quality of life: A randomized controlled trial on patients on sick leave because of burnout. *BMC Complementary and Alternative Medicine*, *18*(1), 1–16. DOI: 10.1186/s12906-018-2141-9 PMID: 29510704

Gross, J. J. (2002). Emotion regulation: Affective, cognitive, and social consequences. *Psychophysiology*, *39*(3), 281–291. DOI: 10.1017/S0048577201393198 PMID: 12212647

Gross, J. J. (2020). The extended process model of emotion regulation: Elaborations, applications, and future directions. *Psychological Inquiry*, *31*(2), 73–90.

Grossman, P. (2015). Mindfulness: Awareness informed by an embodied ethic. *Mindfulness*, *6*(1), 17–22. DOI: 10.1007/s12671-014-0372-5

Guendelman, S., Medeiros, S., & Rampes, H. (2017). Mindfulness and emotion regulation: Insights from neurobiological, psychological, and clinical studies. *Frontiers in Psychology*, *8*, 220. DOI: 10.3389/fpsyg.2017.00220 PMID: 28321194

Guha, D. (2005). Vivekananda's conception of normative ethics and resolution of ethical problems in business. *Management and Labour Studies*, *30*(2), 203–217. DOI: 10.1177/0258042X0503000204

Gundi, M., Kaikobad, R., & Sharma, S. (2025). Diversity in approaches in community-based mental health interventions in India: A narrative review and synthesis. *Global Mental Health (Cambridge, England), 12*, e89. DOI: 10.1017/gmh.2025.10046 PMID: 40895823

Gururaja, C., Rangaprakash, D., & Deshpande, G. (2020). Research Trends in the Application of Yoga to Human Health: A Data Science Approach. *International Journal of Public Mental Health and Neurosciences, 7*(1), 8–13. https://www.ncbi.nlm.nih.gov/pmc/articles/PMC8455111/ PMID: 34553079

Gusha, K. Ç., Shala, I., & Kalo, R. (2017). Current problems in the mental health field. *European Journal of Social Sciences Education and Research, 11*(1), 136–139. DOI: 10.26417/ejser.v11i1.p136-139

Gu, X., Hof, P. R., Friston, K. J., & Fan, J. (2013). Anterior insular cortex and emotional awareness. *The Journal of Comparative Neurology, 521*(15), 3371–3388. DOI: 10.1002/cne.23368 PMID: 23749500

Guz, A. (1997). Brain, breathing and breathlessness. *Respiration Physiology, 109*(3), 197–204. DOI: 10.1016/S0034-5687(97)00050-9 PMID: 9342797

Hackett, J. D. (2014). Values anchoring: Strengthening the link between values and activist behaviors. *Social Influence, 9*(4), 245–260. DOI: 10.1080/15534510.2013.787117

Haddad, G. G., & Farber, J. P. (1991). *Developmental neurobiology of breathing*.

Haller, H., Mitzinger, D., & Cramer, H. (2023). The integration of yoga breathing techniques in cognitive behavioral therapy for post-traumatic stress disorder: A pragmatic randomized controlled trial. *Frontiers in Psychiatry, 14*(April), 1–12. DOI: 10.3389/fpsyt.2023.1101046 PMID: 37139325

Hall, G. C. N., Ibaraki, A. Y., Huang, E. R., Marti, C. N., & Stice, E. (2016). A Meta-Analysis of Cultural Adaptations of Psychological Interventions. *Behavior Therapy, 47*(6), 993–1014. DOI: 10.1016/j.beth.2016.09.005 PMID: 27993346

Hanh, T. N. (2013). *Peace of mind: Becoming fully present*. Parallax Press.

Han, Y.-M. Y., Chen, H., Lee, T. M. C., & Chan, C. C. H. (2023). Neurobiological effects of mind–body exercise: A systematic review and meta-analysis. *Scientific Reports, 13*(17432), 10948. Advance online publication. DOI: 10.1038/s41598-023-37309-4 PMID: 37415072

Hari, S. D. (2015). Concepts in Vedanta applicable to scientific explanation of consciousness. *Scientific GOD Journal, 6*(4), 30–45.

Harrison, O. K., Köchli, L., Marino, S., Luechinger, R., Hennel, F., Brand, K., Hess, A. J., Frässle, S., Iglesias, S., Vinckier, F., Petzschner, F. H., Harrison, S. J., & Stephan, K. E. (2021). Interoception of breathing and its relationship with anxiety. *Neuron, 109*(24), 4080–4093.e8. DOI: 10.1016/j.neuron.2021.09.045 PMID: 34672986

Harris, R. (2023). Vivekananda: Indian swami and global guru. *Religions, 14*(8), 1041. DOI: 10.3390/rel14081041

Hart, C. E., & Tracy, B. L. (2008). Yoga as Steadiness Training: Effects on Motor Variability in Young Adults. *Journal of Strength and Conditioning Research, 22*(5), 1659–1669. DOI: 10.1519/JSC.0b013e31818200dd PMID: 18714217

Hartfiel, N., Havenhand, J., Khalsa, S. B., Clarke, G., & Krayer, A. (2011). The effectiveness of yoga for the improvement of well-being and resilience to stress in the workplace. *Scandinavian Journal of Work, Environment & Health, 37*(1), 70–76. DOI: 10.5271/sjweh.2916 PMID: 20369218

Hasenkamp, W., & Barsalou, L. W. (2012). Effects of Meditation Experience on Functional Connectivity of Distributed Brain Networks. *Frontiers in Human Neuroscience, 6*, 38. DOI: 10.3389/fnhum.2012.00038 PMID: 22403536

Hassan, M. ul, Shahnawaz, F., Imam, A., & Khan, J. (2012). Effect of yoga and exercise on job burnout and job satisfaction on doctors. *Indian Journal of Positive Psychology, 3*(3), 309–313. DOI: 10.15614/ijpp/2012/v3i3/49751

Hayes, S. C., & Hofmann, S. G. (2021). *Process-based CBT: The science and core clinical competencies of cognitive behavioral therapy*. Context Press.

Hayes, S. C., Luoma, J. B., Bond, F. W., Masuda, A., & Lillis, J. (2006a). Acceptance and commitment therapy: Model, processes and outcomes. *Behaviour Research and Therapy, 44*(1), 1–25. DOI: 10.1016/j.brat.2005.06.006 PMID: 16300724

Hayes, S. C., Villatte, M., Levin, M., & Hildebrandt, M. (2011). Open, aware, and active: Contextual approaches as an emerging trend in the behavioral and cognitive therapies. *Annual Review of Clinical Psychology, 7*(1), 141–168. DOI: 10.1146/annurev-clinpsy-032210-104449 PMID: 21219193

Hecht, F. M., & Crane, R. S. (2025). Intervention Fidelity in Mindfulness-Based Research and Practice: Overview of the Special Collection and State of the Field. *Global Advances in Integrative Medicine and Health, 14*, 27536130251349453. DOI: 10.1177/27536130251349453 PMID: 40520822

Heine, S. (2017). animi Velut Respirant. *Comparative Literature, 69*(4), 355–369. DOI: 10.1215/00104124-4260409

Heine, S. (2018). Ebb and Flow: Breath-Writing from Ancient Rhetoric to Jack Kerouac and Allen Ginsberg. *Palgrave Studies in Literature. Science & Medicine*, •••, 91–112. DOI: 10.1007/978-3-319-99948-7_5

Hendriks, T., de Jong, J., & Cramer, H. (2022). The effects of yoga on positive mental health among healthy adults: A systematic review and meta-analysis. *Journal of Alternative and Complementary Medicine (New York, N.Y.)*, *28*(5), 386–398. PMID: 28437149

Henigsberg, N., Kalember, P., Petrović, Z. K., & Šečić, A. (2019). Neuroimaging research in posttraumatic stress disorder – Focus on amygdala, hippocampus and prefrontal cortex. *Progress in Neuro-Psychopharmacology & Biological Psychiatry*, *90*, 37–42. DOI: 10.1016/j.pnpbp.2018.11.003 PMID: 30419321

Hermans, E. J., Henckens, M. J. A. G., Joëls, M., & Fernández, G. (2014). Dynamic adaptation of large-scale brain networks in response to acute stressors. *Trends in Neurosciences*, *37*(6), 304–314. DOI: 10.1016/j.tins.2014.03.006 PMID: 24766931

Herrero de Jáuregui, M. (2015). The construction of inner religious space in wandering religion of classical Greece. *Numen*, *62*(3), 331–358. DOI: 10.1163/15685276-12341395

He, X., Wang, X., Steger, M. F., Ji, L., Jing, K., Liu, M., & Ye, B. (2023). Meaning in life and psychological distress: A meta-analysis. *Journal of Research in Personality*, *104*, 104381. DOI: 10.1016/j.jrp.2023.104381

Hickey, W. S. (2010). Meditation as Medicine: A Critique. *Cross Currents*, *60*(2), 168–184. DOI: 10.1111/j.1939-3881.2010.00118.x

Hoffmann, T. C., Glasziou, P. P., Boutron, I., Milne, R., Perera, R., Moher, D., Altman, D. G., Barbour, V., Macdonald, H., Johnston, M., Lamb, S. E., Dixon-Woods, M., McCulloch, P., Wyatt, J. C., Chan, A.-W., & Michie, S. (2014). Better reporting of interventions: Template for Intervention Description and Replication (TIDieR) checklist and guide. *BMJ (Clinical Research Ed.)*, *348*(mar07 3), g1687. DOI: 10.1136/bmj.g1687 PMID: 24609605

Hofmann, S. G., Grossman, P., & Hinton, D. E. (2011). Loving-kindness and compassion meditation: Potential for psychological interventions. *Clinical Psychology Review*, *31*(7), 1126–1132. DOI: 10.1016/j.cpr.2011.07.003 PMID: 21840289

Hofmann, S. G., Sawyer, A. T., Witt, A. A., & Oh, D. (2010). The effect of mindfulness-based therapy on anxiety and depression: A meta-analytic review. *Journal of Consulting and Clinical Psychology*, *78*(2), 169–183. DOI: 10.1037/a0018555 PMID: 20350028

Hogan, C. (2013). Chronic stress: An approach to management in general practice. *Australian Family Physician*, *42*(3), 155–159. PMID: 23971061

Hollick, M. (2006). *The science of oneness: A worldview for the twenty-first century*. O Books.

Hölzel, B. K., Carmody, J., Vangel, M., Congleton, C., Yerramsetti, S. M., Gard, T., & Lazar, S. W. (2011). Mindfulness practice leads to increases in regional brain gray matter density. *Psychiatry Research*, *191*(1), 36–43. DOI: 10.1016/j.pscychresns.2010.08.006 PMID: 21071182

Hölzel, B. K., Lazar, S. W., Gard, T., Schuman-Olivier, Z., Vago, D. R., & Ott, U. (2011). How does mindfulness meditation work? Proposing mechanisms of action from a conceptual and neural perspective. *Perspectives on Psychological Science*, *6*(6), 537–559. DOI: 10.1177/1745691611419671 PMID: 26168376

Homma, I., & Masaoka, Y. (2008a). Breathing rhythms and emotions. *Experimental Physiology*, *93*(9), 1011–1021. DOI: 10.1113/expphysiol.2008.042424 PMID: 18487316

Hong, Q. N., Pluye, P., Fàbregues, S., Bartlett, G., Boardman, F., Cargo, M., Dagenais, P., Gagnon, M.-P., Griffiths, F., Nicolau, B., O'Cathain, A., Rousseau, M.-C., & Vedel, I. (2018). *Mixed Methods Appraisal Tool (MMAT), version 2018 User guide*. McGill University, Department of Family Medicine.

Hopko, D. R., Lejuez, C. W., Ruggiero, K. J., & Eifert, G. H. (2003). Contemporary behavioral activation treatments for depression: Procedures, principles, and progress. *Clinical Psychology Review*, *23*(5), 699–717. DOI: 10.1016/S0272-7358(03)00070-9 PMID: 12971906

Hume, L. (2002). Ancestral power: The dreaming, consciousness, and Aboriginal Australians. *Choice Reviews Online, 40*(08), 40-4683-40–4683. DOI: 10.5860/CHOICE.40-4683

Hutcherson, C. A., Seppala, E. M., & Gross, J. J. (2008). Loving-kindness meditation increases social connectedness. *Emotion (Washington, D.C.)*, *8*(5), 720–724. DOI: 10.1037/a0013237 PMID: 18837623

Iordanova, R., & Reddivari, A. K. R. (2025). Neuroanatomy, Medulla Oblongata. In *StatPearls*. https://www.ncbi.nlm.nih.gov/pubmed/20483389

Irigaray, L. (2002). *Between east and west: From singularity to community*. Columbia University Press.

Iyengar, B. K. S. (1995). *Light on Yoga: The Bible of Modern Yoga - Its Philosophy and Practice - By the World's Foremost Teacher*. Knopf Doubleday Publishing Group.

Jagadeesan, T., R, A., R, K., Jain, T., Allu, A. R., Selvi G, T., Maveeran, M., & Kuppusamy, M. (2022). Effect of Bhramari Pranayama intervention on stress, anxiety, depression and sleep quality among COVID 19 patients in home isolation. *Journal of Ayurveda and Integrative Medicine*, *13*(3), 100596. DOI: 10.1016/j.jaim.2022.100596 PMID: 35693195

Jamieson, S. D., & Tuckey, M. R. (2017). Mindfulness interventions in the workplace: A critique of the current state of the literature. *Journal of Occupational Health Psychology*, *22*(2), 180–193. DOI: 10.1037/ocp0000048 PMID: 27643606

Janson-Bjerklie, S., Carrieri, V. K., & Hudes, M. (1986). The sensations of pulmonary dyspnea. *Nursing Research*, *35*(3), 154–161.

Jennings, P. A., DeMauro, A. A., & Mischenko, P. (2019). Cultivating Awareness and Resilience in Education. In Ivtzan, I. (Ed.), *Handbook of Mindfulness-Based Programmes* (1st ed., pp. 219–230). Routledge., DOI: 10.4324/9781315265438-18

Jerath, R., Crawford, M. W., Barnes, V. A., & Harden, K. (2015). Self-regulation of breathing as a primary treatment for anxiety. *Applied Psychophysiology and Biofeedback*, *40*(2), 107–115.

Jerath, R., Crawford, M. W., Barnes, V. A., & Harden, K. (2015). Self-Regulation of Breathing as a Primary Treatment for Anxiety. *Applied Psychophysiology and Biofeedback*, *40*(2), 107–115. DOI: 10.1007/s10484-015-9279-8 PMID: 25869930

Jerath, R., Edry, J. W., Barnes, V. A., & Jerath, V. (2006). Physiology of long pranayamic breathing: Neural respiratory elements may provide a mechanism that explains how slow deep breathing shifts the autonomic nervous system. *Medical Hypotheses*, *67*(3), 566–571. DOI: 10.1016/j.mehy.2006.02.042 PMID: 16624497

Jijina, P., Vasa, V., & Biswas, U. N. (2020). Construct description of Samatva from the Bhagavad Gita: Implications for holistic well-being. *Purushartha: A Journal of Management. Ethics and Spirituality*, *13*(2), 1–12.

Ji, M. (2023). *The origin of mindfulness revisited: A conceptual and historical review*. Lecture Notes in Education Psychology and Public Media., DOI: 10.54254/2753-7048/25/20230273

Jones, S. M. W., Guthrie, K. A., Reed, S. D., Landis, C. A., Sternfeld, B., LaCroix, A. Z., Dunn, A., Burr, R. L., & Newton, K. M. (2016). A yoga & exercise randomized controlled trial for vasomotor symptoms: Effects on heart rate variability. *Complementary Therapies in Medicine*, *26*, 66–71. DOI: 10.1016/j.ctim.2016.03.001 PMID: 27261984

Joshi, M., & Telles, S. (2009). A Nonrandomized Non-Naive Comparative Study of the Effects of Kapalabhati and Breath Awareness on Event-Related Potentials in Trained Yoga Practitioners. *Journal of Alternative and Complementary Medicine (New York, N.Y.)*, *15*(3), 281–285. DOI: 10.1089/acm.2008.0250 PMID: 19243275

Ju, X., Liu, H., Xu, J., Hu, B., Jin, Y., & Lu, C. (2024). Effect of Yoga Intervention on Problem Behavior and Motor Coordination in Children with Autism. *Behavioral Sciences (Basel, Switzerland)*, *14*(2), 116. DOI: 10.3390/bs14020116 PMID: 38392469

Kabat-Zinn, J. (2003). Mindfulness-based interventions in context: past, present, and future.

Kabat-Zinn, J. (1994). *Wherever You Go, There You Are: Mindfulness Meditation in Everyday Life*. Hachette Books.

Kabat-Zinn, J. (2003). Mindfulness-based interventions in context: Past, present, and future. *Clinical Psychology : a Publication of the Division of Clinical Psychology of the American Psychological Association*, *10*(2), 144–156. DOI: 10.1093/clipsy.bpg016

Kabat-Zinn, J. (2012). *Mindfulness for beginners: Reclaiming the present moment-and your life*. No Title.

Kachroo, M. J., & Deguire, D. (2024). Braiding Indigenous Yoga. *Indigenous Religious Traditions*, *2*(1), 27–46. DOI: 10.1558/irt.27583

Kaiser, N., & Butler, E. (2021). Introducing social breathing: A model of engaging in relational systems. *Frontiers in Psychology*, *12*, 571298.

Kalisch, R., Baker, D. G., Basten, U., Boks, M. P., Bonanno, G. A., Brummelman, E., Chmitorz, A., Fernàndez, G., Fiebach, C. J., Galatzer-Levy, I., Geuze, E., Groppa, S., Helmreich, I., Hendler, T., Hermans, E. J., Jovanovic, T., Kubiak, T., Lieb, K., Lutz, B., & Kleim, B. (2017). The resilience framework as a strategy to combat stress-related disorders. *Nature Human Behaviour*, *1*(11), 784–790. DOI: 10.1038/s41562-017-0200-8 PMID: 31024125

Kalyani, B. G., Venkatasubramanian, G., Arasappa, R., Rao, N. P., Kalmady, S. V., Behere, R. V., Rao, H., Vasudev, M. K., & Gangadhar, B. N. (2011). Neurohemodynamic correlates of "Om" chanting: A pilot fMRI study. *International Journal of Yoga*, *4*(1), 3–6. DOI: 10.4103/0973-6131.78171 PMID: 21654968

Kapoor, S. (2002). *Encyclopaedia of Vedanta philosophy*. Concept Publishing Company.

Karatsoreos, I. N., & McEwen, B. S. (2013). Resilience and vulnerability: A neurobiological perspective. *F1000prime Reports*, *5*. Advance online publication. DOI: 10.12703/P5-13 PMID: 23710327

Kariuki-Nyuthe, C., & Stein, D. J. (2015). Anxiety and related disorders and physical illness. In *Advances in Psychiatry*. DOI: 10.1159/000365538

Kauffman, K. P. (2015). Emotional sentience and the nature of phenomenal experience. *Progress in Biophysics and Molecular Biology*, *119*(3), 545–562. DOI: 10.1016/j.pbiomolbio.2015.08.003 PMID: 26272799

Kavitha, N., Pal, P., Pal, G. K., Bharadwaj, B., & Nanda, N. (2024). Effects of Slow Breathing Exercises on Cardiac Autonomic Functions in Anxiety Disorder—A Randomised Control Trial. *Annals of Neurosciences*, 09727531241266094. Advance online publication. DOI: 10.1177/09727531241266094 PMID: 39544659

Kelly, A., & Garland, E. L. (2016). Trauma-Informed Mindfulness-Based Stress Reduction for Female Survivors of Interpersonal Violence: Results From a Stage I RCT: TI-MBSR for IPV Survivors. *Journal of Clinical Psychology*, *72*(4), 311–328. DOI: 10.1002/jclp.22273 PMID: 27002222

Kenny, M., Luck, P., & Koerbel, L. (2020). Tending the Field of Mindfulness-Based Programs: The Development of International Integrity Guidelines for Teachers and Teacher Training. *Global Advances in Health and Medicine : Improving Healthcare Outcomes Worldwide*, *9*, 2164956120923975. DOI: 10.1177/2164956120923975 PMID: 32426180

Keshavan, M. S., & Bhargav, H. (2025). Dhyana yoga, the path of meditative being: Psychotherapeutic insights from the East. *Asian Journal of Psychiatry*, *108*, 104483. DOI: 10.1016/j.ajp.2025.104483 PMID: 40279762

Keyes, C. L. M. (2002). The mental health continuum: From languishing to flourishing in life. *Journal of Health and Social Behavior*, *43*(2), 207–222. DOI: 10.2307/3090197 PMID: 12096700

Khoury, B., Sharma, M., Rush, S. E., & Fournier, C. (2015). Mindfulness-based stress reduction for healthy individuals: A meta-analysis. *Journal of Psychosomatic Research*, *78*(6), 519–528. DOI: 10.1016/j.jpsychores.2015.03.009 PMID: 25818837

Khoury, B., Sharma, M., Rush, S. E., & Fournier, C. (2022). Mindfulness-based stress reduction for healthy individuals: A meta-analysis. *Journal of Health Psychology*, *27*(4), 894–906.

Kim, D., Lee, J., Park, M. K., & Ko, S. H. (2024). Recent developments in wearable breath sensors for healthcare monitoring. *Communications Materials*, *5*(1), 1–14. DOI: 10.1038/s43246-024-00480-w

King, A. P., & Fresco, D. M. (2019). A neurobehavioral account for decentering as the salve for the distressed mind. *Current Opinion in Psychology*, *28*, 280–286. DOI: 10.1016/j.copsyc.2019.02.009 PMID: 31059966

King, S., Quist-Møller, S., & Fjorback, L. O. (2022). Arts and Mindfulness Education for Human Flourishing. In *Arts and Mindfulness Education for Human Flourishing* (pp. 238–257). Routledge., DOI: 10.4324/9781003158790-18

Kirby, J. N., Tellegen, C. L., & Steindl, S. R. (2017). A meta-analysis of compassion-based interventions: Current state of knowledge and future directions. *Behavior Therapy*, *48*(6), 778–792. DOI: 10.1016/j.beth.2017.06.003 PMID: 29029675

Kishore, D. M., Bindu, S., & Manjunath, N. K. (2022). Estimation of Yoga Postures Using Machine Learning Techniques. *International Journal of Yoga*, *15*(2), 137–143. DOI: 10.4103/ijoy.ijoy_97_22 PMID: 36329766

Kjaer, T. W., Bertelsen, C., Piccini, P., Brooks, D., Alving, J., & Lou, H. C. (2002). Increased dopamine tone during meditation-induced change of consciousness. *Brain Research. Cognitive Brain Research*, *13*(2), 255–259. DOI: 10.1016/S0926-6410(01)00106-9 PMID: 11958969

Klimecki, O. M., Leiberg, S., Ricard, M., & Singer, T. (2014). Differential pattern of functional brain plasticity after compassion and empathy training. *Social Cognitive and Affective Neuroscience*, *9*(6), 873–879. DOI: 10.1093/scan/nst060 PMID: 23576808

Klukan, K., & Lunsford, D. (2024). Trauma-Informed Yoga: A Scoping Review. *Occupational Therapy in Mental Health*, *40*(4), 430–454. DOI: 10.1080/0164212X.2023.2276148

Knoblauch, S. H. (2017). The Fluidity of Emotions and Clinical Vulnerability: A Field of Rhythmic Tensions. *Psychoanalytic Perspectives*, *14*(3), 283–308. DOI: 10.1080/1551806X.2017.1342421

Knoblauch, S. H. (2019). Fluidity of emotions and vulnerability in the therapeutic situation: A field of rhythmic tensions. *Psyche*, *73*(4), 235–263.

Kop, W. J., Synowski, S. J., Newell, M. E., Schmidt, L. A., Waldstein, S. R., & Fox, N. A. (2011). Autonomic nervous system reactivity to positive and negative mood induction: The role of acute psychological responses and frontal electrocortical activity. *Biological Psychology*, *86*(3), 230–238. DOI: 10.1016/j.biopsycho.2010.12.003 PMID: 21182891

Kornfield, J. (with Internet Archive). (2008). *The wise heart: A guide to the universal teachings of Buddhist psychology*. New York : Bantam Books. http://archive.org/details/wiseheartguideto0000korn_q5q7

Kowall, J. (2014). The vicious cycle of self-identification. *Scientific GOD Journal*, *5*(2), 119–127.

Kowiański, P., Lietzau, G., Czuba, E., Waśkow, M., Steliga, A., & Moryś, J. (2018). BDNF: A Key Factor with Multipotent Impact on Brain Signaling and Synaptic Plasticity. *Cellular and Molecular Neurobiology*, *38*(3), 579–593. DOI: 10.1007/s10571-017-0510-4 PMID: 28623429

Krishna, B. H., Pal, P., Pal, G. K., Balachander, J., Jayasettiaseelon, E., Sreekanth, Y., Sridhar, M. G., & Gaur, G. S. (2014). Effect of yoga therapy on heart rate, blood pressure and cardiac autonomic function in heart failure. *Journal of Clinical and Diagnostic Research : JCDR*, *8*(1), 14. https://www.ncbi.nlm.nih.gov/pmc/articles/PMC3939525/ PMID: 24596712

Krishna, D., Nilesh, S., & Amit, K. (2024). Neurobiological Correlates of Breathing Practices on Cognitive Functions : A Narrative Review. *An Intternational Biannual Refereed Journal of Life Siences*, *19*(2), 85–92. DOI: 10.5281/zenodo.15077455

Krygier, J. R., Heathers, J. A. J., Shahrestani, S., Abbott, M., Gross, J. J., & Kemp, A. H. (2013). Mindfulness meditation, well-being, and heart rate variability: A preliminary investigation into the impact of intensive vipassana meditation. *International Journal of Psychophysiology*, *89*(3), 305–313. DOI: 10.1016/j.ijpsycho.2013.06.017 PMID: 23797150

Kuan, T. (2009). Rethinking non-self: A new perspective from the Ekottarika Āgama. *Buddhist Studies Review*, *26*(2), 155–166. DOI: 10.1558/bsrv.v26i2.155

Kumar, A., & Kumar, S. (2013). Karma Yoga: A path towards work in positive psychology. *Indian Journal of Psychiatry*, *55*(6, S2), 266–270. DOI: 10.4103/0019-5545.105511 PMID: 23858246

Kumar, S., Sinha, P., Dutt, V., & Bhat, A. A. (2023). Real-time fMRI neurofeedback training of amygdala activity in patients with major depressive disorder: A randomized controlled trial. *Biological Psychiatry, 93*(8), 683–691.

Kuppusamy, M., Kamaldeen, D., Pitani, R., Amaldas, J., Ramasamy, P., Shanmugam, P., & Vijayakumar, V. (2020). Effects of yoga breathing practice on heart rate variability in healthy adolescents: A randomized controlled trial. *Integrative Medicine Research, 9*(1), 28–32. DOI: 10.1016/j.imr.2020.01.006 PMID: 32025489

Kuzucu, Y. (2016). Do anger control and social problem-solving mediate relationships between difficulties in emotion regulation and aggression in adolescents? *Educational Sciences: Theory & Practice, 16*(3), 915–933. DOI: 10.12738/estp.2016.3.0003

Laborde, S., Mosley, E., & Thayer, J. F. (2017). Heart rate variability and cardiac vagal tone in psychophysiology: Recommendations for experiment planning, data analysis, and data reporting. *Frontiers in Psychology, 8*, 213. DOI: 10.3389/fpsyg.2017.00213 PMID: 28265249

Laplaud, N., Perrochon, A., Gallou-Guyot, M., Moens, M., Goudman, L., David, R., Rigoard, P., & Billot, M. (2023). Management of post-traumatic stress disorder symptoms by yoga: An overview. *BMC Complementary Medicine and Therapies, 23*(1), 1–15. DOI: 10.1186/s12906-023-04074-w PMID: 37480017

Lattie, E. G., Adkins, E. C., Winquist, N., Stiles-Shields, C., Wafford, Q. E., & Graham, A. K. (2019). Digital mental health interventions for depression, anxiety, and enhancement of psychological well-being among college students: Systematic review. *Journal of Medical Internet Research, 21*(7), e12869. DOI: 10.2196/12869 PMID: 31333198

Lazar, S. W., Kerr, C. E., Wasserman, R. H., Gray, J. R., Greve, D. N., Treadway, M. T., McGarvey, M., Quinn, B. T., Dusek, J. A., Benson, H., Rauch, S. L., Moore, C. I., & Fischl, B. (2005). Meditation experience is associated with increased cortical thickness. *Neuroreport, 16*(17), 1893–1897. DOI: 10.1097/01.wnr.0000186598.66243.19 PMID: 16272874

Lecercle, J.-J., & Riley, D. (2004). A voice without a mouth: Inner speech. In *The force of language* (pp. 19–35). Palgrave Macmillan., DOI: 10.1057/9780230503793_2

Lederer, A. M., & Hoban, M. T. (2022). The development of the American College Health Association-National College Health Assessment III: An improved tool to assess and enhance the health and well-being of college students. *Journal of American College Health, 70*(6), 1606–1610. DOI: 10.1080/07448481.2020.1834401 PMID: 33400616

LeDoux, J. (2003). The emotional brain, fear, and the amygdala. *Cellular and Molecular Neurobiology*, *23*(4–5), 727–738. DOI: 10.1023/A:1025048802629 PMID: 14514027

LeDoux, J. E. (2000). Emotion circuits in the brain. *Annual Review of Neuroscience*, *23*(1), 155–184. DOI: 10.1146/annurev.neuro.23.1.155 PMID: 10845062

Lee, M., Moon, W., & Kim, J. (2014). Effect of Yoga on Pain, Brain-Derived Neurotrophic Factor, and Serotonin in Premenopausal Women with Chronic Low Back Pain. *Evidence-Based Complementary and Alternative Medicine, 2014*(1). DOI: 10.1155/2014/203173

Lee, C.-H., & Park, S. R. (2023). Reviewing the concept of disidentification in the context of psychotherapy. *Culture and Convergence*, *45*(6), 427–445. DOI: 10.33645/cnc.2023.06.45.06.427

Lee, E. E., Torous, J., De Choudhury, M., Depp, C. A., Graham, S. A., Kim, H.-C., Paulus, M. P., Krystal, J. H., & Jeste, D. V. (2021). Artificial Intelligence for Mental Health Care: Clinical Applications, Barriers, Facilitators, and Artificial Wisdom. *Biological Psychiatry: Cognitive Neuroscience and Neuroimaging*, *6*(9), 856–864. DOI: 10.1016/j.bpsc.2021.02.001 PMID: 33571718

Lefebvre, V. A. (2001). Streams of consciousness and acts of awareness. In *Principia Cybernetica* (pp. 497–514). Springer., DOI: 10.1007/978-94-017-0691-9_36

Lehrer, P. M., & Gevirtz, R. (2014). Heart rate variability biofeedback: How and why does it work? *Frontiers in Psychology*, *5*, 756.

Lehrer, P., Kaur, K., Sharma, A., Shah, K., Huseby, R., Bhavsar, J., & Zhang, Y. (2020). Heart Rate Variability Biofeedback Improves Emotional and Physical Health and Performance: A Systematic Review and Meta Analysis. *Applied Psychophysiology and Biofeedback*, *45*(3), 109–129. DOI: 10.1007/s10484-020-09466-z PMID: 32385728

Leow, Y., Rashid, N. L. B. A., Klainin-Yobas, P., Zhang, Z., Wu, X. V., ... (2023). Effectiveness of mindfulness-based interventions on mental, cognitive outcomes and neuroplastic changes in older adults with mild cognitive impairment: A systematic review and meta-analysis. *Journal of Advanced Nursing*. https://pubmed.ncbi.nlm.nih.gov/37248564

Levertov, D. (1992). *New & selected essays* (Vol. 749). New Directions Publishing.

Levine, P. A. (2010). *In an unspoken voice: How the body releases trauma and restores goodness*. North Atlantic Books.

Ley, R. (1999). The modification of breathing behavior: Pavlovian and operant control in emotion and cognition. *Behavior Modification, 23*(3), 441–479.

Li, J., Cochrane, K. A., & Leshed, G. (2024). Beyond Meditation: Understanding Everyday Mindfulness Practices and Technology Use Among Experienced Practitioners. *Proceedings of the ACM on Human-Computer Interaction, 8*(CSCW2), 1–29. DOI: 10.1145/3687023

Lim, S.-A., & Cheong, K.-J. (2015). Regular Yoga Practice Improves Antioxidant Status, Immune Function, and Stress Hormone Releases in Young Healthy People: A Randomized, Double-Blind, Controlled Pilot Study. *Journal of Alternative and Complementary Medicine (New York, N.Y.), 21*(9), 530–538. DOI: 10.1089/acm.2014.0044 PMID: 26181573

Linardon, J., Cuijpers, P., Carlbring, P., Messer, M., & Fuller-Tyszkiewicz, M. (2021). The efficacy of app-supported smartphone interventions for mental health problems: A meta-analysis of randomized controlled trials. *World Psychiatry; Official Journal of the World Psychiatric Association (WPA), 20*(3), 388–398. PMID: 31496095

Linklater, K. (2006). Freeing the natural voice: Imagery and art in the practice of voice and language (Revised & expanded ed.). Drama Publishers / Quite Specific Media Group.

Liu, L., Liu, C., Tang, L., Wang, X., & Feng, Q. (2025). From contemplation to serenity: How yoga meditation improves the mental health of female college students? *Frontiers in Psychology, 16*, 1545943. Advance online publication. DOI: 10.3389/fpsyg.2025.1545943 PMID: 40129498

Liu, S., Ye, M., Pao, G. M., Song, S. M., Jhang, J., Jiang, H., Kim, J.-H., Kang, S. J., Kim, D.-I., & Han, S. (2021). Divergent brainstem opioidergic pathways that coordinate breathing with pain and emotions. *Neuron, 110*(5), 857–873.e9. Advance online publication. DOI: 10.1016/j.neuron.2021.11.029 PMID: 34921781

Löchner, J., Carlbring, P., Schuller, B., Torous, J., & Sander, L. B. (2025). Digital interventions in mental health: An overview and future perspectives. *Internet Interventions : the Application of Information Technology in Mental and Behavioural Health, 40*, 100824. DOI: 10.1016/j.invent.2025.100824 PMID: 40330743

Long, J. D. (2020). A complex ultimate reality: The metaphysics of the four yogas. *Religions, 11*(12), 655. DOI: 10.3390/rel11120655

Long, J. D. (2024). On Swami Vivekananda and caste prejudice: Ethical implications of the experience of non-duality. *Religions, 15*(8), 889. DOI: 10.3390/rel15080889

Luders, E., Thompson, P. M., Kurth, F., Hong, J.-Y., Phillips, O. R., Wang, Y., Gutman, B. A., Chou, Y.-Y., Narr, K. L., & Toga, A. W. (2013). Global and regional alterations of hippocampal anatomy in long-term meditation practitioners. *Human Brain Mapping*, *34*(12), 3369–3375. DOI: 10.1002/hbm.22153 PMID: 22815233

Luders, E., Toga, A. W., Lepore, N., & Gaser, C. (2009). The underlying anatomical correlates of long-term meditation: Larger hippocampal and frontal volumes of gray matter. *NeuroImage*, *45*(3), 672–678. DOI: 10.1016/j.neuroimage.2008.12.061 PMID: 19280691

Lukoff, K., Lyngs, U., Gueorguieva, S., Dillman, E. S., Hiniker, A., & Munson, S. A. (2020). From Ancient Contemplative Practice to the App Store: Designing a Digital Container for Mindfulness. *Proceedings of the 2020 ACM Designing Interactive Systems Conference*, 1551–1564. DOI: 10.1145/3357236.3395444

Lutz, A., Greischar, L. L., Rawlings, N. B., Ricard, M., & Davidson, R. J. (2004). Long-term meditators self-induce high-amplitude gamma synchrony during mental practice. *Proceedings of the National Academy of Sciences of the United States of America*, *101*(46), 16369–16373. DOI: 10.1073/pnas.0407401101 PMID: 15534199

Lutz, A., Slagter, H. A., Dunne, J. D., & Davidson, R. J. (2008). Attention regulation and monitoring in meditation. *Trends in Cognitive Sciences*, *12*(4), 163–169. DOI: 10.1016/j.tics.2008.01.005 PMID: 18329323

Lutz, J., Herwig, U., Opialla, S., Hittmeyer, A., Jäncke, L., Rufer, M., Grosse Holtforth, M., & Brühl, A. B. (2014). Mindfulness and emotion regulation—An fMRI study. *Social Cognitive and Affective Neuroscience*, *9*(6), 776–785. DOI: 10.1093/scan/nst043 PMID: 23563850

Lyons, K. E., & DeLange, J. (2016). Mindfulness Matters in the Classroom: The Effects of Mindfulness Training on Brain Development and Behavior in Children and Adolescents. In Schonert-Reichl, K. A., & Roeser, R. W. (Eds.), *Handbook of Mindfulness in Education* (pp. 271–283). Springer New York., DOI: 10.1007/978-1-4939-3506-2_17

Machida, S., Sunagawa, M., Takahashi, T., & Hiroshima University, Blueberry lodge 206, Koyama719, Gotemba, Shizuoka, Japan. (2018). Oxytocin Release during the Meditation of Altruism andAppreciation (Arigato-Zen): Machida S et al. Oxytocin release stimulated by the meditation. *International Journal of Neurology Research*, *4*(1), 364–370. DOI: 10.17554/j.issn.2313-5611.2018.04.75

Madaio, J. (2017). Rethinking Neo-Vedānta: Swami Vivekananda and the selective historiography of Advaita Vedānta. *Religions*, *8*(6), 101. DOI: 10.3390/rel8060101

Magomedova, A., & Fatima, G. (2025). Mental Health and Well-Being in the Modern Era: A Comprehensive Review of Challenges and Interventions. *Cureus, 17*(1), 1–16. DOI: 10.7759/cureus.77683 PMID: 39974249

Maharaj, A. (2017). Swami Vivekananda's Vedāntic critique of Schopenhauer's doctrine of the will. *Philosophy East & West, 67*(4), 1013–1031. DOI: 10.1353/pew.2017.0098

Maharaj, A. (2019). Śivajñāne jīver sevā: Reexamining Swami Vivekananda's practical Vedānta in the light of Sri Ramakrishna. *Journal of Dharma Studies, 2*(2), 175–187. DOI: 10.1007/s42240-019-00046-x

Maheshkumar, K., Dilara, K., Ravishankar, P., Julius, A., Padmavathi, R., Poonguzhali, S., & Venugopal, V. (2022). Effect of six months pranayama training on stress-induced salivary cortisol response among adolescents-Randomized controlled study. *Explore (New York, N.Y.), 18*(4), 463–466. DOI: 10.1016/j.explore.2021.07.005 PMID: 34366293

Mahoney, M. J. (2003). *Constructive Psychotherapy: A Practical Guide*. Guilford Press.

Maity, S., Abbaspour, R., Bandelow, S., Pahwa, S., Alahdadi, T., Shah, S., Chhetri, P., Jha, A., Nauhria, S., Nath, R., Nayak, N., & Nauhria, S. (2024). The psychosomatic impact of Yoga in medical education: A systematic review and meta-analysis. *Medical Education Online, 29*(1), 2364486. Advance online publication. DOI: 10.1080/10872981.2024.2364486 PMID: 38861675

Maluleke, A. (2024). Exploring Ubuntu-Based Research Methodologies in Southern African Bantu People's Embodied Movements: Ethical Considerations, Community-Based Strategies, and Philosophy. *Conversations Across the Field of Dance Studies, 43*(0). Advance online publication. DOI: 10.3998/conversations.5950

Manna, A., Raffone, A., Perrucci, M. G., Nardo, D., Ferretti, A., Tartaro, A., Londei, A., Del Gratta, C., Belardinelli, M. O., & Romani, G. L. (2010). Neural correlates of focused attention and cognitive monitoring in meditation. *Brain Research Bulletin, 82*(1–2), 46–56. DOI: 10.1016/j.brainresbull.2010.03.001 PMID: 20223285

Marchand, W. R. (2014). Neural mechanisms of mindfulness and meditation: Evidence from neuroimaging studies. *World Journal of Radiology, 6*(7), 471–479. DOI: 10.4329/wjr.v6.i7.471 PMID: 25071887

Marshall, J. E. (2012). Prophylactic effects of mindfulness: The role of mindfulness in the treatment of anxiety. [No DOI available]. *Journal of Clinical Psychology Practice, 3*(1), 22–31.

Martinez, L., Chen, Y., Rodriguez, A., & Patel, N. (2022). Trauma-informed yoga for healthcare workers during COVID-19: A randomized controlled trial. *Journal of Occupational Health Psychology*, *27*(3), 298–308.

Masten, A. S., & Motti-Stefanidi, F. (2020). Multisystem Resilience for Children and Youth in Disaster: Reflections in the Context of COVID-19. *Adversity and Resilience Science*, *1*(2), 95–106. DOI: 10.1007/s42844-020-00010-w PMID: 32838305

Matsumoto, N., & Mochizuki, S. (2018). Why do people overthink? A longitudinal investigation of a meta-cognitive model and uncontrollability of rumination. *Behavioural and Cognitive Psychotherapy*, *46*(2), 129–143. DOI: 10.1017/S1352465818000103 PMID: 29510773

McCrimmon, D. R., Mitchell, G. S., & Alheid, G. F. (2008). Overview: The neurochemistry of respiratory control. *Respiratory Physiology & Neurobiology*, *164*(1-2), 1–2. DOI: 10.1016/j.resp.2008.07.021 PMID: 18721910

McKenna, J. F. (2006). The meaningfulness of mental health as being within a world of apparently meaningless being. In *New perspectives in psychotherapy* (pp. 233–249). Springer., DOI: 10.1007/1-4020-3737-6_20

McKibben, E. (2025). Mind-Stuff and Withdrawal of the Senses: Toward an Interpretation of Pratyahara in Contemporary Postural Yoga. *Health*, *29*(1), 83–99. DOI: 10.1177/13634593231222450 PMID: 38311913

McLeod, C., & Boyes, M. (2021). The Effectiveness of Social-Emotional Learning Strategies and Mindful Breathing with Biofeedback on the Reduction of Adolescent Test Anxiety. *Canadian Journal of Education*, *44*(3), 815–847. DOI: 10.53967/cje-rce.v44i3.4869

Medhananda, S. (2022). *Swami Vivekananda's Vedāntic cosmopolitanism*. Oxford University Press., DOI: 10.1093/oso/9780197624463.001.0001

Meduri, A. (Ed.). (2005). *Rukmini Devi Arundale, 1904-1986: A visionary architect of Indian culture and the performing arts*. Motilal Banarsidass Publishing House.

Mehta, N. (2011). Mind-body Dualism: A critique from a Health Perspective. *Mens Sana Monographs*, *9*(1), 202–209. DOI: 10.4103/0973-1229.77436 PMID: 21694971

Meissner, M., Cantell, M. H., Steiner, R., & Sanchez, X. (2016). Evaluating Emotional Well-Being after a Short-Term Traditional Yoga Practice Approach in Yoga Practitioners with an Existing Western-Type Yoga Practice. *Evidence-Based Complementary and Alternative Medicine : eCAM*, *2016*(1), 7216982. DOI: 10.1155/2016/7216982 PMID: 27123033

Meister, K., & Juckel, G. (2018). A Systematic Review of Mechanisms of Change in Body-Oriented Yoga in Major Depressive Disorders. *Pharmacopsychiatry*, *51*(3), 73–81. DOI: 10.1055/s-0043-111013 PMID: 28571077

Melnychuk, M. C., Dockree, P. M., O'Connell, R. G., Murphy, P. R., Balsters, J. H., & Robertson, I. H. (2018). Coupling of respiration and attention via the locus coeruleus: Effects of meditation and pranayama. *Psychophysiology*, *55*(9), e13091. Advance online publication. DOI: 10.1111/psyp.13091 PMID: 29682753

Mendo, B., Gonçalves, M., Lopes, L., Matos, L. C., & Machado, J. (2022). Can Yoga, Qigong, and Tai Chi Breathing Work Support the Psycho-Immune Homeostasis during and after the COVID-19 Pandemic? A Narrative Review. *Health Care*, *10*(10), 1934. DOI: 10.3390/healthcare10101934 PMID: 36292380

Mennin, D. S., Ellard, K. K., Fresco, D. M., & Gross, J. J. (2013). United we stand: Emphasizing commonalities across cognitive-behavioral therapies. *Behavior Therapy*, *44*(2), 234–248. DOI: 10.1016/j.beth.2013.02.004 PMID: 23611074

Merleau-Ponty, M. (1962). An unpublished work by Maurice Merleau-Ponty. *Revue de Metaphysique et de Morale*, *67*(4), 401–409.

Meuret, A. E., Kroll, J., & Ritz, T. (2019). Panic disorder comorbidity with medical conditions and treatment implications. *Annual Review of Clinical Psychology*, *15*, 309–340. PMID: 28375724

Meuret, A. E., Rosenfield, D., Seidel, A., Bhaskara, L., & Hofmann, S. G. (2010). Respiratory and cognitive mediators of treatment change in panic disorder: Evidence for intervention specificity. *Journal of Consulting and Clinical Psychology*, *78*(5), 691.

Mewhinney, M. (2023). The Rhythm of Breath in Natsume Sōseki's Recollecting and Such. *Literature*, *3*(1), 94–111. DOI: 10.3390/literature3010008

Miao, C., Gao, Y., Li, X., Zhou, Y., Chung, J. W., & Smith, G. D. (2023). The effectiveness of mindfulness yoga on patients with major depressive disorder: A systematic review and meta-analysis of randomized controlled trials. *BMC Complementary Medicine and Therapies*, *23*(1), 313. DOI: 10.1186/s12906-023-04141-2 PMID: 37684609

Michaelsen, M. M., Adolph, D., Schinköthe, A., Witthöft, M., & Wessa, M. (2023). Mindfulness-based and mindfulness-informed interventions at the workplace: A meta-analysis of randomized controlled trials. *Mindfulness*, *14*, 1271–1304. DOI: 10.1007/s12671-023-02130-7 PMID: 37362186

Michalsen, A., Grossman, P., Acil, A., Langhorst, J., Lüdtke, R., Esch, T., Stefano, G. B., & Dobos, G. J. (2005). Rapid stress reduction and anxiolysis among distressed women as a consequence of a three-month intensive yoga program. *Medical Science Monitor, 11*(12), CR555–CR561. https://www.ncbi.nlm.nih.gov/pubmed/16319785 PMID: 16319785

Miehls, D. (2011). Surrender as a developmental achievement in couple systems. *Psychoanalytic Social Work, 18*(1), 34–49. DOI: 10.1080/15228878.2011.561706

Mishra, S. K., Singh, P., Bunch, S., & Zhang, R. (2012). The therapeutic value of yoga in neurological disorders. *Annals of Indian Academy of Neurology, 15*(4), 247–254. DOI: 10.4103/0972-2327.104328 PMID: 23349587

Mishra, V. (2014). Ethical responsibility and the spectres of demonic sacralisation in Swami Vivekananda. In *The guru question* (pp. 199–214). Routledge., DOI: 10.4324/9781315819112-14

Mitra, S. (2000). The discourse vanishes: Revolution and resilience in Indian politics. *Contemporary South Asia, 9*(3), 327–339. DOI: 10.1080/713658755

Mitsea, E., Drigas, A., & Skianis, C. (2024). Artificial Intelligence, Immersive Technologies, and Neurotechnologies in Breathing Interventions for Mental and Emotional Health: A Systematic Review. *Electronics (Basel), 13*(12), 2253. DOI: 10.3390/electronics13122253

Mittal, G., Pathania, M., Bhardwaj, P., Dhar, M., Khapre, M., & Mittal, S. (2025). An Exploratory Randomised Trial to Assess the Effect of Nadi Shodhan Pranayama as an Adjunct Versus Standard Non-pharmacological Management in Hypertensives. *Annals of Neurosciences*, 09727531251318810. Advance online publication. DOI: 10.1177/09727531251318810 PMID: 40242728

Montgomery, J. D. (2000). The self as a fuzzy set of roles, role theory as a fuzzy system. *Sociological Methodology, 30*(1), 261–314. DOI: 10.1111/0081-1750.00081

Mooneyham, B. W., Mrazek, M. D., Mrazek, A. J., Mrazek, K. L., Ihm, E. D., & Schooler, J. W. (2017). An Integrated Assessment of Changes in Brain Structure and Function of the Insula Resulting from an Intensive Mindfulness-Based Intervention. *Journal of Cognitive Enhancement: Towards the Integration of Theory and Practice, 1*(3), 327–336. DOI: 10.1007/s41465-017-0034-3

Mrazek, M. D., Dow, B., Richelle, J., Pasch, A. M., Godderis, N., Pamensky, T. A., Rutila, B. A., & Mrazek, A. J. (2024). Aspects of acceptance: Building a shared conceptual understanding. *Frontiers in Psychology, 15*, 1423976. DOI: 10.3389/fpsyg.2024.1423976 PMID: 38974104

Mulla, Z. R., & Krishnan, V. R. (2014). Karma-yoga: The Indian model of moral development. *Journal of Business Ethics*, *123*(2), 341–351. DOI: 10.1007/s10551-013-1842-8

Munns, L., Spark, N., Crossland, A., & Preston, C. (2024). The effects of yoga-based interventions on postnatal mental health and well-being: A systematic review. *Heliyon*, *10*(3), e25455. DOI: 10.1016/j.heliyon.2024.e25455 PMID: 38322903

Murphy, J., Brewer, R., Catmur, C., & Bird, G. (2022). Interoception and psychopathology: A developmental neuroscience perspective. *Developmental Cognitive Neuroscience*, *58*, 101168. PMID: 28081519

Myers, M. W. (2000). *Brahman: A comparative theology*. Fordham University Press.

Nagar, P. (2024). Karma Yoga and management practice. *Gurugram University Business Review*, *1*, 1–12.

Nair, A. K., & Kutty, B. M. (2017). Meditation, cognitive reserve and the neural basis of consciousness. In *Meditation and Neuroscience* (pp. 37–56). https://doi.org/DOI: 10.1007/978-981-10-5777-9_3

Nair, S. (2007). *Restoration of Breath*. https://doi.org/DOI: 10.1163/9789401205177

Natarajan, A. (2023). Heart rate variability during mindful breathing meditation. *Frontiers in Physiology*, *14*, 1017350. DOI: 10.3389/fphys.2022.1017350 PMID: 36756034

National Institute of Mental Health and Neuro Sciences. (2016). *National Mental Health Survey of India, 2015–16: Prevalence, patterns and outcomes*. NIMHANS Publication.

National Institute of Mental Health. (2024). *Mental illness statistics*. https://www.nimh.nih.gov/health/statistics/mental-illness

Nautiyal, S., Rayal, S. P., & Bhardwaj, A. K. (2024). The effect of Om Chanting, Bhramari Pranayama, and Nadi Shodhana Pranayama on cognitive functions among medical students: An experimental trial. *Yoga Mimamsa*, *56*(1), 21–26. DOI: 10.4103/ym.ym_13_24

Navarro-Haro, M. V., López-Del-Hoyo, Y., Campos, D., Linehan, M. M., Hoffman, H. G., García-Palacios, A., Modrego-Alarcón, M., Borao, L., & García-Campayo, J. (2017). Meditation experts try Virtual Reality Mindfulness: A pilot study evaluation of the feasibility and acceptability of Virtual Reality to facilitate mindfulness practice in people attending a Mindfulness conference. *PLoS One*, *12*(11), e0187777. DOI: 10.1371/journal.pone.0187777 PMID: 29166665

Naveen, G. H., Thirthalli, J., Rao, M. G., Varambally, S., Christopher, R., & Gangadhar, B. N. (2013). Positive therapeutic and neurotropic effects of yoga in depression: A comparative study. *Indian Journal of Psychiatry*, *55*(7, Suppl 3), S400–S404. https://journals.lww.com/indianjpsychiatry/fulltext/2013/55003/positive_therapeutic_and_neurotropic_effects_of.17.aspx. DOI: 10.4103/0019-5545.116313 PMID: 24049208

Nayan Rishi, N. (2024). Bridging the Science Between Yogic Postures (Asanas) and Neurophysiology: A Narrative Review. *Journal of Cancer Research and Cellular Therapeutics, 8*(4), 01–04. DOI: 10.31579/2640-1053/198

Nayyar, R., Yadav, P., Baral, R., Raina, M., & Jena, L. K. (2024). Unveiling the past, present and future of workplace spirituality research: A systematic literature review of 15 years. *The International Journal of Organizational Analysis*. Advance online publication. DOI: 10.1108/IJOA-04-2024-4438

Neacsiu, A. D.. (2018). Neural effects of mindfulness-based interventions on patients with major depressive disorder: A systematic review. *Neuroscience and Biobehavioral Reviews*, *95*, 500–513. https://pubmed.ncbi.nlm.nih.gov/29548932

Neff, K. (with Internet Archive). (2011). *Self-compassion: The proven power of being kind to yourself.* New York : William Morrow. http://archive.org/details/self compassionpr0000neff

Newcombe, S. (2009). The Development of Modern Yoga: A Survey of the Field. *Religion Compass*, *3*(6), 6. Advance online publication. DOI: 10.1111/j.1749-8171.2009.00171.x

Newman, M. G., Basterfield, C., Erickson, T. M., Caulley, E., Przeworski, A., & Llera, S. J. (2022). Psychotherapeutic treatments for generalized anxiety disorder: Cognitive and behavioral therapies, enhancement strategies, and emerging efforts. *Expert Review of Neurotherapeutics*, *22*(9), 751–770. DOI: 10.1080/14737175.2022.2125800 PMID: 36107159

Ng, H. Y. H., Wu, C. W., Huang, F. Y., Cheng, Y. T., Guu, S. F., Huang, C. M., Hsu, C. F., Chao, Y. P., Jung, T. P., & Chuang, C. H. (2021). Mindfulness Training Associated With Resting-State Electroencephalograms Dynamics in Novice Practitioners via Mindful Breathing and Body-Scan. *Frontiers in Psychology*, *12*(October), 748584. Advance online publication. DOI: 10.3389/fpsyg.2021.748584 PMID: 34777144

Nivethitha, L., Mooventhan, A., & Manjunath, N. (2016). Effects of various Prā āyāma on cardiovascular and autonomic variables. *Ancient Science of Life*, *36*(2), 72. DOI: 10.4103/asl.ASL_178_16 PMID: 28446827

Nivette, S., Mascret, N., & Augé, S. (2021). Effects of coherent breathing on anxiety, blood pressure, and cortisol levels: A systematic review. *Applied Psychology. Health and Well-Being, 13*(4), 923–942.

Northoff, G., Magioncalda, P., Martino, M., Lee, H. C., Tseng, Y. C., & Lane, T. (2021). Too fast or too slow? Time and neuronal variability in bipolar disorder—A combined theoretical and empirical investigation. *Schizophrenia Bulletin, 47*(1), 54–70. DOI: 10.1093/schbul/sbx050 PMID: 28525601

Nourollahimoghadam, E., Gorji, S., Gorji, A., & Khaleghi Ghadiri, M. (2021). Therapeutic role of yoga in neuropsychological disorders. *World Journal of Psychiatry, 11*(10), 754–773. DOI: 10.5498/wjp.v11.i10.754 PMID: 34733640

Novaes, M. M., Palhano-Fontes, F., Onias, H., Andrade, K. C., Lobão-Soares, B., Arruda-Sanchez, T., Kozasa, E. H., Santaella, D. F., & de Araujo, D. B. (2020). Effects of Yoga Respiratory Practice (Bhastrika pranayama) on Anxiety, Affect, and Brain Functional Connectivity and Activity: A Randomized Controlled Trial. *Frontiers in Psychiatry, 11*(May), 1–13. DOI: 10.3389/fpsyt.2020.00467 PMID: 32528330

Nuss, P. (2015). Anxiety disorders and GABA neurotransmission: A disturbance of modulation. *Neuropsychiatric Disease and Treatment, 11*, 165–175. DOI: 10.2147/NDT.S58841 PMID: 25653526

Oei, N. Y. L., Veer, I. M., Wolf, O. T., Spinhoven, P., Rombouts, S. A. R. B., & Elzinga, B. M. (2012). Stress shifts brain activation towards ventral affective areas during emotional distraction. *Social Cognitive and Affective Neuroscience, 7*(6), 653–662. DOI: 10.1093/scan/nsr024 PMID: 21498384

Ong, I. (2021). Treating Complex Trauma Survivors: A Trauma-Sensitive Yoga (TSY)-Informed Psychotherapeutic Approach. *Journal of Creativity in Mental Health, 16*(2), 182–195. DOI: 10.1080/15401383.2020.1761498

Ong, N. Y., Teo, F. J. J., Ee, J. Z. Y., Tan, J. X., Goh, H. K., & Lee, J. C. (2024). Effectiveness of mindfulness-based interventions on the well-being of healthcare workers: A systematic review and meta-analysis. *General Psychiatry, 37*(3), e101115. DOI: 10.1136/gpsych-2023-101115 PMID: 38737894

Page, M. J., McKenzie, J. E., Bossuyt, P. M., Boutron, I., Hoffmann, T. C., Mulrow, C. D., Shamseer, L., Tetzlaff, J. M., Akl, E. A., Brennan, S. E., Chou, R., Glanville, J., Grimshaw, J. M., Hróbjartsson, A., Lalu, M. M., Li, T., Loder, E. W., Mayo-Wilson, E., McDonald, S., & Moher, D. (2021). The PRISMA 2020 statement: An updated guideline for reporting systematic reviews. *BMJ (Clinical Research Ed.), 372*(71), n71. Advance online publication. DOI: 10.1136/bmj.n71 PMID: 33782057

Pal, D. K., Bhalla, A., Bammidi, S., Telles, S., Kohli, A., Kumar, S., Devi, P., Kaur, N., Sharma, K., Kumar, R., Malik, N., Thakur, V., Bhargava, G. G., Goyal, A. K., Devi, G., Chauhan, S., Singh, G., Ahmad, S., Joshi, M., & Anand, A. (2017). Can Yoga-Based Diabetes Management Studies Facilitate Integrative Medicine in India Current Status and Future Directions. *Integrative Medicine International*, *4*(3–4), 125–141. DOI: 10.1159/000479816

Pal, G. K., Velkumary, S., & Madanmohan, A. (2004). Effect of short-term practice of breathing exercises on autonomic functions in normal human volunteers. *The Indian Journal of Medical Research*, *120*(2), 115–121. PMID: 15347862

Pallathadka, H., & Roy, P. D. (2025). Transcendent unity and social transformation: A comprehensive analysis of Swami Vivekananda's philosophical legacy and contemporary relevance. *Stallion Journal for Multidisciplinary Associated Research Studies*, *4*(3), 91–109. DOI: 10.55544/sjmars.4.3.9

Pallvi, K., & Jhajharia, P. (2025). Exploring trends in workplace spirituality through bibliometric analysis. *SN Business & Economics*, *5*(9), 108. Advance online publication. DOI: 10.1007/s43546-025-00883-y

Palmer, P. J. (with Internet Archive). (2010). *The heart of higher education: A call to renewal : transforming the academy through collegial conversations*. San Francisco : Jossey-Bass. http://archive.org/details/heartofhigheredu0000palm

Palmieri, A., Fernandez, K. C., Cariolato, Y., Kleinbub, J. R., Salvatore, S., & Gross, J. J. (2022). Emotion regulation in psychodynamic and cognitive behaviour therapy: An integrative perspective. *Clinical*, 2022(2). https://doi.org/DOI: 10.36131/cnfioritieditore20220204

Pal, R., Adhikari, D., Heyat, M. B. B., Ullah, I., & You, Z. (2023). Yoga Meets Intelligent Internet of Things: Recent Challenges and Future Directions. *Bioengineering (Basel, Switzerland)*, *10*(4), 459. DOI: 10.3390/bioengineering10040459 PMID: 37106646

Pandurangi, A., Keshavan, M., Ganapathy, V., & Gangadhar, B. (2017). Yoga: Past and Present. *The American Journal of Psychiatry*, *174*(1), 16–17. DOI: 10.1176/appi.ajp.2016.16080853 PMID: 28040996

Park, C. L., Finkelstein-Fox, L., Groessl, E., Elwy, A. R., & Lee, S. Y. (2020). Exploring How Different Types of Yoga Change Psychological Resources and Emotional Well-Being across a Single Session. *Complementary Therapies in Medicine*, *49*, 102354. DOI: 10.1016/j.ctim.2020.102354 PMID: 32147083

Partners, W. (2021). Trauma Sensitive Yoga. *CHWP*, (August), 2.

Pascoe, M. C., De Manincor, M. J., Hallgren, M., Baldwin, P. A., Tseberja, J., & Parker, A. G. (2021). Psychobiological mechanisms underlying the mental health benefits of yoga-based interventions: A narrative review. *Mindfulness*, *12*(12), 2877–2889. DOI: 10.1007/s12671-021-01736-z

Pascoe, M. C., Thompson, D. R., Jenkins, Z. M., & Ski, C. F. (2017). Mindfulness mediates the physiological markers of stress: Systematic review and meta-analysis. *Journal of Psychiatric Research*, *95*, 156–178. DOI: 10.1016/j.jpsychires.2017.08.004 PMID: 28863392

Pascoe, M. C., Thompson, D. R., & Ski, C. F. (2017). Yoga, mindfulness-based stress reduction and stress-related physiological measures: A meta-analysis. *Psychoneuroendocrinology*, *86*, 152–168. DOI: 10.1016/j.psyneuen.2017.08.008 PMID: 28963884

Pascoe, M., & Bauer, I. (2015). A systematic review of randomised control trials on the effects of yoga on stress measures and mood. *Journal of Psychiatric Research*, *68*, 270–282. DOI: 10.1016/j.jpsychires.2015.07.013 PMID: 26228429

Patañjali. (2009). *The Yoga Sūtras of Patañjali*, translated and commented by Edwin F. Bryant. North Point Press.

Patla, I. (2025). *Addressing self-esteem in mental health: A systematic review* (Doctoral dissertation, California Southern University).

Payne, P., Levine, P. A., & Crane-Godreau, M. A. (2015). Somatic experiencing: Using interoception and proprioception as core elements of trauma therapy. *Frontiers in Psychology*, *6*, 93. DOI: 10.3389/fpsyg.2015.00093 PMID: 25699005

Perez-Diaz, O., Góngora, D., González-Mora, J. L., Rubia, K., Barrós-Loscertales, A., & Hernández, S. E. (2024). Enhanced amygdala–anterior cingulate white matter structural connectivity in Sahaja Yoga Meditators. *PLoS One*, *19*(3), e0301283. DOI: 10.1371/journal.pone.0301283 PMID: 38547155

Pérezts, M., Fotaki, M., Shymko, Y., & Islam, G. (2025). Breathe and let breathe: Breathing as a political model of organizing. *Organization*, *32*(1), 136–153.

Permadhi, A. K., & Marhaeni, A. A. I. N. (2019). Effect of understanding the teaching of Karma Yoga and empowerment of poor family resource management. *International Journal of Sciences, Basic and Applied Research*, *45*(1), 256–269.

Pernet, C. R., Belov, N., Delorme, A., & Zammit, A. (2021). Mindfulness-related changes in grey matter: A systematic review and meta-analysis. *Brain Imaging and Behavior*, *15*(6), 3056–3076. DOI: 10.1007/s11682-021-00453-4 PMID: 33624219

Peterman, A. H., Fitchett, G., Brady, M. J., Hernandez, L., & Cella, D. (2002). Measuring spiritual well-being in people with cancer: The Functional Assessment of Chronic Illness Therapy–Spiritual Well-Being Scale (FACIT-Sp). *Annals of Behavioral Medicine*, *24*(1), 49–58. DOI: 10.1207/S15324796ABM2401_06 PMID: 12008794

Phatak, A. A., Wieland, F. G., Vempala, K., Volkmar, F., & Memmert, D. (2021). Artificial Intelligence Based Body Sensor Network Framework—Narrative Review: Proposing an End-to-End Framework using Wearable Sensors, Real-Time Location Systems and Artificial Intelligence/Machine Learning Algorithms for Data Collection, Data Mining and. *Sports Medicine - Open*, *7*(1), 79. Advance online publication. DOI: 10.1186/s40798-021-00372-0 PMID: 34716868

Phelps, J., & Manipod, V. (2012). Treating anxiety by discontinuing antidepressants: A case series. *Medical Hypotheses*, *79*(4), 477–479. DOI: 10.1016/j.mehy.2012.05.029 PMID: 22698959

Philippe, T. J., Sikder, N., Jackson, A., Koblanski, M. E., Liow, E., Pilarinos, A., & Vasarhelyi, K. (2022). Digital health interventions for delivery of mental health care: Systematic and comprehensive meta-review. *JMIR Mental Health*, *9*(5), e35159. DOI: 10.2196/35159 PMID: 35551058

Philippi, C. L., Weible, E., Ehlers, A., Walsh, E. C., Hoks, R. M., Birn, R. M., & Abercrombie, H. C. (2024). Effects of cortisol administration on heart rate variability and functional connectivity across women with different depression histories. *Behavioural Brain Research*, *463*, 114923. DOI: 10.1016/j.bbr.2024.114923 PMID: 38408523

Philippot, P., Chapelle, G., & Blairy, S. (2002). Respiratory feedback in the generation of emotion. *Cognition and Emotion*, *16*(5), 605–627. DOI: 10.1080/02699930143000392

Piet, J., & Hougaard, E. (2011). The effect of mindfulness-based cognitive therapy for prevention of relapse in recurrent major depressive disorder: A systematic review and meta-analysis. *Clinical Psychology Review*, *31*(6), 1032–1040. DOI: 10.1016/j.cpr.2011.05.002 PMID: 21802618

Pillay, Y., Ziff, K., & Bhat, C. S. (2008). Vedānta personality development: A model to enhance the cultural competence of psychotherapists. *International Journal of Hindu Studies*, *12*(3), 273–291. DOI: 10.1007/s11407-008-9057-9

Pise, V., Pradhan, B., & Gharote, M. (2018). Effect of yoga practices on psycho-motor abilities among intellectually disabled children. *Journal of Exercise Rehabilitation*, *14*(4), 581–585. DOI: 10.12965/jer.1836290.145 PMID: 30276177

Pomerantz, A. M. (2020). *Clinical psychology: Science, practice, and diversity* (5th ed.). SAGE Publications.

Popova, N. K., & Naumenko, V. S. (2019). Neuronal and behavioral plasticity: The role of serotonin and BDNF systems tandem. *Expert Opinion on Therapeutic Targets, 23*(3), 227–239. DOI: 10.1080/14728222.2019.1572747 PMID: 30661441

Porges, S. W. (2011). *The polyvagal theory: Neurophysiological foundations of emotions, attachment, communication, and self-regulation* (pp. xvii, 347). W. W. Norton & Company.

Porges, S. W. (2007). The polyvagal perspective. *Biological Psychology, 74*(2), 116–143. DOI: 10.1016/j.biopsycho.2006.06.009 PMID: 17049418

Porges, S. W. (2011). *The polyvagal theory: Neurophysiological foundations of emotions, attachment, communication, and self-regulation.* Norton.

Posner, M. I., Rothbart, M. K., & Tang, Y.-Y. (2015). Enhancing attention through training. *Current Opinion in Behavioral Sciences, 4*, 1–5. DOI: 10.1016/j.cobeha.2014.12.008

Powers, J., & LaBar, K. S. (2019). Regulating emotion through distancing: A taxonomy, neurocognitive model, and supporting meta-analysis. *Neuroscience and Biobehavioral Reviews, 103*, 124–138. DOI: 10.1016/j.neubiorev.2018.04.023 PMID: 30502352

Prabhu, H. R. A., & Bhat, P. (2013). Mind and consciousness in Yoga–Vedanta: A comparative analysis with Western psychological concepts. *Indian Journal of Psychiatry, 55*(6, S2), 338–342. DOI: 10.4103/0019-5545.105524 PMID: 23858252

Pradhan, B. (2015). Yoga: Original Concepts and History. In *Yoga and Mindfulness Based Cognitive Therapy* (pp. 3–36). Springer International Publishing. DOI: 10.1007/978-3-319-09105-1_1

Pradhan, B. (2019). *Yoga and mindfulness-based cognitive therapy.* Springer.

Pragya, S. U., Mehta, N. D., Abomoelak, B., Uddin, P., Veeramachaneni, P., Mehta, N., Moore, S., Jean-Francois, M., Garcia, S., Pragya, S. C., & Mehta, D. I. (2021). Effects of Combining Meditation Techniques on Short-Term Memory, Attention, and Affect in Healthy College Students. *Frontiers in Psychology, 12*, 607573. Advance online publication. DOI: 10.3389/fpsyg.2021.607573 PMID: 33746830

Primack, B. A., Shensa, A., Sidani, J. E., Whaite, E. O., Lin, L. Y., Rosen, D., Colditz, J. B., Radovic, A., & Miller, E. (2017). Social Media Use and Perceived Social Isolation Among Young Adults in the U.S. *American Journal of Preventive Medicine*, *53*(1), 1–8. DOI: 10.1016/j.amepre.2017.01.010 PMID: 28279545

Prpa, M., Stepanova, E. R., Schiphorst, T., Riecke, B. E., & Pasquier, P. (2020). Inhaling and Exhaling: How Technologies Can Perceptually Extend our Breath Awareness. *Proceedings of the 2020 CHI Conference on Human Factors in Computing Systems*. DOI: 10.1145/3313831.3376183

Prpa, M., Tatar, K., Françoise, J., Riecke, B., Schiphorst, T., & Pasquier, P. (2018). Attending to Breath: Exploring how the cues in a virtual environment guide the attention to breath and shape the quality of experience to support mindfulness. *Proceedings of the 2018 Designing Interactive Systems Conference*, 71–84. DOI: 10.1145/3196709.3196765

Purser, R., & Order, C. P. is a professor of management at S. F. S. U. H. is an ordained teacher in the K. B. T., Cranks, co-host of the podcast T. M., Loy, D., & Teacher, C. (2013, July 1). *Beyond McMindfulness*. HuffPost. https://www.huffpost.com/entry/beyond-mcmindfulness_b_3519289

Purser, R. E. (2019). *McMindfulness: How Mindfulness Became the New Capitalist Spirituality*. Repeater Books.

Putnam, R. D. (2000). *Bowling alone: The collapse and revival of American community*. Touchstone Books/Simon & Schuster., DOI: 10.1145/358916.361990

Radhakrishnan, S., & Moore, C. A. (Eds.). (1957). *A Sourcebook in Indian Philosophy*. Princeton University Press.

Rahman, S., & Singh, K. (2020). Acute effects of 4-7-8 breathing technique on anxiety and physiological parameters: A randomized controlled trial. *International Journal of Yoga*, *13*(2), 144–148. PMID: 32669769

Rahrig, H., Vago, D. R., Passarelli, M. A., Auten, A., Lynn, N. A., & Brown, K. W. (2022). Meta-analytic evidence that mindfulness training alters resting state default mode network connectivity. *Scientific Reports*, *12*(1), 1–13. DOI: 10.1038/s41598-022-15195-6 PMID: 35851275

Rajkumar, R. P. (2024). Are There Biological Correlates of Response to Yoga-Based Interventions in Depression? A Critical Scoping Review. *Brain Sciences*, *14*(6), 543. DOI: 10.3390/brainsci14060543 PMID: 38928543

Rajneesh, B. S., & Neiman, S. C. (2001). *Awareness: The key to living in balance: Insights for a new way of living*. Osho International Foundation.

Rambachan, A. (2017). That from which all words return: The distinctive methods of language utilization in Advaita Vedānta. In *Language, cognition, and consciousness in Indian philosophy* (pp. 173–195). https://doi.org/DOI: 10.1007/978-3-319-64165-2_9

Rambachan, A. (2006). *The Advaita Worldview: God, World, and Humanity*. SUNY Press. DOI: 10.1353/book5101

Ram-Prasad, C. (2002). *Advaita epistemology and metaphysics: An outline of Indian non-realism*. Routledge.

Ramsundarsingh, S. (2019). Vedanta and social work practice. *Social Thought, 38*(1), 68–92.

Ren, B., Yuan, Q., Cha, S., Liu, S., Zhang, J., & Guo, G. (2025). Maladaptive Neuroplasticity Under Stress: Insights into Neuronal and Synaptic Changes in the Prefrontal Cortex. *Molecular Neurobiology, 0123456789*(11), 15227–15249. Advance online publication. DOI: 10.1007/s12035-025-05152-5 PMID: 40545507

Ressler, K. J. (2010). Amygdala Activity, Fear, and Anxiety: Modulation by Stress. *Biological Psychiatry, 67*(12), 1117–1119. DOI: 10.1016/j.biopsych.2010.04.027 PMID: 20525501

Roberts, A. C., & Mulvihill, K. G. (2024). Multiple faces of anxiety: A frontal lobe perspective. *Trends in Neurosciences, 47*(9), 708–721. DOI: 10.1016/j.tins.2024.07.001 PMID: 39127569

Robinson, D. N., Hopke, T., & Massey-Abernathy, A. (2023). Learning to relax: The impact of brief biofeedback training and gentle yoga on salivary cortisol reduction. *Current Psychology (New Brunswick, N.J.), 42*(9), 6980–6989. DOI: 10.1007/s12144-021-02036-4

Rocha, K. K. F., Ribeiro, A. M., Rocha, K. C. F., Sousa, M. B. C., Albuquerque, F. S., Ribeiro, S., & Silva, R. H. (2012). Improvement in physiological and psychological parameters after 6 months of yoga practice. *Consciousness and Cognition, 21*(2), 843–850. DOI: 10.1016/j.concog.2012.01.014 PMID: 22342535

Rochet-Capellan, A., & Fuchs, S. (2014). Take a breath and take the turn: How breathing meets turns in spontaneous dialogue. *Philosophical Transactions of the Royal Society of London. Series B, Biological Sciences, 369*(1658).

Roemer, L., & Orsillo, S. M. (2009). *Mindfulness- and acceptance-based behavioral therapies in practice* (pp. xii, 244). The Guilford Press.

Roemer, L., Orsillo, S. M., & Salters-Pedneault, K. (2021). Efficacy of an acceptance-based behavior therapy for generalized anxiety disorder: Evaluation in a randomized controlled trial. *Journal of Consulting and Clinical Psychology*, *89*(3), 173–185. PMID: 19045976

Ross, D. S., & Vasantha, S. (2014). A conceptual study on impact of stress on work-life balance. *Sai Om Journal of Commerce & Management*, *1*(1), 1–8.

Rudolph, K. (2021). Ethical Considerations in Trauma-Informed Care. *The Psychiatric Clinics of North America*, *44*(4), 521–535. DOI: 10.1016/j.psc.2021.07.001 PMID: 34763786

Ruggiero, V., Dell'Acqua, C., Cremonese, E., Giraldo, M., & Patron, E. (2025). Under the surface: Low cardiac vagal tone and poor interoception in young adults with subclinical depressive symptoms. *Journal of Affective Disorders*, *375*, 1–9. DOI: 10.1016/j.jad.2025.01.057 PMID: 39826615

Rush, A. J., Trivedi, M. H., Wisniewski, S. R., Nierenberg, A. A., Stewart, J. W., Warden, D., Niederehe, G., Thase, M. E., Lavori, P. W., Lebowitz, B. D., McGrath, P. J., Rosenbaum, J. F., Sackeim, H. A., Kupfer, D. J., Luther, J., & Fava, M. (2006). Acute and longer-term outcomes in depressed outpatients requiring one or several treatment steps: A STAR*D report. *The American Journal of Psychiatry*, *163*(11), 1905–1917. DOI: 10.1176/ajp.2006.163.11.1905 PMID: 17074942

Saha, R. (2025). The Exciting Frontier of Neuroplasticity: Innovations in Brain Health and Recovery. *Journal of Behavioral and Brain Science*, *15*(03), 47–80. DOI: 10.4236/jbbs.2025.153003

Saito, H., Iwai, Y., Yamano, A., Matsushita, K., Yokoyama, H., Nakazawa, K., & Ito, S. (2025). Comparing muscle coordination patterns in yoga-focused exercises with those in standard stabilization exercises. *Journal of Bodywork and Movement Therapies*, *44*, 245–250. DOI: 10.1016/j.jbmt.2025.05.059 PMID: 40954586

Saleem, Y., Noushad, S., Ahmed, S., & Ansari, B. (2025). Psychophysiological Biomarkers for the Effects of Yoga as an Alternative Therapy among Healthcare Professionals with Chronic Low Back Pain: A Randomized Controlled Trial. *Journal of Nature and Science of Medicine*, *8*(1), 74–80. DOI: 10.4103/jnsm.jnsm_39_24

Santiago, P. N., & Gall, T. L. (2016). Acceptance and Commitment Therapy as a spiritually integrated psychotherapy. *Counseling and Values*, *61*(2), 239–255. DOI: 10.1002/cvj.12040

Santomauro, D. F., Mantilla Herrera, A. M., Shadid, J., Zheng, P., Ashbaugh, C., Pigott, D. M., Abbafati, C., Adolph, C., Amlag, J. O., Aravkin, A. Y., Bang-Jensen, B. L., Bertolacci, G. J., Bloom, S. S., Castellano, R., Castro, E., Chakrabarti, S., Chattopadhyay, J., Cogen, R. M., Collins, J. K., & Ferrari, A. J. (2021). Global prevalence and burden of depressive and anxiety disorders in 204 countries and territories in 2020 due to the COVID-19 pandemic. *Lancet, 398*(10312), 1700–1712. DOI: 10.1016/S0140-6736(21)02143-7 PMID: 34634250

Santos, B. de S. (2014). *Epistemologies of the South: Justice Against Epistemicide*. Routledge.

Saoji, A. A., Raghavendra, B. R., & Manjunath, N. K. (2019). Effects of yogic breath regulation: A narrative review of scientific evidence. *Journal of Ayurveda and Integrative Medicine, 10*(1), 50–58. DOI: 10.1016/j.jaim.2017.07.008 PMID: 29395894

Saraswati, S. S., & Alston, A. J. (1997). *The method of the Vedanta: A critical account of the Advaita tradition*. State University of New York Press.

Sarkar, M. C. (2021). The concept of practical Vedanta philosophy of Swami Vivekananda and human development: An analytical study. *International Journal of Multidisciplinary Educational Research, 1*(5), 17–20.

Satchidananda, S. (with Internet Archive). (1990). *The yoga sutras of Patanjali*. Yogaville, Va.: Integral Yoga Publications. http://archive.org/details/yogasutrasofpata0000satc

Satyananda Saraswati, S. (1996). *Asana, pranayama, mudra, bandha* (Rev. ed.). Yoga Publications Trust.

Schmalzl, L., Powers, C., Blom, E. H., & Kerr, C. (2015). *Neurophysiological and neurocognitive mechanisms underlying the effects of yoga-based practices : towards a comprehensive theoretical framework*. 9(May), 1–19. DOI: 10.3389/fnhum.2015.00235

Schneiderman, N., Ironson, G., & Siegel, S. D. (2005). STRESS AND HEALTH: Psychological, Behavioral, and Biological Determinants. *Annual Review of Clinical Psychology, 1*(1), 607–628. DOI: 10.1146/annurev.clinpsy.1.102803.144141 PMID: 17716101

Schober, P. (2018). The Introduction of Yoga Recovery on Physiological and Psychological Stress and Performance in NCAA Athletes [University of Montana Missoula, Montana]. In *Graduate Student Theses, Dissertations, & Professional Papers*. https://scholarworks.umt.edu/etd/11141/

Schulz, K. F., Altman, D. G., & Moher, D. (2010). CONSORT 2010 statement: Updated guidelines for reporting parallel group randomised trials. *BMJ (Clinical Research Ed.)*, *340*(mar23 1), c332. DOI: 10.1136/bmj.c332 PMID: 20332509

Sedlmeier, P., Eberth, J., Schwarz, M., Zimmermann, D., Haarig, F., Jaeger, S., & Kunze, S. (2012). The psychological effects of meditation: A meta-analysis. *Psychological Bulletin*, *138*(6), 1139–1171. DOI: 10.1037/a0028168 PMID: 22582738

Seeley, W. W., Menon, V., Schatzberg, A. F., Keller, J., Glover, G. H., Kenna, H., Reiss, A. L., & Greicius, M. D. (2007). Dissociable intrinsic connectivity networks for salience processing and executive control. *The Journal of Neuroscience : The Official Journal of the Society for Neuroscience*, *27*(9), 2349–2356. DOI: 10.1523/JNEUROSCI.5587-06.2007 PMID: 17329432

Segal, Z. V., Williams, J. M. G., & Teasdale, J. D. (2002). *Mindfulness-based cognitive therapy for depression: A new approach to preventing relapse* (pp. xiv, 351). Guilford Press.

Sengupta, P. (2012). Health impacts of yoga and pranayama: A state-of-the-art review. *International Journal of Preventive Medicine*, *3*(7), 444.

Sengupta, P. (2012). Health Impacts of Yoga and Pranayama: A State-of-the-Art Review. *International Journal of Preventive Medicine*, *3*(7), 444–458. https://www.ncbi.nlm.nih.gov/pubmed/22891145 PMID: 22891145

Seth, A. K. (2013). Interoceptive inference, emotion, and the embodied self. *Trends in Cognitive Sciences*, *17*(11), 565–573. DOI: 10.1016/j.tics.2013.09.007 PMID: 24126130

Sezer, I., Pizzagalli, D. A., & Sacchet, M. D. (2022). Resting-state fMRI functional connectivity and mindfulness in clinical and non-clinical contexts: A review and synthesis. *Neuroscience and Biobehavioral Reviews*, *135*, 104583. DOI: 10.1016/j.neubiorev.2022.104583 PMID: 35202647

Shaffer, F., McCraty, R., & Zerr, C. L. (2014). A healthy heart is not a metronome: An integrative review of the heart's anatomy and heart rate variability. *Frontiers in Psychology*, *5*, 1040.

Shafir, T. (2016). Using Movement to Regulate Emotion: Neurophysiological Findings and Their Application in Psychotherapy. *Frontiers in Psychology*, *7*. Advance online publication. DOI: 10.3389/fpsyg.2016.01451 PMID: 27721801

Shah, M. (2021). Acceptance-based therapies and Asian philosophical traditions: Similarities and differences in the concept of acceptance. *Journal of Rational-Emotive & Cognitive-Behavior Therapy*, *39*(3), 457–475. DOI: 10.1007/s10942-020-00355-2

Shao, R., Man, I. S. C., & Lee, T. M. C. (2024). The Effect of Slow-Paced Breathing on Cardiovascular and Emotion Functions: A Meta-Analysis and Systematic Review. *Mindfulness*, *15*(1), 1–18. DOI: 10.1007/s12671-023-02294-2

Shapiro, S. L., Brown, K. W., & Astin, J. (2011). Toward the integration of meditation into higher education: A review of research evidence. *Teachers College Record*, *113*(3), 493–528. DOI: 10.1177/016146811111300306

Sharma, A., Barrett, M. S., Cucchiara, A. J., Gooneratne, N. S., & Thase, M. E. (2017). A Breathing-Based Meditation Intervention for Patients With Major Depressive Disorder Following Inadequate Response to Antidepressants: A Randomized Pilot Study. *The Journal of Clinical Psychiatry*, *78*(1), e59–e63. DOI: 10.4088/JCP.16m10819 PMID: 27898207

Sharma, D. K. (2017). Yoga and meditation: Integral correlation is a bit of mystery. *Journal of Applied Consciousness Studies*, *5*(2), 42–47. https://journals.lww.com/joacs/fulltext/2017/05020/yoga_and_meditation__integral_correlation_is_a_bit.4.aspx

Sharma, D., & Sharma, B. R. (2024). The Impact of Yoga and Meditation on Mental and Physical Well-being. *Journal of Ayurveda and Integrated Medical Sciences*, *9*(5), 144–153. DOI: 10.21760/jaims.9.5.23

Sharma, R. R., & Cooper, C. (2016). Indian approaches to coping with stress and burnout. In *Executive burnout* (pp. 163–220). Emerald Group Publishing. DOI: 10.1108/978-1-78635-286-620161010

Sharma, S. (2004). Vedanta as ved-ananta: A new unfolding of universal spiritual consciousness. *Social Science Research Network*. https://doi.org/DOI: 10.2139/ssrn.3188289

Sharratt, L. (2023). *Who I am and how I feel: The role of identity and self-concept in psychological distress* (Doctoral dissertation, Aston University).

Shier, M. L., & Turpin, A. (2017). A Multi-Dimensional Conceptual Framework for Trauma-Informed Practice in Addictions Programming. *Journal of Social Service Research*, *43*(5), 609–623. DOI: 10.1080/01488376.2017.1364318

Shih, C. H., Tomita, N., Lukic, Y. X., Reguera, Á. H., Fleisch, E., & Kowatsch, T. (2019). Breeze: Smartphone-based acoustic real-time detection of breathing phases for a gamified biofeedback breathing training. *Proceedings of the ACM on Interactive, Mobile, Wearable and Ubiquitous Technologies*, *3*(4), 1–30.

Shirane, H. (2012). *Traditional Japanese literature: An anthology, beginnings to 1600*. Columbia University Press.

Siegel, D. J. (2010). *Mindsight: The new science of personal transformation* (pp. xviii, 314). Bantam Books.

Siew, S., Grant, J., Lim, T. H., & Chia, Y. (2023). Mindfulness-based randomized controlled trials and structural brain change: A meta-analysis. *Scientific Reports, 13*(22055). Advance online publication. DOI: 10.1038/s41598-023-51492-1

Silveira, K., & Smart, C. M. (2020). Cognitive, physical, and psychological benefits of yoga for acquired brain injuries: A systematic review of recent findings. *Neuropsychological Rehabilitation, 30*(7), 1388–1407. DOI: 10.1080/09602011.2019.1583114 PMID: 30789008

Šimić, G., Tkalčić, M., Vukić, V., Mulc, D., Španić, E., Šagud, M., Olucha-Bordonau, F. E., Vukšić, M., & Hof, P. R. (2021). Understanding emotions: Origins and roles of the amygdala. *Biomolecules, 11*(6), 1–58. DOI: 10.3390/biom11060823 PMID: 34072960

Singh, B. D. (1999). Relevance of Nishkama Karma Yoga in today's business world. *Vision: The Journal of Business Perspective, 3*(2), 35–42. DOI: 10.1177/097226299900300205

Singh, P., Ravi Prakash, S., Awadhesh Kumar, S., & Anita, P. (2024). *The science of yoga*. Book Saga Publications. DOI: 10.60148/TheScience_of_Yoga

Singh, R. K. (2015). To each his God: An Upanishadic approach to religion. *Journal of Indian Council of Philosophical Research, 32*(2), 221–232. DOI: 10.1007/s40961-015-0017-7

Singh, R., Kumar, A., Sharma, M., & Patel, S. (2022). Rapid neuroplastic changes in anxiety disorders following mindfulness intervention: The MIND study. *Journal of Psychiatric Research, 148*, 267–276.

Singh, S. P. (2022). Sakshi and dhyana: The origin of mindfulness-based therapies. *BJPsych Bulletin, 46*(4), 216–220. DOI: 10.1192/bjb.2022.39 PMID: 35796539

Skivington, K., Matthews, L., Simpson, S. A., Craig, P., Baird, J., Blazeby, J. M., Boyd, K. A., Craig, N., French, D. P., McIntosh, E., Petticrew, M., Rycroft-Malone, J., White, M., & Moore, L. (2021). A new framework for developing and evaluating complex interventions: Update of Medical Research Council guidance. *BMJ (Clinical Research Ed.), 374*(2061), n2061. Advance online publication. DOI: 10.1136/bmj.n2061 PMID: 34593508

Škof, L., & Holmes, E. A. (Eds.). (2013). *Breathing with Luce Irigaray*. Bloomsbury Publishing Plc., DOI: 10.5040/9781472547965

Slonim, T. (2014). The Polyvagal Theory: Neuropsychological Foundations of Emotions, Attachment, Communication, & Self-Regulation. *International Journal of Group Psychotherapy*, *64*(4), 593–600. DOI: 10.1521/ijgp.2014.64.4.593

Solano Durán, P., Morales, J.-P., & Huepe, D. (2024). Interoceptive awareness in a clinical setting: The need to bring interoceptive perspectives into clinical evaluation. *Frontiers in Psychology*, *15*, 1244701. Advance online publication. DOI: 10.3389/fpsyg.2024.1244701 PMID: 38933585

Solomon, H. (2021). Living on borrowed breath: Respiratory distress, social breathing, and the vital movement of ventilators. *Medical Anthropology Quarterly*, *35*(1), 102–119.

Sonawane, M. A., Lee, A. K., Gaikwad, S., Almeida, G. J., Darby, N. T., Calderon, T., Ramirez, A. G., Hughes, D. C., & Patel, D. I. (2025). Therapeutic Yoga Enhances Neuroplasticity and Metabolic Regulation Through Elevated Plasma Brain-Derived Neurotrophic Factor (BDNF) and Ghrelin in a Heterogeneous Cancer Survivor Population. *Integrative Cancer Therapies*, *24*, 15347354251385572. i.org/10.1177/15347354251385573. DOI: 10.1177/15347354251385573 PMID: 41128015

Sousa, T., & Neves, P. (2021). Two tales of rumination and burnout: Examining the effects of boredom and overload. *Applied Psychology*, *70*(3), 1018–1044. DOI: 10.1111/apps.12257

Southwick, S. M., & Charney, D. S. (2012). *Resilience: The science of mastering life's greatest challenges*. Cambridge University Press. DOI: 10.1017/CBO9781139013857

Spiteri, D. (2012). Does the adoption of an in-depth questioning approach promote self-reflexivity? Its application to the social work education context. *Social Work & Society*, *10*(1), 1–14.

Srinivasan, R., & Aithal, P. S. (2025). Seven Branches of Yoga : Exploring the Unique Methodologies, Practices, and Spiritual Goals. In *Yoga & Naturopathy Practices and their Relevance to the 21st Century* (pp. 665–1061). Poornaprajna Publication. DOI: 10.5281/zenodo.14928194

Steger, M. F., Frazier, P., Oishi, S., & Kaler, M. (2006). The Meaning in Life Questionnaire: Assessing the presence of and search for meaning in life. *Journal of Counseling Psychology*, *53*(1), 80–93. DOI: 10.1037/0022-0167.53.1.80

Steiner-Adair, C., & Barker, T. (2013). *The big disconnect: Protecting childhood and family relationships in the digital age*. HarperCollins.

Sterne, J. A. C., Hernán, M. A., Reeves, B. C., Savović, J., Berkman, N. D., Viswanathan, M., Henry, D., Altman, D. G., Ansari, M. T., Boutron, I., Carpenter, J., Chan, A.-W., Churchill, R., Deeks, J. J., Hróbjartsson, A., Kirkham, J. J., Jüni, P., Loke, Y. K., Pigott, T. D., & Higgins, J. P. T. (2016). ROBINS-I: A tool for assessing risk of bias in non-randomised studies of interventions. *BMJ (Clinical Research Ed.)*, *355*, i4919. DOI: 10.1136/bmj.i4919 PMID: 27733354

Sterne, J. A. C., Savović, J., Page, M. J., Elbers, R. G., Blencowe, N. S., Boutron, I., Cates, C. J., Cheng, H.-Y., Corbett, M. S., Eldridge, S. M., Emberson, J. R., Hernán, M. A., Hopewell, S., Hróbjartsson, A., Junqueira, D. R., Jüni, P., Kirkham, J. J., Lasserson, T., Li, T., & Higgins, J. P. T. (2019). RoB 2: A revised tool for assessing risk of bias in randomised trials. *BMJ (Clinical Research Ed.)*, *366*, l4898. DOI: 10.1136/bmj.l4898 PMID: 31462531

Stevens, C. F. (1999). Memory: From Mind to Molecules. *Nature Medicine*, *5*(12), 1343–1344. DOI: 10.1038/70903 PMID: 10581065

Stevens, J. P., Sheridan, A. R., Bernstein, H. B., Baker, K., Lansing, R. W., Schwartzstein, R. M., & Banzett, R. B. (2019). A Multidimensional Profile of Dyspnea in Hospitalized Patients. *Chest*, *156*(3), 507–517. DOI: 10.1016/j.chest.2019.04.128 PMID: 31128117

Stone, L. (2008, July 24). Continuous Partial Attention—Not the Same as Multi-Tasking. *Bloomberg.Com*. https://www.bloomberg.com/news/articles/2008-07-23/continuous-partial-attention-not-the-same-as-multi-tasking

Streeter, C. C., Gerbarg, P. L., Saper, R. B., Ciraulo, D. A., & Brown, R. P. (2020). Effects of yoga on the autonomic nervous system, gamma-aminobutyric-acid, and allostasis in epilepsy, depression, and post-traumatic stress disorder. *Medical Hypotheses*, *78*(5), 571–579. DOI: 10.1016/j.mehy.2012.01.021 PMID: 22365651

Streeter, C. C., Whitfield, T. H., Owen, L., Rein, T., Karri, S. K., Yakhkind, A., Perlmutter, R., Prescot, A., Renshaw, P. F., Ciraulo, D. A., & Jensen, J. E. (2010). Effects of Yoga Versus Walking on Mood, Anxiety, and Brain GABA Levels: A Randomized Controlled MRS Study. *Journal of Alternative and Complementary Medicine (New York, N.Y.)*, *16*(11), 1145–1152. DOI: 10.1089/acm.2010.0007 PMID: 20722471

Sukhsohale, N. D., Phatak, M. S., Sukhsohale, S. D., & Agrawal, S. B. (2012). Does Raja Yoga meditation bring out physiological and psychological general well-being among practitioners. *International Journal of Collaborative Research on Internal Medicine & Public Health*, *4*(12), 1908–1915.

Sullivan, M. B., Erb, M., Schmalzl, L., Moonaz, S., Taylor, J. N., & Porges, S. W. (2018). Yoga therapy and polyvagal theory: The convergence of traditional wisdom and contemporary neuroscience for self-regulation and resilience. *Frontiers in Human Neuroscience*, *12*(February), 1–15. DOI: 10.3389/fnhum.2018.00067 PMID: 29535617

Suls, J., & Rothman, A. (2004). Evolution of the biopsychosocial model: Prospects and challenges for health psychology. *Health Psychology: Official Journal of the Division of Health Psychology, American Psychological Association*, *23*(2), 119–125. DOI: 10.1037/0278-6133.23.2.119 PMID: 15008654

Sweatt, J. D. (2016). Neural plasticity and behavior – sixty years of conceptual advances. *Journal of Neurochemistry*, *139*(S2), 179–199. DOI: 10.1111/jnc.13580 PMID: 26875778

Syamala, D. H. (2018). The universal self and the individual self in Vedanta. *Philosophy and Cosmology*, *21*, 72–80. DOI: 10.29202/phil-cosm/21/7

Szulczewski, M. T. (2022). Transcutaneous Auricular Vagus Nerve Stimulation Combined With Slow Breathing: Speculations on Potential Applications and Technical Considerations. *Neuromodulation*, *25*(3), 380–394. DOI: 10.1111/ner.13458 PMID: 35396070

Tabor, A., Bateman, S., Scheme, E. J., & schraefel, . (2022). Comparing heart rate variability biofeedback and simple paced breathing to inform the design of guided breathing technologies. *Frontiers of Computer Science*, *4*, 926649. Advance online publication. DOI: 10.3389/fcomp.2022.926649

Tang, Y. Y., Tang, R., & Posner, M. I. (2021). Mechanisms of white matter changes induced by meditation. *Proceedings of the National Academy of Sciences of the United States of America*, *118*(2), e2016976118. PMID: 22689998

Tang, Y.-Y., Hölzel, B. K., & Posner, M. I. (2015). The neuroscience of mindfulness meditation. *Nature Reviews. Neuroscience*, *16*(4), 213–225. DOI: 10.1038/nrn3916 PMID: 25783612

Tang, Y.-Y., Ma, Y., Wang, J., Fan, Y., Feng, S., Lu, Q., Yu, Q., Sui, D., Rothbart, M. K., Fan, M., & Posner, M. I. (2007). Short-term meditation training improves attention and self-regulation. *Proceedings of the National Academy of Sciences of the United States of America*, *104*(43), 17152–17156. DOI: 10.1073/pnas.0707678104 PMID: 17940025

Tang, Y.-Y., & Posner, M. I. (2009). Attention training and attention state training. *Trends in Cognitive Sciences, 13*(5), 222–227. DOI: 10.1016/j.tics.2009.01.009 PMID: 19375975

Tanzer, M., Derome, M., Morosan, L., Salaminios, G., & Debbané, M. (2021). Cortical thickness of the insula and prefrontal cortex relates to externalizing behavior: Cross-sectional and prospective findings. *Development and Psychopathology, 33*(4), 1437–1447. DOI: 10.1017/S0954579420000619 PMID: 32638690

Taren, A. A., Creswell, J. D., & Gianaros, P. J. (2013). Dispositional mindfulness co-varies with smaller amygdala and caudate volumes in community adults. *PLoS One, 8*(5), e64574. DOI: 10.1371/journal.pone.0064574 PMID: 23717632

Tataranu, L. G., & Rizea, R. E. (2025). Neuroplasticity and Nervous System Recovery: Cellular Mechanisms, Therapeutic Advances, and Future Prospects. *Brain Sciences, 15*(4), 1–21. DOI: 10.3390/brainsci15040400 PMID: 40309875

Taylor, A. G., Goehler, L. E., Galper, D. I., Innes, K. E., & Bourguignon, C. (2010). Top-Down and Bottom-Up Mechanisms in Mind-Body Medicine: Development of an Integrative Framework for Psychophysiological Research. *Explore (New York, N.Y.), 6*(1), 29–41. DOI: 10.1016/j.explore.2009.10.004 PMID: 20129310

Teasdale, J. D., Moore, R. G., Hayhurst, H., Pope, M., Williams, S., & Segal, Z. V. (2002). Metacognitive awareness and prevention of relapse in depression: Empirical evidence. *Journal of Consulting and Clinical Psychology, 70*(2), 275–287. DOI: 10.1037/0022-006X.70.2.275 PMID: 11952186

Telles, S., Nagarathna, R., & Nagendra, H. R. (1994). Breathing through a particular nostril can alter metabolism and autonomic activities. *Indian Journal of Physiology and Pharmacology, 38*(2), 133–137. https://www.ncbi.nlm.nih.gov/pubmed/8063359 PMID: 8063359

Telles, S., Singh, N., Bhardwaj, A. K., Kumar, A., & Balkrishna, A. (2013). Effect of yoga or physical exercise on physical, cognitive and emotional measures in children: A randomized controlled trial. *Child and Adolescent Psychiatry and Mental Health, 7*(1), 37. DOI: 10.1186/1753-2000-7-37 PMID: 24199742

Thanalakshmi, J., Maheshkumar, K., Kannan, R., Sundareswaran, L., Venugopal, V., & Poonguzhali, S. (2020). Effect of Sheetali pranayama on cardiac autonomic function among patients with primary hypertension - A randomized controlled trial. *Complementary Therapies in Clinical Practice, 39*, 101138. DOI: 10.1016/j.ctcp.2020.101138 PMID: 32379673

Thayer, J. F., Ahs, F., Fredrikson, M., Sollers, J. J.III, & Wager, T. D. (2012). A meta-analysis of heart rate variability and neuroimaging studies: Implications for heart rate variability as a marker of stress and health. *Neuroscience and Biobehavioral Reviews, 36*(2), 747–756. DOI: 10.1016/j.neubiorev.2011.11.009 PMID: 22178086

Thayer, J. F., & Lane, R. D. (2000). A model of neurovisceral integration in emotion regulation and dysregulation. *Journal of Affective Disorders, 61*(3), 201–216.

Thirthalli, J., Naveen, G., Rao, M., Varambally, S., Christopher, R., & Gangadhar, B. (2013). Cortisol and antidepressant effects of yoga. *Indian Journal of Psychiatry, 55*(7), 405. DOI: 10.4103/0019-5545.116315 PMID: 24049209

Thomas, J., & Harden, A. (2008). Methods for the thematic synthesis of qualitative research in systematic reviews. *BMC Medical Research Methodology, 8*(1), 45. DOI: 10.1186/1471-2288-8-45 PMID: 18616818

Thompson, R., & Rodriguez, M. (2021). Loving-kindness meditation effects on serotonin and dopamine: A PET imaging study. *NeuroImage, 234*, 117965.

Tolahunase, M. R., Sagar, R., Faiq, M., & Dada, R. (2018). *Yoga- and meditation-based lifestyle intervention increases neuroplasticity and reduces severity of major depressive disorder : A randomized controlled trial. 36*, 423–442. DOI: 10.3233/RNN-170810

Tolahunase, M., Sagar, R., & Dada, R. (2017). Impact of Yoga and Meditation on Cellular Aging in Apparently Healthy Individuals: A Prospective, Open-Label Single-Arm Exploratory Study. *Oxidative Medicine and Cellular Longevity, 2017*(1), 7928981. Advance online publication. DOI: 10.1155/2017/7928981 PMID: 28191278

Treves, I. N., Kucyi, A. K., Tierney, A. O., Balkind, E., Whitfield-Gabrieli, S., Schuman-Olivier, Z., Gabrieli, J. D. E., & Webb, C. A. (2025). Dynamic functional connectivity signatures of focused attention on the breath in adolescents. *Cerebral Cortex (New York, N.Y.), 35*(2), bhaf024. Advance online publication. DOI: 10.1093/cercor/bhaf024 PMID: 39995218

Tricco, A. C., Lillie, E., Zarin, W., O'Brien, K. K., Colquhoun, H., Levac, D., Moher, D., Peters, M. D. J., Horsley, T., Weeks, L., Hempel, S., Akl, E. A., Chang, C., McGowan, J., Stewart, L., Hartling, L., Aldcroft, A., Wilson, M. G., Garritty, C., & Straus, S. E. (2018). PRISMA extension for scoping reviews (PRISMA-ScR): Checklist and explanation. *Annals of Internal Medicine, 169*(7), 467–473. DOI: 10.7326/M18-0850 PMID: 30178033

Trivedi, N. (2025). Positive mental health: A correlated study of the consciousness-based Advait Vedanta and modern psychotherapy. *Journal of Psychology and Neuroscience*. DOI: 10.47485/2693-2490.1100

Troy, A. S., Willroth, E. C., Shallcross, A. J., Giuliani, N. R., Gross, J. J., & Mauss, I. B. (2023). Psychological Resilience: An Affect-Regulation Framework. *Annual Review of Psychology*, *74*(1), 547–576. DOI: 10.1146/annurev-psych-020122-041854 PMID: 36103999

Tsaknaki, V. (2021, June). The breathing wings: An autobiographical soma design exploration of touch qualities through shape-change materials. In *Proceedings of the 2021 ACM Designing Interactive Systems Conference* (pp. 1266-1279).

Twenge, J. M., & Campbell, W. K. (2018). Associations between screen time and lower psychological well-being among children and adolescents: Evidence from a population-based study. *Preventive Medicine Reports*, *12*, 271–283. DOI: 10.1016/j.pmedr.2018.10.003 PMID: 30406005

Twenge, J. M., & Campbell, W. K. (2021). The age of entitlement: How casual sex, digital anxiety, and modern narcissism are reshaping our culture. *Personality and Social Psychology Review*, *25*(3), 234–252.

Udupa, K., & Sathyaprabha, T. N. (2018). *Influence of Yoga on the Autonomic Nervous System*., DOI: 10.4018/978-1-5225-2788-6.ch005

Uebelacker, L. A., Epstein-Lubow, G., Gaudiano, B. A., Tremont, G., Battle, C. L., & Miller, I. W. (2010). Hatha yoga for depression: Critical review of the evidence for efficacy, plausible mechanisms of action, and directions for future research. *Journal of Psychiatric Practice*, *16*(1), 22–33. DOI: 10.1097/01.pra.0000367775.88388.96 PMID: 20098228

Upadhya, Y. (2025). A Comprehensive Exploration of the Holistic Healing Power of Yoga. *Journal of Rapti Babai Campus*, *5*(1), 152–163. DOI: 10.3126/jrbc.v5i1.78102

Urrutia, J., Anderson, B. T., Belouin, S. J., Berger, A., Griffiths, R. R., Grob, C. S., Henningfield, J. E., Labate, B. C., Maier, L. J., Maternowska, M. C., Weichold, F., Yaden, D. B., & Magar, V. (2023). Psychedelic Science, Contemplative Practices, and Indigenous and Other Traditional Knowledge Systems: Towards Integrative Community-Based Approaches in Global Health. *Journal of Psychoactive Drugs*, *55*(5), 523–538. DOI: 10.1080/02791072.2023.2258367 PMID: 37747281

Vago, D. R., & Silbersweig, D. A. (2012). Self-awareness, self-regulation, and self-transcendence (S-ART): A framework for understanding the neurobiological mechanisms of mindfulness. *Frontiers in Human Neuroscience, 6*, 296. DOI: 10.3389/fnhum.2012.00296 PMID: 23112770

Vali, K. M., & Azeem, M. (2025). Psycho-cultural sensitivity in Indian context: Integrating traditional knowledge with modern mental health practices. *International Journal for Multidisciplinary Research, 7*(4), 52014. Advance online publication. DOI: 10.36948/ijfmr.2025.v07i04.52014

van Aalst, J., Ceccarini, J., Demyttenaere, K., Sunaert, S., & Van Laere, K. (2020). What Has Neuroimaging Taught Us on the Neurobiology of Yoga? A Review. *Frontiers in Integrative Neuroscience, 14*(July), 1–16. DOI: 10.3389/fnint.2020.00034 PMID: 32733213

Van der Kolk, B. (2014). The body keeps the score: Brain, mind, and body in the healing of trauma. *New York, 3*, 14-211.

van der Kolk, B. A. (2014). *The body keeps the score: Brain, mind, and body in the healing of trauma* (pp. xvi, 443). Viking.

van der Veer, P. (1989). The power of detachment: Disciplines of body and mind in the Ramanandi order. *American Ethnologist, 16*(3), 517–536. DOI: 10.1525/ae.1989.16.3.02a00030

van Loon, A. W. G., Creemers, H. E., Okorn, A., Vogelaar, S., Miers, A. C., Saab, N., Westenberg, P. M., & Asscher, J. J. (2022). The effects of school-based interventions on physiological stress in adolescents: A meta-analysis. *Stress and Health, 38*(2), 187–209. DOI: 10.1002/smi.3081 PMID: 34275188

Vancampfort, D., Stubbs, B., Van Damme, T., Smith, L., Hallgren, M., Schuch, F., Deenik, J., Rosenbaum, S., Ashdown-Franks, G., Mugisha, J., & Firth, J. (2020). The efficacy of meditation-based mind-body interventions for mental disorders: A meta-review of 17 meta-analyses of randomized controlled trials. *Journal of Psychiatric Research, 134*, 181–191. DOI: 10.1016/j.jpsychires.2020.12.048 PMID: 33388701

Vandenberghe, L., & de Sousa, A. C. A. (2006). Mindfulness nas terapias cognitivas e comportamentais. *Revista Brasileira de Terapias Cognitivas, 2*(1), 37–46. DOI: 10.5935/1808-5687.20060004

Varambally, S., Venkatasubramanian, G., Govindaraj, R., Shivakumar, V., Mullapudi, T., Christopher, R., Debnath, M., Philip, M., Bharath, R. D., & Gangadhar, B. (2019). Yoga and schizophrenia—A comprehensive assessment of neuroplasticity. *Medicine, 98*(43), e17399. DOI: 10.1097/MD.0000000000017399 PMID: 31651843

Varela Francisco, J., Evan, T., & Eleanor, R. (1991). The embodied mind: Cognitive science and human experience.

Varela, F. J., Thompson, E., & Rosch, E. (1991). *The Embodied Mind: Cognitive Science and Human Experience*. MIT Press. DOI: 10.7551/mitpress/6730.001.0001

Varma, R. (2025). Meditation and mindfulness in Indian philosophical traditions. *ShodhSamajik: Journal of Social Studies*, *2*(1), 1–7. DOI: 10.29121/ShodhSamajik.v2.i1.2025.10

Varne, S. R., & A, B. P. (2023). A systematic review on molecular, bio-chemical, and pathophysiological mechanisms of yoga, pranayama and meditation causing beneficial effects in various health disorders. *Indian Journal of Integrative Medicine*, *3*(4), 87–96. https://www.mansapublishers.com/ijim/article/view/4284

Varne, S. R., & Balaji, P. A. (2023). A systematic review on molecular, bio-chemical, and pathophysiological mechanisms of yoga, pranayama and meditation causing beneficial effects in various health disorders. *Molecular Mechanisms of Yogic Practices in Health and Disease*, *3*(4), 1–11.

Veerakannan, S. (2025). Yoga Effects on Brain Health: A Systematic Review of the Current Literature. *Aathiyoga Indian Journal of Ancient Medicine and Yoga*, *5*(1), 1–21.

Verhaeghen, P. (2017). The Self-Effacing Buddhist: No(t)-Self in Early Buddhism and Contemplative Neuroscience. *Contemporary Buddhism*, *18*(1), 21–36. DOI: 10.1080/14639947.2017.1297344

Verma, R. K. (2025). Mind and moksha: Integrating Vedantic wisdom and contemporary psychology for a unified approach to self and well-being. *Human Arenas*, 1–24.

Verma, R. K. (2025). Mind and Moksha: Integrating Vedantic Wisdom and Contemporary Psychology for a Unified Approach to Self and Well-Being. *Human Arenas*, *0123456789*. Advance online publication. DOI: 10.1007/s42087-025-00488-9

Verrier, M. M. (2021). A psychospiritual exploration of the transpersonal self as the ground of healing. *Religions*, *12*(9), 725. DOI: 10.3390/rel12090725

Verzili, B., Cerasa, A., & Quattrone, A. (2023). Yoga and neuropsychiatric aging: A systematic review and meta-analysis. *Neuroscience and Biobehavioral Reviews*, *150*(105223). Advance online publication. DOI: 10.1016/j.neubiorev.2023.105223 PMID: 37598905

Videbech, P. (2000). PET measurements of brain glucose metabolism and blood flow in major depressive disorder: A critical review. *Acta Psychiatrica Scandinavica, 101*(1), 11–20. DOI: 10.1034/j.1600-0447.2000.101001011.x PMID: 10674946

Vigo, D., Thornicroft, G., & Atun, R. (2016). Estimating the true global burden of mental illness. *The Lancet. Psychiatry, 3*(2), 171–178. DOI: 10.1016/S2215-0366(15)00505-2 PMID: 26851330

Villemure, C., Eko, M., Cotton, V. A., & Bushnell, M. C. (2014). Insular Cortex Mediates Increased Pain Tolerance in Yoga Practitioners. *Cerebral Cortex (New York, N.Y.), 24*(10), 2732–2740. DOI: 10.1093/cercor/bht124 PMID: 23696275

Vinay, A., Venkatesh, D., & Ambarish, V. (2016). Impact of short-term practice of yoga on heart rate variability. *International Journal of Yoga, 9*(1), 62. DOI: 10.4103/0973-6131.171714 PMID: 26865773

Vinu, W., Kabeer, D. A., Kumar G, V., Safad, A. K., & Manibharathi, G. (2025). Yoga-based interventions for enhancing psychological well-being in postpartum women: A randomized controlled trial. *Journal of Bodywork and Movement Therapies, 42*, 1177–1185. DOI: 10.1016/j.jbmt.2025.02.007 PMID: 40325654

Virgili, M. (2015). Mindfulness-Based Interventions Reduce Psychological Distress in Working Adults: A Meta-Analysis of Intervention Studies. *Mindfulness, 6*(2), 326–337. DOI: 10.1007/s12671-013-0264-0

Vishnubhotla, R. V., Radhakrishnan, R., Kveraga, K., Deardorff, R., Ram, C., Pawale, D., Wu, Y. C., Renschler, J., Subramaniam, B., & Sadhasivam, S. (2021). Advanced Meditation Alters Resting-State Brain Network Connectivity Correlating With Improved Mindfulness. *Frontiers in Psychology, 12*(November), 1–11. DOI: 10.3389/fpsyg.2021.745344 PMID: 34867626

Vivekananda, S. (1940/1942/1944). *Letters of Swami Vivekananda*. Advaita Ashram.

Vivekananda, S. (1896). *Practical Vedanta: Part 1*. Advaita Ashram.

Vivekananda, S. (1899). *Speeches and writings of Swami Vivekananda*. G. A. Natesan & Co.

Vivekananda, S. (1944). *Lectures from Colombo to Almora*. Advaita Ashram.

Vivekananda, S. (1947). *Work and its secret*. Advaita Ashram.

Vivekananda, S. (1951). *The complete works of Swami Vivekananda* (Vol. 8). Advaita Ashram.

Vivekananda, S. (1985). *The complete works of Swami Vivekananda: Abridged edition*. Advaita Ashrama.

Vivekananda, S., & Madhurananda, S. (2016). *Bhagavad Gita as viewed by Swami Vivekananda*. Advaita Ashrama.

Vivekaprana, P. (2014). Vivekananda and the inner quest of humanity. *International Journal of Development Issues, 13*(3), 227–241. DOI: 10.1108/IJDI-06-2014-0042

Vlemincx, E., Abelson, J. L., Lehrer, P. M., Davenport, P. W., Van Diest, I., & Van den Bergh, O. (2013). Respiratory variability and sighing: A psychophysiological reset model. *Biological Psychology, 93*(1), 24–32. DOI: 10.1016/j.biopsycho.2012.12.001 PMID: 23261937

Vollbehr, N., Schmidt, A., Bartels-Velthuis, A., Ostafin, B., & Hoenders, H. (2023). The ethics of yoga in (mental) healthcare: Beyond the traditional Eightfold path. *Complementary Therapies in Medicine, 102979*, 102979. Advance online publication. DOI: 10.1016/j.ctim.2023.102979 PMID: 37640167

Voltmer, K., Hondrich, F., & von Salisch, M. (2023). Daily breath-based mindfulness exercises in a randomized controlled trial improve primary school children's performance in arithmetic. *Scientific Reports, 13*(1), 1–13. DOI: 10.1038/s41598-023-49354-0 PMID: 38092836

von Leupoldt, A., Mertz, C., Kegat, S., Burmester, S., & Dahme, B. (2006). The impact of emotions on the sensory and affective dimension of perceived dyspnea. *Psychophysiology, 43*(4), 382–386. DOI: 10.1111/j.1469-8986.2006.00415.x PMID: 16916434

Vorkapic, C. F. (2016). Yoga and mental health: A dialogue between ancient wisdom and modern psychology. *International Journal of Yoga, 9*(2), 104–105. DOI: 10.4103/0973-6131.171720 PMID: 26865774

Voss, S., Cerna, J., & Gothe, N. P. (2023). Yoga Impacts Cognitive Health: Neurophysiological Changes and Stress Regulation Mechanisms. *Exercise and Sport Sciences Reviews, 51*(2), 73–81. DOI: 10.1249/JES.0000000000000311 PMID: 36342265

Vyas, B., & Vyas, R. (2017). *Contemporizing Raj Yoga: Neuroscience and Practices*. Dr. Bhaskar Vyas. https://books.google.com/books?hl=en&lr=&id=SY3vDwAAQBAJ&oi=fnd&pg=PR1&dq=Synchronization+through+Yoga:+Connecting+the+Physical+and+Mental+Realms&ots=Y3xKy8uG7R&sig=cOoP0g8Y9sxJezNoN8ZCjrUCP_s

Vyasa. (2006). *The Bhagavadgita* (S. Radhakrishnan, Trans. & Comm.). New Delhi: HarperCollins Publishers India. (Original work composed ca. 2nd century BCE) https://www.verywellmind.com/mindfulness-based-cognitive-therapy-1067396_ https://www.britannica.com/science/neuroplasticity https://positivepsychology.com/history-of-mindfulness/

Wadhen, V., & Cartwright, T. (2021). Feasibility and outcome of an online streamed yoga intervention on stress and wellbeing of people working from home during COVID-19. *Work (Reading, Mass.)*, *69*(2), 331–349. DOI: 10.3233/WOR-205325 PMID: 34120925

Wagner, C., & Cáceres-Melillo, R. (2023). Mindfulness-Based Cognitive Therapy (MBCT) and Mindfulness-Based Stress Reduction (MBSR) in the treatment of Post-Traumatic Stress Disorder (PTSD): A literature review. *Salud Mental*, *46*(1), 35–42. DOI: 10.17711/SM.0185-3325.2023.005

Walker, G., & Flaherty, B. (2024). Cuing Safety in the Law School Classroom: Using a Polyvagal Theory Framework in Support of Trauma-Informed Teaching Practices. *SSRN*, *53*(1). Advance online publication. DOI: 10.2139/ssrn.5009275

Watkins, E., & Teasdale, J. D. (2004). Adaptive and maladaptive self-focus in depression. *Journal of Affective Disorders*, *82*(1), 1–8. DOI: 10.1016/j.jad.2003.10.006 PMID: 15465571

Wayne, P. M., & Kaptchuk, T. J. (2008). Challenges inherent to t'ai chi research: Part I—t'ai chi as a complex multicomponent intervention. *The Journal of Alternative and Complementary Medicine: Paradigm, Practice, and Policy Advancing Integrative Health*, *14*(1), 95–102.

Weick, K. E., & Sutcliffe, K. M. (2006). Mindfulness and the Quality of Organizational Attention. *Organization Science*, *17*(4), 514–524. DOI: 10.1287/orsc.1060.0196

Wells, A. (2000). *Emotional disorders and metacognition: Innovative cognitive therapy* (pp. ix, 236). John Wiley & Sons Ltd.

Wenger, E., & Kühn, S. (2021). Neuroplasticity. In *Cognitive Training* (pp. 69–83). Springer International Publishing., DOI: 10.1007/978-3-030-39292-5_6

Weng, H. Y., Fox, A. S., Shackman, A. J., Stodola, D. E., Caldwell, J. Z. K., Olson, M. C., Rogers, G. M., & Davidson, R. J. (2013). Compassion Training Alters Altruism and Neural Responses to Suffering. *Psychological Science*, *24*(7), 1171–1180. DOI: 10.1177/0956797612469537 PMID: 23696200

Whittemore, R., & Knafl, K. (2005). The integrative review: Updated methodology. *Journal of Advanced Nursing*, *52*(5), 546–553. DOI: 10.1111/j.1365-2648.2005.03621.x PMID: 16268861

Wielgosz, J., Goldberg, S. B., Kral, T. R., Dunne, J. D., & Davidson, R. J. (2019). Mindfulness meditation and psychopathology. *Annual Review of Clinical Psychology*, *15*(1), 285–316. DOI: 10.1146/annurev-clinpsy-021815-093423 PMID: 30525995

Williams, A. (2020). Twenge, J. M. (2017). iGen: Why Today's Super-Connected Kids Are Growing Up Less Rebellious, More Tolerant, Less Happy and Completely Unprepared for Adulthood. New York, NY: Atria. ISBN: 978-1-5011-5201-6 paperback. 342 pp. *Family and Consumer Sciences Research Journal*, *48*(3), 290–293. DOI: 10.1111/fcsr.12345

Woodyard, C. (2011). Exploring the therapeutic effects of yoga and its ability to increase quality of life. *International Journal of Yoga*, *4*(2), 49. DOI: 10.4103/0973-6131.85485 PMID: 22022122

World Health Organization. (2017). *Depression and Other Common Mental Disorders*. https://www.who.int/publications/i/item/depression-global-health-estimates

World Health Organization. (2022). Mental disorders fact sheet. https://www.who.int/news-room/fact-sheets/detail/mental-disorders

World Health Organization. (2022). *Mental disorders*. https://www.who.int/news-room/fact-sheets/detail/mental-disorders

World Health Organization. (2022). *World mental health report: Transforming mental health for all*. https://www.who.int/publications/i/item/9789240049338

World Health Organization. (2022). *World mental health report: Transforming mental health for all*. World Health Organization.

World Health Organization. (2025, September 2). *Over a billion people living with mental health conditions – services require urgent scale-up*. https://www.who.int/news/item/02-09-2025-over-a-billion-people-living-with-mental-health-conditions-services-require-urgent-scale-up

Worsley, J. D., Pennington, A., & Corcoran, R. (2022). Supporting mental health and wellbeing of university and college students: A systematic review of review-level evidence of interventions. *PLoS One*, *17*(7), e0266725. DOI: 10.1371/journal.pone.0266725 PMID: 35905058

Wright, R. W., & Strawn, B. D. (2010). Grief, hope, and prophetic imagination: Psychoanalysis and Christian tradition in dialogue. *Journal of Psychology and Christianity, 29*(3), 195–205.

Wu, Y., Wang, L., Tao, M., Cao, H., Yuan, H., Ye, M., Chen, X., Wang, K., & Zhu, C. (2023). Changing trends in the global burden of mental disorders from 1990 to 2019 and predicted levels in 25 years. *Epidemiology and Psychiatric Sciences, 32*, e63. DOI: 10.1017/S2045796023000756 PMID: 37933540

Wu, Y., Yan, D., & Yang, J. (2023). Effectiveness of yoga for major depressive disorder: A systematic review and meta-analysis. *Frontiers in Psychiatry, 14*, 1138205. DOI: 10.3389/fpsyt.2023.1138205 PMID: 37032928

Xiong, J., Lipsitz, O., Nasri, F., Lui, L. M. W., Gill, H., Phan, L., Chen-Li, D., Iacobucci, M., Ho, R., Majeed, A., & McIntyre, R. S. (2020). Impact of COVID-19 pandemic on mental health in the general population: A systematic review. *Journal of Affective Disorders, 277*, 55–64. DOI: 10.1016/j.jad.2020.08.001 PMID: 32799105

Yang, Y., Cao, D., Lyu, T., & Gao, W. (2023). Meta-analysis of a mindfulness yoga exercise intervention on depression – based on intervention studies in China. *Frontiers in Psychology, 14*, 1283172. Advance online publication. DOI: 10.3389/fpsyg.2023.1283172 PMID: 38148781

Yarrow, T., Candea, M., Trundle, C., & Cook, J. (2015). *Detachment: Essays on the limits of relational thinking*. Manchester University Press.

Yeung, A., Chan, J. S. M., Cheung, J. C., & Zou, L. (2018). Qigong and Tai-Chi for Mood Regulation. *Focus (San Francisco, Calif.), 16*(1), 40–47. DOI: 10.1176/appi.focus.20170042 PMID: 31975898

Yii, A. C., & Koh, M. S. (2013). A review of psychological dysfunction in asthma: Affective, behavioral and cognitive factors. *The Journal of Asthma : Official Journal of the Association for the Care of Asthma, 50*(9), 915–921.

Yoo, J. (2019). Learning to Write Through an Awareness of Breath. *Qualitative Inquiry, 107780041984653*. Advance online publication. DOI: 10.1177/1077800419846533

Yoshihara, K., Hiramoto, T., Sudo, N., & Kubo, C. (2011). Profile of mood states and stress-related biochemical indices in long-term yoga practitioners. *BioPsychoSocial Medicine, 5*(1), 6. DOI: 10.1186/1751-0759-5-6 PMID: 21635790

Zaccaro, A., Piarulli, A., Laurino, M., Garbella, E., Menicucci, D., Neri, B., Gemignani, A., & Palombo, D. (2018). How breath-control can change your life: A systematic review on psychophysiological correlates of slow breathing. *Frontiers in Human Neuroscience, 12*, 353. DOI: 10.3389/fnhum.2018.00353 PMID: 30245619

Zamorano, A. M., Cifre, I., Montoya, P., Riquelme, I., & Kleber, B. (2017). *Insula-Based Networks in Professional Musicians : evidence for Increased Functional Connectivity during Resting State fMRI. 00*(March). DOI: 10.1002/hbm.23682

Zatorre, R. J., Fields, R. D., & Johansen-Berg, H. (2012). Plasticity in gray and white: Neuroimaging changes in brain structure during learning. *Nature Neuroscience, 15*(4), 528–536. DOI: 10.1038/nn.3045 PMID: 22426254

Zenner, C., Herrnleben-Kurz, S., & Walach, H. (2014). Mindfulness-based interventions in schools-a systematic review and meta-analysis. *Frontiers in Psychology, 5*, 603. DOI: 10.3389/fpsyg.2014.00603 PMID: 25071620

Zhao, C. Y. (2025). Exploring "Who am I": The potential of applying the Indian Vedanta philosophical practice of self-enquiry in psychotherapy. *Humanities & Social Sciences Communications, 12*(1), 1–10. DOI: 10.1057/s41599-025-04387-w

Zhu, L., Li, L., Li, X., & Wang, L. (2022). Mind–Body Exercises for PTSD Symptoms, Depression, and Anxiety in Patients With PTSD: A Systematic Review and Meta-Analysis. *Frontiers in Psychology, 12*, 738211. Advance online publication. DOI: 10.3389/fpsyg.2021.738211 PMID: 35153889

Zilverstand, A., Parvaz, M. A., & Goldstein, R. Z. (2022). Neuroimaging cognitive reappraisal in clinical populations to define neural targets for enhancing emotion regulation: A systematic review. *NeuroImage, 151*, 105–118. DOI: 10.1016/j.neuroimage.2016.06.009 PMID: 27288319

Zimmermann, A. C., Morgan, W. J., & Morgan, W. J. (2016). A time for silence? Its possibilities for dialogue and for reflective learning. *Studies in Philosophy and Education, 35*(1), 37–54. DOI: 10.1007/s11217-015-9485-0

Zotey, V., Andhale, A., Shegekar, T., & Juganavar, A. (2023). Adaptive Neuroplasticity in Brain Injury Recovery: Strategies and Insights. *Cureus, 15*(9). Advance online publication. DOI: 10.7759/cureus.45873 PMID: 37885532

Zylowska, L., Ackerman, D. L., Yang, M. H., Futrell, J. L., Horton, N. L., Hale, T. S., Pataki, C., & Smalley, S. L. (2008). Mindfulness meditation training in adults and adolescents with ADHD: A feasibility study. *Journal of Attention Disorders, 11*(6), 737–746. DOI: 10.1177/1087054707308502 PMID: 18025249

About the Contributors

Shubhangni Jain aspires to explore more aspects of psychology further in the field of education & hone their knowledge further. Also, it will allow them to interact with fresh minds with whom they would be able to share & demonstrate knowledge both theoretical and empirical. As an entry-level psychologist, they intend to contribute to the development and progress of the esteemed organization. They are confident that they possess excellent communication skills, attitude & mindset related to various aspects of the field with good interpersonal skills, which are required for the job. They are also confident that they have good knowledge of psychological research methods and practices, including clinical psychology work experience in solving psychological problems

Shweta Sharma is hardworking and passionate with strong psychological teaching and research skills, eager to secure an assistant professor position. Proficient in psychological testing (diagnosis), implementing therapeutic plans, and Research writing skills such as writing Research papers, synopses, books, and research projects with good communication skills. Proficient in Hindi and English language. Proficient with various word processing, spreadsheet, and presentation software. Thorough understanding of software related to data analysis and other technological skills required for teaching and research. They are also a quality life coach, Creative artist, YouTuber, and who loves to create content about Quality life (@qualityoflifewellnessservi1136) and loves to think outside of the box while creating new concepts and ideas.

Akanksha Singh is an accomplished psychologist, academician, and researcher whose work seamlessly integrates teaching excellence, rigorous scholarship, and sustained professional engagement. She currently serves as an Assistant Professor of Psychology at the Chitkara School of Psychology and Counselling, Chitkara University, Punjab, where she actively contributes to teaching, research, academic administration, and community-oriented initiatives. Dr. Singh holds a Ph.D. in

Psychology from Amity University Uttar Pradesh, Lucknow, with her doctoral specialization in forensic victimology. Her doctoral research marked the beginning of a focused and impactful scholarly trajectory examining LGBTQIA+ victimization, minority stress, heterosexist experiences, and the psychological consequences of social exclusion, legal processes, and systemic bias. Complementing her doctoral training, she earned a Master's degree in Clinical Psychology from Indira Gandhi National Open University (IGNOU) and an M.Sc. in Forensic Science from Banaras Hindu University, Varanasi. Her early academic grounding in chemistry and zoology further strengthened her empirical and analytical orientation, enabling her to bridge psychological science with forensic investigation, criminology, and mental health practice. With extensive teaching experience across central and private universities, Dr. Singh has taught a wide range of undergraduate and postgraduate courses including forensic psychology, victimology, gender psychology, social psychology, abnormal psychology, neuropsychology, criminology, research methodology, counselling skills, and scientific communication. In addition to classroom teaching, she has contributed to academic administration as an Examination Co-coordinator, reflecting her commitment to institutional responsibilities and academic quality assurance. A defining feature of Dr. Singh's professional profile is her strong and consistent research output. She has published extensively in reputed, peer-reviewed journals indexed in Scopus, Web of Science, and PubMed, including Sexuality & Culture, Annals of Neurosciences, and Cureus. Her research addresses critical themes such as minority stress, victim-blaming, domestic violence, substance use disorders, cognitive styles, and emotional regulation, with a strong emphasis on culturally sensitive and methodologically rigorous approaches. Her scholarship contributes not only to theoretical advancement but also to policy-relevant and practice-oriented discourse in psychology and criminology. Beyond journal publications, Dr. Singh has authored scholarly book chapters with international publishers such as Bloomsbury (UK) and IGI Global, engaging with ethical considerations in gender-inclusive research and the psychosocial impact of the COVID-19 pandemic on marginalized populations. She is currently editing an international volume titled Improving Mental Well-Being at the Intersection of Mindfulness, Meditation, and Yoga with IGI Global, reflecting her growing engagement with integrative, preventive, and interdisciplinary approaches to mental health. Dr. Singh's academic and research excellence has been recognized through multiple prestigious accolades. She has qualified the UGC-NET in Forensic Science on several occasions and is a recipient of both the Junior Research Fellowship (JRF) and Senior Research Fellowship (SRF) awarded by the University Grants Commission. She has received a Best Paper Award at an international conference and holds a copyright for the Hindi translation and cultural adaptation of the Daily Heterosexist Experiences Questionnaire, highlighting her contribution to developing culturally responsive psychometric tools for the Indian context. An active and visible member of the academic community, Dr. Singh has presented her research at numerous national and international conferences, including the World Conference on Criminology and the Annual Conference of the Indian Association of Clinical Psychologists. Her conference engagements consistently foreground issues of victimization, minority stress, emotional regulation, and social well-being, positioning her as a credible and emerging voice in contemporary psychological and criminological research. Alongside her academic and research roles, Dr. Singh has been actively involved in extension and community initiatives, including LGBTQIA+ counselling and support services and large-scale tele-counselling during the COVID-19 pandemic. These engagements underscore her commitment to translating research into practice and ensuring that psychological knowledge remains socially responsive, ethical, and inclusive. Through her integrated contributions to teaching, research, professional service, and community engagement, Dr. Akanksha Singh represents a new generation of psychologists who effectively bridge science and society. Her work continues to advance understanding in the areas of victimology, gender and sexuality, and mental health, while mentoring students and contributing meaningfully to the academic and professional psychology landscape in India and beyond.

***

Tashi Ongmu Bhutia is a distinguished academician in the field of Physical Education, currently serving at the Government B.Ed. College, Soreng, Sikkim. She began her academic journey at the prestigious Lakshmibai National Institute of Physical Education (LNIPE), Gwalior, where she completed both her Bachelor of Physical Education (B.P.Ed.) and Master of Physical Education (M.P.Ed.) with excellence. Driven by a passion for research and academic growth, she pursued her doctoral studies at the University of Delhi, earning a Ph.D. in Physical Education. Over the years, Dr. Bhutia has contributed significantly to promoting physical education, sports, and wellness through her teaching, mentorship, and scholarly pursuits. Her academic background and professional dedication reflect her commitment to advancing the standards of teacher education in Sikkim. Known for her expertise, discipline, and inspiring approach, she continues to shape the future of aspiring educators while fostering holistic development through physical education.

Bonasu Sesha Kavitha, is an Assistant Professor of Psychology at GITAM University, Visakhapatnam, India. She holds a M.A. Ph.D. in Psychology from Andhra University and a Master of Performing Arts (M.P.A) in Dance (Kuchipudi) from Potti Sriramulu Telugu University. She is UGC NET qualifed in both Psychology and Dance. She has two decades of work experience in the fields of Teaching, Research and Counseling. Her teaching interests include General Psychology, Abnormal Psychology, Clinical Psychology, Counseling and Psychotherapy, Personality Theories, Neuropsychology and Positive psychology. Dr. Kavita's research interests focus on mental health and well-being, with particular emphasis on exploring activities that promote mental health and well-being, counseling interventions, and psychological adjustment across populations. She has been involved in funded research projects related to HIV/AIDS program evaluation and Institutional assessment of NACP conducted through the Institute of Health Systems, Hyderabad. Beyond her teaching and research, she actively provides mental health counseling and career guidance. Her interdisciplinary interests also connect psychology with performing arts, dance in particular, and well-being.

Anindita Das is an esteemed Associate Professor at the Lakshmibai National Institute of Physical Education (LNIPE), Gwalior, with a distinguished career in teaching, research, and sports. Since joining LNIPE in 2007, she has been actively engaged in teaching core subjects such as Health Education, Physiology, and Football (practical). Dr. Das has made significant academic contributions through her authorship of numerous research papers in Scopus, patents, books and chapters in the field of physical education and sports sciences. She has published over twenty research articles in reputed national and international journals and has presented her work at a wide array of conferences. Notably, she presented papers at the Pre-Olympic Congress in Liverpool, UK (2012) and the World Congress on Kinanthropometry in Santiago, Chile (2018). A recipient of international training, Dr. Das completed a 3-month International Coaching Course (ICC) in General Conditioning at Semmelweis University, Budapest, Hungary, in 2009, further enriching her academic and practical expertise. Beyond academics, Dr. Das is a former athlete who has passionately contributed to women's football. She was a four-time member of her university's intervarsity women's football team and won a bronze medal in the All India Intervarsity Women Football Tournament in 2002. She also represented Madhya Pradesh in the National Women's Football Championship and played a key role when her team participated in the 1st Khelo India University Games (KIUG) held in Bhubaneswar, Odisha, in February 2020. Dr. Das continues to inspire students and peers alike with her commitment to excellence in physical education, research, and sports development.

Hitakshi Dutta is a distinguished academic and management expert, currently serving as Professor and Associate Director of the Internal Quality Assurance Cell (IQAC) at Chandigarh University, Mohali. Her areas of expertise include Human Resource Management, organizational effectiveness, and employee engagement. She has extensive experience in academic leadership, quality assurance, and outcome-based education, contributing significantly to institutional excellence and continuous improvement initiatives. Dr. Dutta's scholarly and professional work focuses on strengthening human capital, enhancing organizational performance, and fostering sustainable workplace practices through strategic HR interventions.

Karuppasamy Govindasamy is a dedicated researcher and academician at Symbiosis International (Deemed University), specializing in exercise physiology, sports science, and physical fitness interventions. With a strong publication record and active involvement in national and international collaborations, he is committed to advancing health and performance through scientific research and education.

Shareef K. K. is a Research Scholar in the Department of Physical Education and Sports, Pondicherry University. My academic interests include sports training methods, physical fitness, and the role of physical activity in promoting health and wellness. My work also explores the integration of yoga for improving mental well-being and physical performance. I am also actively engaged in research focusing on performance enhancement, exercise physiology, and contemporary trends in physical education.

Ibnu Noufal Kambitta Valappil is a committed researcher and academic in the field of physical education and sports sciences. He completed his Ph.D. from Pondicherry University, where his research primarily focused on resistance training, plyometrics, and yoga-based interventions aimed at enhancing physical fitness and performance outcomes. With a growing footprint in the domain of sports science, Dr. Ibnu Noufal has authored 17 research articles exploring a range of topics including training adaptations, physiological responses, and performance metrics in athletic populations. His scholarly contributions include 15 papers indexed in Scopus (Q2 and Q3 journals) and 3 publications indexed in the Web of Science, reflecting the quality and impact of his research. He continues to engage in evidence-based exploration to advance knowledge in the areas of exercise science, athletic performance, and holistic wellness, particularly within resistance and yogic training paradigms.

Debajit Karmakar, is a distinguished research scholar and accomplished academic in the field of Physical Education and Sports Science. Currently pursuing his Ph.D. at the prestigious Lakshmibai National Institute of Physical Education (LNIPE), Gwalior, he has established himself as a prolific researcher. Mr. Karmakar completed his educational journey with remarkable academic excellence, earning his B.A./B.Sc. (Hons) in Physical Education from Visva-Bharati University, Santiniketan, followed by his B.P.Ed. from the same institution where he topped in his class. His Master's degree in Physical Education is from LNIPE, and he subsequently qualified UGC NET-JRF & WBSET examinations, demonstrating his academic prowess. A specialist in football and sports psychology, Mr. Karmakar has made significant contributions to academic literature with extensive publications in Scopus & Web of Science indexed journals. His research focuses on mental training, performance psychology, and innovative training methodologies. He has authored multiple books on sports psychology and performance enhancement, while also serving as editor for several academic publications. Mr. Karmakar's innovative spirit extends to intellectual properties also. His athletic background includes participation in various inter-university championships in and NCC activities. Beyond research, he actively contributes to the sports community through conference presentations, workshops, and certifications in coaching and sports science. His expertise spans statistical analysis, research methodology, and sports technology, making him a valuable asset to the academic and sporting communities. With proficiency in multiple software platforms for research and data analysis, Mr. Karmakar continues to advance the field of sports science through his doctoral research and ongoing scholarly contributions. Currently based in Gwalior, he remains committed to utilizing his knowledge and skills for the development of Physical Education and Sports.

Akshay Korol is a Senior Research Fellow at the National Institute of Technology, Puducherry, specializing in exercise physiology and biomechanics. Research passion lies at the intersection of yoga, sports science, and emerging technologies. With a strong foundation in scientific inquiry and practical application and explores how yogic principles can enhance athletic performance, recovery, and neuromuscular efficiency across various sports disciplines. By integrating traditional wisdom with modern tools such as surface electromyography (sEMG).

Aravind M K, currently affiliated with the Department of Physical Education & Sports, Pondicherry University, India. As a dedicated scholar and author in the field of physical education and sports sciences, I am actively engaged in research and academic contributions that enhance the understanding of athletic performance, yoga, sports training methodologies, and health promotion

Raj Madhu is a Research Scholar in the Department of Educational Studies at the Central University of Jammu. He holds an M.A. in Education from the University of Kalyani and has successfully qualified for the Junior Research Fellowship (NET-JRF). His research interests encompass Educational Philosophy, Educational Technology, Inclusive Education, and the Indian Knowledge System (IKS), reflecting his commitment to advancing innovative and inclusive educational practices.

Atisha Mandal is a dedicated scholar and emerging professional in the field of Physical Education and Sports Sciences. She possesses a strong academic foundation and a keen interest in sport pedagogy, fitness education, and holistic athlete development. Her academic journey reflects consistent engagement in both theoretical and practical dimensions of physical education, with emphasis on health, wellness, and performance enhancement. She is a Research Scholar at the Lakshmibai National Institute of Physical Education (LNIPE), Gwalior, where she is actively involved in advanced research and scholarly activities. Ms. Mandal regularly participates in academic seminars, workshops, and research-oriented programs, contributing to knowledge generation and professional development. With a strong commitment to academic excellence, she aspires to make meaningful contributions to physical education, sports training, and health promotion through research, teaching, and community engagement.

Asit Mantry is a Professor and Head of the Department of Educational Studies at the Central University of Jammu, India. With over 17 years of academic and administrative experience. He holds a Ph.D. and M.Phil. in Education from Kurukshetra University and has qualified the UGC-NET. His research interests include educational leadership, integral education, action research, and teacher education. Prof. Mantry has authored and edited multiple books, published over 40 research articles in reputed national and international journals, and guided several M.Ed. and Ph.D. scholars. He is also a life member of the Indian Association of Teacher Education (IATE) and serves on several academic and administrative committees at CUJ.

Elayaraja Masilamani is a Professor in the Department of Physical Education & Sports, Pondicherry University, with 25 years of academic and research experience in physical education and sports sciences. His research focuses on the physiology of sports training, predictors of human performance, fundamental movement skills, and the application of yoga for physical and mental health and wellness. He has demonstrated excellence in research supervision, having guided 15 Ph.D. and 35 M.Phil. scholars to date. Dr. Elayaraja has contributed to over 32 Scopus-indexed journal articles, accumulating 189 citations, with an h-index of 5 and an i10-index of 3, and is actively involved in peer review for several reputed journals in exercise science and sports research. He received the Best Ph.D. Thesis Award from Annamalai University in 2009 and the UGC Research Award for 2016–2018. His teaching and research excellence have also been recognized with the Best Teacher Award by Pondicherry University in 2012, 2015, 2016, 2017, and 2018. In addition to his academic accomplishments, Dr. Elayaraja holds sports specializations in Tennis, Ball Badminton, Cricket, and Athletics, and is a certified AITA Level I

Coach, ITF Level I official, and has qualified the FSTO examination conducted by the Athletics Federation of India (AFI). His academic journey is marked by a sustained commitment to high-impact research, mentoring, and advancing the science of human performance and sports training.

Ashif N K is a Research Scholar in the Department of Physical Education and Sports, Pondicherry University. Research interests include exercise science, fitness assessment, and the impact of training methods on athletic performance. I am also involved in exploring the applications of yoga and mindfulness practices in enhancing physical and mental health.

Kritika Ohri is a PhD Research Scholar at the University School of Business, Chandigarh University, Mohali, specializing in Human Resource Management and Organizational Behaviour. Her research focuses on the intersection of workplace spirituality, emotional resilience, employee engagement, and organizational effectiveness in the digital era, with particular emphasis on mental well-being at work. She explores how spiritually informed values and analytical approaches can support employees navigating complex work-life transitions, has developed conceptual frameworks such as the Soulful Work model, which integrates spiritual intelligence and ethical perspectives to foster meaningful and resilient work experiences, especially for women professionals. She has substantial experience in advanced research methodologies, including (PLS-SEM), bibliometric and scientometric analysis, and systematic literature reviews.Published nine scholarly contributions, including research papers in Scopus.

Sohom Saha is a passionate academic and sports psychology professional, currently pursuing his Ph.D. in Physical Education at Lakshmibai National Institute of Physical Education (LNIPE), Gwalior. He completed his Master of Physical Education (M.P.Ed.) from LNIPE, Gwalior with distinction, following his Bachelor of Physical Education (B.P.Ed.) and Bachelor of Arts (B.A.) in Physical Education from Visva-Bharati University, Shantiniketan, West Bengal. His areas of specialization include Sports Psychology, Volleyball, and Yoga, where he combines both scientific knowledge and practical expertise. Throughout his academic journey, Mr. Saha has actively participated in national-level sports events, including the All-India Inter-University Yoga and Ball Badminton Championships. He has also secured championships in NCC Inter-Battalion Football and Badminton tournaments. In addition to his athletic pursuits, he has contributed extensively to sports research, with multiple publications in reputed Scopus Indexed, Web of Science and peer-reviewed journals. His research interests focus on emotional resilience, psychological well-being, performance optimization, and contemporary trends in sports psychology. Beyond academics and athletics, Mr. Saha has authored several books on sports psychology and technology in sports. He is an active reviewer for leading international journals and a member of the Sports Psychology Association of India. His work reflects a deep commitment to promoting inclusivity, mental toughness, and holistic development in the field of sports. Through his scholarly contributions and practical experience, he aspires to inspire future generations of athletes, educators, and researchers in building a more inclusive and psychologically enriched sporting world.

Piyali Sarkar is an Assistant Principal at Barabisha High School (H.S.), has 14 years of academic and administrative experience. She holds a B.Sc., M.Sc., and Ph.D. in Education from Lovely Professional University under the guidance of Dr. Sonia Sharma, Associate Professor, LPU. Sarkar's research interests include education, educational psychology, higher education, and educational technology, women education. She has more than 27 published (10 under publications UGC CARE) in her account, her research papers have published in Scopus and various ISBN Books, ISSN National and International journals/peer reviewed journals/UGC approved journals/conferences. She has attended more than 5 workshops sponsored by UGC, HRDC, ICSSR. She has attended more than 15 conferences/seminars including international and national with paper presentations and publications as well as a participant.

Deepanjali Sharma is a dedicated scholar in the field of Physical Education and Sports Sciences. She completed her Bachelor of Physical Education (B.P.Ed.) from the Indira Gandhi Institute of Physical Education & Sports Sciences and earned her Master of Physical Education (M.P.Ed.) from the Laxmibai National Institute of Physical Education (LNIPE). She has demonstrated strong academic commitment through her continued engagement in higher education and research. Currently, she is pursuing her Ph.D. in Physical Education at LNIPE, Gwalior, where her research interests focus on advancing scientific knowledge in physical education, sports training, and performance enhancement. Her academic interests include pedagogy in physical education, sports science applications, and evidence-based training methodologies. She aspires to contribute to teaching, research, and professional practice in physical education and sports sciences through rigorous scholarship and innovation.

Pallvi Sharma is a research scholar in the Department of Educational Studies at the Central University of Jammu. She has done a Master in Science (Chemistry) from the Hemvati Nandan Bahuguna Grahwal University, Uttarakhand and also Master in Education (M.Ed) from the Central University of Jammu. She has also qualified

Junior Research Fellowship (NET-JRF). Her research area encompass Educational Philosophy, Indian Knowledge System, Educational Psychology, Mental Health, Education of Chemistry, reflecting her commitment to advancing the innovative and integrated educational practices.

Mahendra Singh is a Professor of Sports Psychology in the Department of Sports Psychology at Lakshmibai National Institute of Physical Education (LNIPE), Gwalior, Madhya Pradesh, under the Ministry of Youth Affairs & Sports, Government of India. He is currently also serving as the Controller of Examinations at LNIPE, Gwalior. He holds B.P.E., M.P.E., M.Phil., and Ph.D. degrees from LNCPE/LNIPE, Gwalior, has qualified UGC NET, and completed various yoga certifications including a Certificate Course in Yoga from Lonavla, Pune, as well as Yoga Pravesh and Yoga Parichaya from LNCPE, Gwalior. He also holds an NCC 'B' Certificate from the 8 MP Battalion, Gwalior. Dr. Singh has been engaged in teaching for over 34 years, including more than 19 years in postgraduate and Ph.D.-level teaching and research. He has extensive administrative experience, having served as Former Incharge Registrar, Former Dean of Academics, Sport Sciences, and Physical Education and Applied Areas, Former Chief Proctor, Former Chairman of the UGC Student Grievance Redressal Cell, Former Nodal Officer for the UGC Grievance Portal, Former HOD of the Department of Sports Psychology at LNIPE, Former Deputy Controller of Examinations, Former HOD of the School of Law at Guru Ghasidas Central University, Bilaspur, Former HOD of the Department of Physical Education at CSJM University, Kanpur, Anti-Ragging Coordinator at GGV, Bilaspur, Warden of various boys' hostels across Engineering, Pharmacy, and other UG/PG courses at CSJM University and Administrative Warden at GGV. He has authored six books on Physical Education, Sports, and Yoga, and published more than 50 research papers in national and international journals, including SCOPUS-indexed journals. Dr. Singh has presented over 35 papers at various national and international conferences/seminars. He is a member of academic bodies of various universities, a continuing member and former Chairperson of the Board of Studies and Departmental Research Committee at LNIPE, and has served as Secretary of the Board of Management at LNIPE. He has frequently been invited as a resource person, chairperson, and keynote speaker at national and international conferences and seminars. Additionally, he has extensive experience as an external examiner, paper setter, and evaluator for UG/PG/Ph.D. courses across various universities and has handled confidential assignments with state public service commissions. Dr. Singh has organized several mega events, sports tournaments, seminars, and conferences, and guided numerous Ph.D. scholars, with several more currently under his supervision. He also serves as the Chief Editor of conference proceedings publications and is on the editorial boards of reputed journals. During his student years, he represented Jiwaji University in Inter-University Tournaments in Basketball and Kho-Kho under AIU, and also participated in M.P. State Inter-University Tournaments in the same sports, along with several other achievements.

Gavoutamane Vasanthi is a Professor in the Department of Physical Education and Sports, Pondicherry University, has over 35 years of teaching experience and a strong academic and research background. She has successfully guided 20 Ph.D. scholars, with 5 currently pursuing their doctoral research under her supervision. Her research contributions are significant, with 60 publications in reputed national and international journals, including 4 papers indexed in Scopus (Q2, Q3, and Q4) and 3 papers indexed in the Web of Science, reflecting the quality and impact of her scholarly work. Her areas of academic expertise include Sports Psychology, Sports Medicine, Measurement and Evaluation, and Volleyball. She has also completed a Postgraduate Diploma in Yoga Education from Bharathiar University and a six-week certification in Table Tennis from Patiala. In addition to her academic roles, she has held key administrative positions such as Head of the Department, Director In-Charge of the Directorate of Sports, and is currently serving as the Head of the Women's Cell at Pondicherry University, continuing her commitment to research, leadership, and institutional development.

Index

A

B

C

D

E

F

H

I

M

N

www.ingramcontent.com/pod-product-compliance
Lightning Source LLC
LaVergne TN
LVHW062332300926
849161LV00007B/1670
9798337341873